Current Topics in Microbiology and Immunology

Volume 354

Current Topics in Microbiology and Immunology

Previously published volumes

Further volumes can be found at www.springer.com

Vol. 326: **Reddy, Anireddy S. N.; Golovkin, Maxim (Eds.)**: Nuclear pre-mRNA processing in plants. 2008
ISBN 978-3-540-76775-6

Vol. 327: **Manchester, Marianne; Steinmetz Nicole F. (Eds.)**: Viruses and Nanotechnology. 2008.
ISBN 978-3-540-69376-5

Vol. 328: **van Etten, (Ed.)**: Lesser Known Large dsDNA Viruses. 2008.
ISBN 978-3-540-68617-0

Vol. 329: **Griffin, Diane E.; Oldstone, Michael B. A. (Eds.)**: Measles. 2009
ISBN 978-3-540-70522-2

Vol. 330: **Griffin, Diane E.; Oldstone, Michael B. A. (Eds.)**: Measles. 2009.
ISBN 978-3-540-70616-8

Vol. 331: **Villiers, E. M. de (Ed.)**: TT Viruses. 2009.
ISBN 978-3-540-70917-8

Vol. 332: **Karasev A. (Ed.)**: Plant produced Microbial Vaccines. 2009.
ISBN 978-3-540-70857-5

Vol. 333: **Compans, Richard W.; Orenstein, Walter A. (Eds.)**: Vaccines for Pandemic Influenza. 2009.
ISBN 978-3-540-92164-6

Vol. 334: **McGavern, Dorian; Dustin, Micheal (Eds.)**: Visualizing Immunity. 2009.
ISBN 978-3-540-93862-0

Vol. 335: **Levine, Beth; Yoshimori, Tamotsu; Deretic, Vojo (Eds.)**: Autophagy in Infection and Immunity. 2009.
ISBN 978-3-642-00301-1

Vol. 336: **Kielian, Tammy (Ed.)**: Toll-like Receptors: Roles in Infection and Neuropathology. 2009.
ISBN 978-3-642-00548-0

Vol. 337: **Sasakawa, Chihiro (Ed.)**: Molecular Mechanisms of Bacterial Infection via the Gut. 2009.
ISBN 978-3-642-01845-9

Vol. 338: **Rothman, Alan L. (Ed.)**: Dengue Virus. 2009.
ISBN 978-3-642-02214-2

Vol. 339: **Spearman, Paul; Freed, Eric O. (Eds.)**: HIV Interactions with Host Cell Proteins. 2009.
ISBN 978-3-642-02174-9

Vol. 340: **Saito, Takashi; Batista, Facundo D. (Eds.)**: Immunological Synapse. 2010.
ISBN 978-3-642-03857-0

Vol. 341: **Bruserud, Øystein (Ed.)**: The Chemokine System in Clinical and Experimental Hematology. 2010.
ISBN 978-3-642-12638-3

Vol. 342: **Arvin, Ann M. (Ed.)**: Varicella-zoster Virus. 2010.
ISBN 978-3-642-12727-4

Vol. 343: **Johnson, John E. (Ed.)**: Cell Entry by Non-Enveloped Viruses. 2010.
ISBN 978-3-642-13331-2

Vol. 344: **Dranoff, Glenn (Ed.)**: Cancer Immunology and Immunotherapy. 2011.
ISBN 978-3-642-14135-5

Vol. 345: **Simon, M. Celeste (Ed.)**: Diverse Effects of Hypoxia on Tumor Progression. 2010.
ISBN 978-3-642-13328-2

Vol. 346: **Christian Rommel; Bart Vanhaesebroeck; Peter K. Vogt (Ed.)**: Phosphoinositide 3-kinase in Health and Disease. 2010.
ISBN 978-3-642-13662-7

Vol. 347: **Christian Rommel; Bart Vanhaesebroeck; Peter K. Vogt (Ed.)**: Phosphoinositide 3-kinase in Health and Disease. 2010.
ISBN 978-3-642-14815-6

Vol. 348: **Lyubomir Vassilev; David Fry (Eds.)**: Small-Molecule Inhibitors of Protein-Protein Interactions. 2011.
ISBN 978-3-642-17082-9

Vol. 349: **Michael Kartin (Ed.)**: NF-kB in Health and Disease. 2011.
ISBN: 978-3-642-16017-2

Vol. 350: **Rafi Ahmed; Tasuku Honjo (Eds.)**: Negative Co-receptors and Ligands. 2011.
ISBN: 978-3-642-19545-7

Vol. 351: **Marcel, B. M. Teunissen (Ed.)**: Intradermal Immunization. 2011.
ISBN: 978-3-642-23689-1

Vol. 352: **Rudolf Valenta; Robert L. Coffman (Eds.)**: Vaccines against Allergies. 2011.
ISBN 978-3-642-20054-0

Pamela A. Kozlowski
Editor

Mucosal Vaccines

Modern Concepts, Strategies, and Challenges

Series editor-in-charge: Hilary Koprowski

Springer

Pamela A. Kozlowski
Louisiana State University Health Sciences Center
Department of Microbiology, Immunology
and Parasitology
533 Bolivar Street
New Orleans, LA 70112
USA

ISSN 0070-217X
ISBN 978-3-642-23692-1 e-ISBN 978-3-642-23693-8
DOI 10.1007/978-3-642-23693-8
Springer Heidelberg Dordrecht London New York

Library of Congress Control Number: 2011942408

Cover design: Deblik, Berlin

Printed on acid-free paper

Springer is part of Springer Science+Business Media (www.springer.com)

Preface

Most pathogens exploit mucosal surfaces for entry into the host, and vaccines which most effectively concentrate immune effectors in tissues at these sites are those which are most likely to provide optimal immune protection: complete blocking of pathogen entry or local elimination of the pathogen in the tissue before it spreads. The superior potential to accomplish this by applying vaccines directly to a mucosal surface is the overarching advantage of mucosal vaccination over conventional intramuscular vaccination. But mucosal vaccine development is challenging because vaccine must be able to penetrate epithelial barriers and to survive luminal innate defenses. The present book collects a group of articles that review advances in mucosal vaccine delivery strategies and formulations. Regulatory issues, safety concerns, and advances in manufacturing are integral components of these reviews.

Success in the development of a mucosal vaccine requires that mucosal tissues be recognized and approached as separate entities. Each is unique overall with regard to its physiological function, luminal defenses, environmental stimuli (including commensals), the types of epithelia present, lymphoid organization, and endocrine influences. Local vaccination typically elicits the greatest immune responses within each compartment, but cross-talk can be negligible. This must be considered when local immunization is impractical and alternative delivery routes are being contemplated. In the first chapter of this volume, Czerkinsky and Holmgren review the mechanisms responsible for regionalization within the mucosal immune system and address other critical factors that should be taken into account when designing and evaluating mucosal vaccines. The mucosal tissues most effectively seeded by antigen-specific lymphocytes after immunization by different routes are reviewed, with an emphasis on the ability to populate numerous distal tissues using the sublingual route, which may have considerable advantages over the nasal route in terms of safety.

Needle-free topical application of antigen with appropriate adjuvant on the skin can also induce mucosal immune responses and may be an ideal delivery strategy for vaccines that are especially susceptible to denaturation in the mucosal lumen. In the following chapter, Lawson, Clements and Freytag review the transcutaneous immunization route and the adjuvants, including toll-like receptor agonists, which have proved effective for inducing mucosal responses using this route. Notably, enterotoxin adjuvants can be safely administered to humans by the transcutaneous route and may be optimal for generating cellular and humoral immunity in the gastrointestinal, respiratory or female genital tract.

Vaccine platforms and formulations for the delivery of mucosal vaccines are the focus of the next five chapters. Yamamoto, Pascual and Kiyono review recently identified molecules that facilitate the delivery of oral or nasal vaccines specifically to intestinal or tonsillar M cells, which may be the most efficient antigen-sampling cells in the body. Schneider-Ohrum and Ross describe the production and use of recombinant noninfectious virus-like particles (VLP) to generate protective immunity against specific viruses or co-expressed foreign antigens, while McNeela and Lavelle review new formulation strategies that improve mucosal uptake of polymer-based microsphere and nanoparticle delivery vehicles. Mason and Herbst-Kralovetz discuss advances in the manufacture of plant-based vaccines and the challenges associated with the development of edible vaccines. In turn, Hickey and Staats discuss the advantages of dry vaccines over liquid formulations for pulmonary or nasal immunization. Invaluable information on the manufacture of powder vaccines, absorption enhancers, mucoadhesives, delivery devices and methods for evaluating safety in the respiratory tract is also included.

The final chapters review two of the greatest challenges in vaccine development: human immunodeficiency virus type 1 (HIV-1) and biodefense weapons. There is no longer any doubt that HIV is a mucosal disease and optimal vaccine-mediated protection will likely require that immune effectors be established not only at mucosal portals of entry but also throughout the gastrointestinal tract, which is home to the largest reservoir of HIV target cells. Belyakov and Ahlers review vaccination strategies that have augmented HIV-specific immunity in the intestinal mucosa and increased the protective efficacy of immunodeficiency virus vaccines. Mantis, Morici and Roy discuss the unique and daunting hurdles facing the development of biodefense vaccines for the numerous microbes and toxins that have been deemed potential biothreats in the respiratory or gastrointestinal tract. It is clear from the reviews in this volume that significant progress has been made in mucosal vaccination strategies over the last decade. However, further basic research on mucosal host defense mechanisms, adjuvants, and delivery vehicles is still needed for the optimal design of mucosal vaccines and prevention of infectious diseases.

New Orleans, 2011 Pam Kozlowski

Contents

Contributors

J. D. Ahlers Division of AIDS, National Institute of Allergy and Infectious Diseases, National Institutes of Health, 6700 Rockledge Drive, Bethesda, MD 20817, USA

I. M. Belyakov Midwest Research Institute, 110 Thomas Johnson Drive, Suite 170, Frederick, MD 21702, USA, e-mail: igorbelyakov@yahoo.com

J. D. Clements Department of Microbiology and Immunology, Tulane University School of Medicine, 1430 Tulane Avenue, New Orleans, LA 70112, USA

C. Czerkinsky International Vaccine Institute, Seoul, South Korea, e-mail: cczerkinsky@ivi.int

L. C. Freytag Department of Microbiology and Immunology, Tulane University School of Medicine, 1430 Tulane Avenue, New Orleans, LA 70112, USA, e-mail: lfreyta@tulane.edu

M. M. Herbst-Kralovetz Center for Infectious Diseases and Vaccinology, Biodesign Institute, Arizona State University, Tempe, AZ, 85287, USA Department of Basic Medical Sciences, University of Arizona College of Medicine-Phoenix, Phoenix, AZ 85004, USA

A. J. Hickey Division of Molecular Pharmaceutics, School of Pharmacy, University of North Carolina, Chapel Hill, NC 27599, USA

J. Holmgren Institute of Biomedicine, Sahlgrenska Academy at Gothenburg University, Göteborg, Sweden

H. Kiyono Division of Mucosal Immunology, Department of Microbiology and Immunology, The Institute of Medical Science, The University of Tokyo, Minato-ku, Tokyo 108-8639, Japan

E. C. Lavelle Adjuvant Research Group, School of Biochemistry and Immunology, Trinity College, Dublin 2, Ireland

L. B. Lawson Department of Microbiology and Immunology, Tulane University School of Medicine, 1430 Tulane Avenue, New Orleans, LA 70112, USA

N. J. Mantis Division of Infectious Diseases, Wadsworth Center, NYDOH, 120 New Scotland Ave, Albany, NY 12208, USA, e-mail: nmantis@wadsworth.org

H. S. Mason School of Life Sciences, Arizona State University, Tempe, AZ 85287, USA

E. A. McNeela Adjuvant Research Group, School of Biochemistry and Immunology, Trinity College, Dublin 2, Ireland, e-mail: mcneele@tcd.ie

L. A. Morici Department of Microbiology and Immunology, Tulane University School of Medicine, 1430 Tulane Ave, New Orleans, LA 70112, USA

D. W. Pascual Department of Immunology and Infectious Diseases, Montana State University, Bozeman, MT 59717, USA

T. M. Ross Center for Vaccine Research, Department of Microbiology and Molecular Genetics, University of Pittsburgh, Pittsburgh, PA, USA, e-mail: tmr15@pitt.edu

C. J. Roy Infectious Disease Aerobiology, Tulane National Primate Research Center, 18703 Three Rivers Rd, Covington, LA 70433, USA

K. Schneider-Ohrum Center for Vaccine Research Department of Microbiology and Molecular Genetics, University of Pittsburgh, Pittsburgh, PA, USA

H. F. Staats Department of Pathology, Duke University Medical Center, Durham, NC 27710, USA, e-mail: Herman.staats@duke.edu

A. L. Thompson Department of Pathology Duke University Medical Center, Durham, NC 27710, USA

S. H. Wang Division of Molecular Pharmaceutics, School of Pharmacy, University of North Carolina, Chapel Hill, NC 27599, USA

M. Yamamoto Department of Oral Immunology, Nihon University School of Dentistry at Matsudo, Matsudo, Chiba 271-8587, Japan, e-mail: yamamoto.masafumi@nihon-u.ac.jp

Mucosal Delivery Routes for Optimal Immunization: Targeting Immunity to the Right Tissues

C. Czerkinsky and J. Holmgren

Abstract The mucosal immune system exhibits a high degree of anatomic compartmentalization related to the migratory patterns of lymphocytes activated at different mucosal sites. The selective localization of mucosal lymphocytes to specific tissues is governed by cellular "homing" and chemokine receptors in conjunction with tissue-specific addressins and epithelial cell-derived chemokines that are differentially expressed in "effector" tissues. The compartmentalization of mucosal immune responses imposes constraints on the selection of vaccine administration route. Traditional routes of mucosal immunization include oral and nasal routes. Other routes for inducing mucosal immunity include the rectal, vaginal, sublingual, and transcutaneous routes. Sublingual administration is a new approach that results in induction of mucosal and systemic T cell and antibody responses with an exceptionally broad dissemination to different mucosae, including the gastrointestinal and respiratory tracts, and the genital mucosa. Here, we discuss how sublingual and different routes of immunization can be used to generate immune responses in the desired mucosal tissue(s).

Contents

C. Czerkinsky (✉)
International Vaccine Institute, Seoul, South Korea
e-mail: cczerkinsky@ivi.int

J. Holmgren
Institute of Biomedicine, Sahlgrenska Academy at Gothenburg University, Göteborg, Sweden

Current Topics in Microbiology and Immunology (2012) 354: 1–18
DOI: 10.1007/82_2010_112

Published Online: 5 November 2010

1 Introduction

The gastrointestinal, respiratory and urogenital tracts, eye conjunctiva, inner ear, and ducts of all the exocrine glands are covered by mucous membranes endowed with powerful mechanical and chemical cleansing mechanisms that repel and degrade most foreign matter (Brandtzaeg and Pabst 2004; Ogra 1999). In addition, a highly specialized innate and adaptive mucosal immune system protects these surfaces, and thereby the body interior, against insults from the environment. In a healthy human adult, this local immune system is estimated to comprise nearly 80% of all lymphocytes, commensurate with the ca. 400 square meters of mucosal surfaces that it has to defend. These immune cells are accumulated in, or in transit between, various mucosa-associated lymphoid tissues (MALTs), which together form the largest mammalian lymphoid organ system. The MALT represents a highly compartmentalized immunological system that functions independently of the systemic immune apparatus. At variance with the systemic immune system, which normally functions in a sterile milieu and can thus afford to respond vigorously to invaders, the MALT guards organs that are replete with foreign matter. Only a limited proportion of these foreign antigens are derived from pathogens; most are commensals, food proteins, and other ingested or inhaled foreign materials. This means that upon encounter with this broad range of antigenic stimuli, the MALT must select appropriate effector mechanisms and regulate their intensity to avoid bystander tissue damage and immunological exhaustion.

There is a great need to develop vaccines against many bacterial and viral pathogens. The majority of microbial pathogens have a mucosal port of entry. Although parenteral vaccination can provide protection in some instances, a mucosal vaccination route is necessary in most cases. In addition, as compared to injectable vaccines, mucosal vaccines would be easier to administer, carry less risk of transmitting infections, and could simplify manufacturing, thereby increasing the potential for local vaccine production in developing countries (Holmgren and Czerkinsky 2005).

In the early days of mucosal immunology, it was thought (based on studies in mice) that immune responses initiated at one mucosal site would be widely disseminated to multiple mucosal tissues. Had this common mucosal immune system existed, it would have meant that immunization of humans by the oral route could be used effectively to induce immune responses not only in the gastrointestinal tract, but also in the airways and the urogenital tract. However, further work has shown that mucosal immune responses are highly compartmentalized, not only between separate mucosal organs (Ogra and Karzon 1969), but also between regions within the same mucosal organ, such as the gut (Holmgren and Czerkinsky 2005; Ogra and Karzon 1969).

In this review, we summarize the anatomical distribution of immune responses after mucosal immunization by different routes. Whenever possible, the information provided is based on findings in humans or non-human primates since studies in mice may give misleading information. Most of our knowledge is from oral or site-specific immunization in the gastrointestinal tract, but some information exists for vaccination by the nasal or vaginal routes. We will also discuss, in some detail, the newer sublingual vaccine delivery approach. When compared with other vaccination routes, the sublingual route offers the potential to produce strong and more broadly disseminated T cell and antibody responses in systemic and mucosal tissues.

2 Mucosal Vaccines: An Unmet Need

Most, perhaps 90%, of all infections are caused by pathogens which have a mucosal portal of entry. There is an urgent need for vaccines that induce effective and long-lasting immunity, especially during infancy and early childhood, against numerous respiratory and enteric pathogens. It is estimated that mucosal respiratory and gastrointestinal infections kill approximately five million children under age five in developing countries and cause more than ten billion disease episodes each year. These diseases negatively impact growth, cognitive function, and quality of life. Similarly, there is a great need for vaccines that can protect against human immunodeficiency virus (HIV) and other sexually transmitted infections that affect millions of adults and adolescents. These conditions have a tremendous negative impact on global health and overall economic development. To date, more than 30 injectable vaccines have been licensed for human use, compared with only a handful of mucosal vaccines. All of these mucosal vaccines are for oral use against enteric infections with the exception of two nasal cold-adapted attenuated influenza vaccines (Table 1).

A large number of pathogens cause or initiate infections in the gastrointestinal tract (e.g. *Helicobacter pylori*, *Vibrio cholerae*, enterotoxigenic *Escherichia coli* (ETEC), *Shigella* spp., *Salmonella* spp., *Clostridium difficile*, polioviruses, rotaviruses and noroviruses). Several other pathogens cause acute or chronic respiratory infections (group A streptococci, *Streptococcus pneumoniae, Haemophilus*

Table 1 Internationally licensed mucosal vaccines currently used in humans

Oral polio virus vaccines (OPV)
Oral live-attenuated typhoid vaccine (Vivotif™)
Oral inactivated B subunit-whole cell cholera vaccine[a] (Dukoral™)
Oral live-attenuated rotavirus vaccines (RotaTeq™ and ROTARIX™)
Nasal cold-adapted live-attenuated influenza vaccine[b] (FluMist™)

[a] Domestically licensed killed whole cell oral cholera vaccines are also used in Vietnam, India, and China
[b] A cold-adapted live-attenuated nasal influenza vaccine is also licensed in Russia since 1961

influenzae, Mycoplasma pneumoniae, influenza virus, respiratory syncytial virus, and *Mycobacterium tuberculosis).* There are also a number of sexually transmitted mucosal pathogens (e.g. HIV, human papillomavirus, *Chlamydia*, *Neisseria gonorrhea* and herpes simplex virus). Collectively, infections caused by these agents represent an enormous challenge toward the development of vaccines which induce protective immunity by either preventing the infectious agent from attaching to and colonizing the mucosal epithelium (non-invasive bacteria) or from penetrating and replicating in the mucosa (viruses and invasive bacteria), or by blocking the binding of microbial toxins to epithelial and other target cells.

2.1 Considerations in Selecting a Mucosal or Parenteral Vaccine Delivery Route

It is highly probable that infection by and inter-person transmission of most mucosal pathogens can be effectively controlled by mucosal vaccines provided these vaccines are rationally designed and formulated to be administered through an appropriate route. However, the nature of the pathogen and of the target mucosal tissue will determine whether the vaccine should be given mucosally or parenterally to be efficacious (Fig. 1). A topical mucosal vaccination route seems to be critical for protection against non-invasive infections at mucosal surfaces and such infections involve pathogens that remain on the apical (luminal) side of mucosal epithelia, i. e. at sites (i) that are poorly accessible to antibodies transudating from blood, and (ii) where blood-derived monomeric IgG or IgA are insufficiently concentrated on the apical cell surface (due to the lack of receptor-mediated transport) or are unstable to function in the external mucosal environment. Cholera and ETEC are typical examples of infections in which vaccine-induced protection appears to be mediated mainly, if not exclusively, by locally produced secretory IgA (S-IgA) antibodies, and is associated with immunological memory.

On the other hand, when infection occurs at mucosal surfaces, such as those in the respiratory and urogenital tract, which are more permeable than the intestines to transudation by serum antibodies, a parenteral route of vaccination may be effective. The same may hold true for enteric infections where the pathogen is first

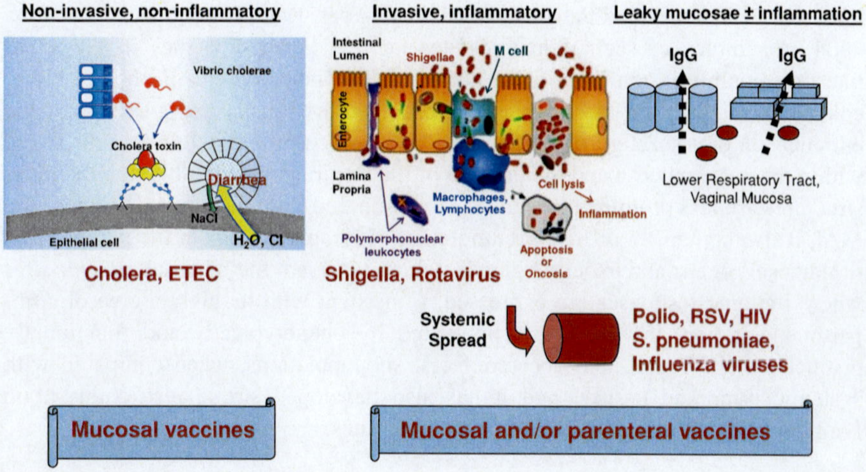

Fig. 1 Different types of mucosal infections and mucosal surfaces may call for different types of vaccines. Mucosal vaccination may be critical for protecting against non-invasive infections at mucosal surfaces that are normally impermeable to serum antibody transudation; V. cholerae and ETEC infections are examples of such infections, where vaccine-induced protection is mediated mainly, if not exclusively, by locally produced SIgA antibodies. Protection against more invasive pathogens or infections at mucosal surfaces that are permeable to transudation by serum antibodies, such as the lower respiratory tract or genital mucosae, may be achieved by either mucosal or parenteral vaccines

translocated across the epithelial barrier and then infects the basolateral side of the epithelium (as with *Shigellae*) or when the pathogen causes disease only after multiplying and producing inflammation in the submucosal tissues (as for *Campylobacter* and most *Salmonella* bacteria). Finally, parenteral vaccines are clearly efficacious for many viral and bacterial infections caused by pathogens that utilize a mucosal portal of entry, but then quickly enter the blood for systemic spread. Typical pathogens in this category for which effective injectable vaccines exist include *S. pneumoniae*, *H. influenzae*, *S. typhi*, poliovirus and influenza virus. It is notable that for the last three, mucosal vaccines are also available.

Taken together, and amid our gaps in knowledge of the mucosal immune system as well as our ability to measure its effector and memory arms, these considerations highlight the challenges to be met by vaccinologists when attempting to design, formulate, and deploy future mucosal vaccines.

3 Compartmentalization and Cell Migration in the Mucosal Immune System

The MALT comprises anatomically defined lymphoid microcompartments, which serve as the principal mucosal *inductive sites* where immune responses are initiated (Brandtzaeg and Pabst 2004; Ishikawa et al. 1999; Kiyono and Fukuyama 2004). Examples of such inductive sites are the Peyer's patches in the small intestine (mainly in the ileum), the abundant lymphoid follicles in the appendix, colon and rectum; the mesenteric lymph nodes, the tonsils and adenoids at the entrance of the aerodigestive tract, and the many lymphoid follicles dispersed within the nasal mucosa and the bronchi of the respiratory tract (although the latter structures are less prominent in humans as compared to some animal species). The MALT also contains a diffuse accumulation of lymphoid cells in the parenchyma of mucosal organs and exocrine glands, which represent the mucosal *effector sites* where immune responses are expressed. Consistent with its high degree of compartmentalization, the MALT is populated by phenotypically and functionally distinct B cell, T cell, and accessory cell subpopulations, when compared with systemic lymphoid tissues; and it has also developed strong restrictions upon lymphoid cell recirculation between mucosal sites.

3.1 Induction of Mucosal Immune Responses

As extensively discussed elsewhere (Fahlen-Yrlid et al. 2009; Iwasaki 2007; Kraehenbuhl and Neutra 2000), antigens may either penetrate or be taken up in mucosal inductive sites through a variety of mechanisms. One such example is the gut where the presence of a mucosal lymphoid follicle influences the adjacent intestinal epithelium by inducing differentiation of M cells (Kraehenbuhl and Neutra 2000). The latter cells, which are most prominent over the Peyer's patches, have special properties for transporting antigens across the epithelial barrier (Jang et al. 2004). Recently, an additional mechanism has been proposed for the uptake of antigens at mucosal surfaces that can occur in the absence of an organized follicle-associated epithelium. This mechanism involves dendritic cells (DCs), which can protrude antigen-sampling dendrites across the intestinal epithelium and into the lumen (Rescigno and Di Sabatino 2009).

Irrespective of sampling mechanism, antigens taken up at a mucosal surface can be ferried to, or directly captured by professional antigen-presenting cells (APCs), and presented to conventional CD4+ and CD8+ $\alpha\beta$ T cells. Certain antigens may also be processed and presented directly by epithelial cells to neighbouring intraepithelial T cells, including T cells with limited repertoire diversity ($\gamma\delta$ T cells and NKT cells). With the majority of antigens, this results in the suppression of specific immunity or "oral tolerance" (Mowat 2003). However, an active immune response may also ensue, depending on the nature of the antigen, the type of APC involved, and the local microenvironment. In general, inflammatory conditions favor the development of productive immune responses, and these responses are triggered by pathogens harboring motifs that are sensed as "danger signals" after binding to Toll-like receptor (TLR) ligands on mucosal APC (Bilsborough and Viney 2004; Rakoff-Nahoum et al. 2004). The stimulation of the mucosal innate immune system is an important reason why pathogens, live-attenuated bacterial or viral vaccines, and killed whole-cell bacterial vaccines induce an immune response rather than tolerance. Selected subunit vaccines may also induce strong immune response by possessing similar or functionally analogous motifs, but subunit vaccines typically need to be delivered with a pro-inflammatory adjuvant to stimulate a strong immune response. In most cases, a mucosal immune response appears to critically depend on appropriate antigen presentation by mucosal DCs, although a mucosal IgA response could be induced in DC-depleted animals when very high amounts of mucosal antigens were given (Fahlen-Yrlid et al. 2009).

3.2 *Tissue-Specific Homing of Mucosal Lymphocytes*

Sensitized mucosal immunocytes, both B and T cells and also IgA plasmablast precursors, leave the site of initial antigen encounter (e.g. Peyer's patch), transit through the lymph, enter the circulation, and then seed selected mucosal sites, preferentially the mucosa of origin, where they differentiate into memory or effector cells. Anatomic affinity of mucosal lymphoid cells appears to be largely determined through site-specific integrins ("homing receptors") and chemokine receptors and complementary tissue-specific endothelial cell adhesion molecules ("addressins") and chemokines which are expressed differentially in the various mucosal tissues (Berg et al. 1989). This explains why mucosal lymphocytes preferentially traffic to mucosal rather than peripheral organs and tissues. For instance, gut-homing IgA B cell precursors, their plasmablast progenitors, and memory T cells express $\alpha4\beta7$ integrin that specifically attaches to MadCAM-1, a tissue-specific addressin that is selectively expressed on the endothelium in the gastrointestinal tract (Kunkel and Butcher 2003).

Mucosal DCs in concert with neighboring epithelial cells play a critical role in this process by programming B and T lymphocytes to express tissue-specific homing receptors (Iwasaki 2007; Johansson-Lindbom et al. 2005; Mora et al. 2003, 2006; Rescigno and Di Sabatino 2009; Stagg et al. 2002). Likewise, chemokines produced by epithelial cells in the local microenvironment promote chemotaxis of immune cells with cognate chemokine receptors (Kunkel et al. 2003; Rescigno and Di Sabatino 2009). For instance, in the gastrointestinal tract, CCL28 selectively attracts IgA B cells and plasmablasts expressing the chemokine receptor CCR10, whereas CCL25 produced by small intestinal epithelia selectively attracts B and T cells expressing the CCR9 receptor from the blood into the small intestinal lamina propria (Kunkel et al. 2003). The tissue-specific imprinting of homing molecules and chemokine receptors on lymphocytes activated in mucosal inductive sites and the selective expression of addressins and chemokines in the target mucosal tissue explains the segregation of mucosal and systemic immune responses as well as the preferential dissemination of mucosal lymphocytes to privileged mucosal sites.

Table 2 Anatomic distribution of mucosal IgA antibody responses after immunization by different routes

	Immunization route					
	Nasal	Sub-lingual	Oral	Rectal	Vaginal	Trans-dermal
Upper respiratory tract	+++	+++	–	–	–	+++
Lower respiratory tract	+/+++[a]	+++	–	–	–	+++
Stomach	–	+[b]	+[b]	–	–	?
Small intestine	–	+++	+++	–	–	+
Colon	–	?	++	++	–	+
Rectum	–	?	±	+++	–	?
Reproductive tract	++	+++	–	–	++/+++[c]	?
Blood	+++	+++	+	+/±	+/±	+++

[a] Strong response only by aerosol administration
[b] Stronger response (+++) in *H. pylori*-infected individuals
[c] Strongest response when immunization is performed during the mid-follicular phase

4 Mucosal Effector Sites Associated with Vaccination Routes

The compartmentalization within the mucosal immune system places constraints on the choice of vaccination route for induction of immune responses at a desired site. Administration of antigens by rectal, vaginal, and more recently sublingual, routes has been explored but only for experimental purposes so far, and mainly for studying S-IgA antibody responses. In general, as summarized in Table 2, the strongest immune response is obtained at the site of initial vaccine exposure and in anatomically adjacent mucosal sites. However, a few notable exceptions have been found that may allow for more practical vaccine administration than would otherwise be possible, especially for infections in the urogenital tract. This has obvious implications for the development and deployment of mucosal vaccines.

4.1 Intestinal, Nasal, and Vaginal Vaccination

Traditional routes of mucosal immunization include the oral and nasal routes. If antigens with inherent immunogenicity are used either alone or co-administered with an effective adjuvant, oral immunization induces a substantial antibody response in mainly the small intestine (and then strongest in the proximal segment), in the ascending colon (Fig. 2), the stomach and in the mammary and salivary glands (Czerkinsky et al. 1991; Eriksson et al. 1998; Jertborn et al. 2001; Johansson et al. 2004; Quiding et al. 1991) (Table 2). Oral immunization is, however, relatively inefficient for evoking an IgA antibody response in the distal segments of the large intestine (Fig. 2), the tonsils, the lower airway mucosa, or

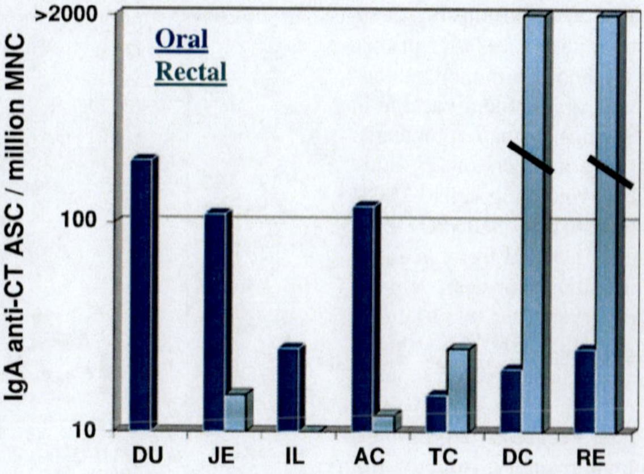

Fig. 2 Compartmentalization of mucosal immunity illustrated by the anatomic segmentation of the intestinal IgA immune response in macaques after oral and rectal immunizations with cholera toxin (two doses two weeks apart). Data are from Eriksson et al. (1998).

the reproductive tract mucosa (Eriksson et al. 1998; Kozlowski et al. 1997; Nardelli-Haefliger et al. 2003; Wassén et al. 1996). Conversely, rectal immunization evokes a strong local antibody response in the rectum, sigmoid colon, and descending colon (although weaker), but little, if any response, in the small intestine and ascending colon (Johansson et al. 2004) (Fig. 2) and distal reproductive tract (Kozlowski et al. 1997, 2002). Vaginal immunization, especially during the mid-follicular phase of the menstrual cycle, similarly induces strong local mucosal immune responses without producing notable distal immune responses (Johansson et al. 2001; Kozlowski et al. 1997, 2002; Wassén et al. 1996).

On the other hand, nasal or tonsillar immunization in humans produces IgA antibodies in the upper airway mucosa and regional nasal or salivary secretions without evoking an immune response in the gut (Quiding-Järbrink et al. 1995, 1997). However, for possible vaccination against HIV and other sexually transmitted infections, nasal immunization has been found to give rise to substantial IgA and IgG antibody responses in the human cervico-vaginal mucosae (Johansson et al. 2001; Kozlowski et al. 2002; Nardelli-Haefliger et al. 2003). The magnitude of the response achieved in the genital mucosa of women after intranasal immunization appears to be fully comparable to that seen when the vaccine is given by topical vaginal application (Johansson et al. 2001; Nardelli-Haefliger et al. 2003).

Apart from the anatomical differences in the dissemination of S-IgA antibody responses induced by oral and nasal immunization, respectively, the kinetics of the responses also appear to be markedly different. Several studies have shown that the intestinal immune response after oral immunization is rapid and relatively short-lived, although it is associated with long-lasting immunological memory. After oral cholera vaccination, data from extensive field trials in developing countries have shown that protection mediated by the acute intestinal IgA response appears to vanish after 6–9 months, but overall protection lasts for several years, consistent with the demonstration of mucosal immunological memory lasting for

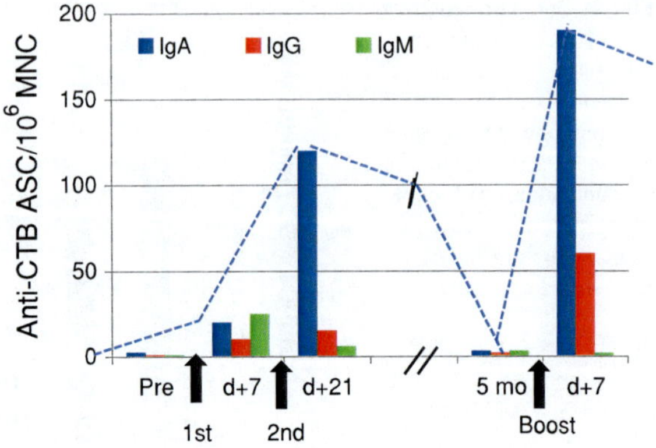

Fig. 3 Local intestinal antibody responses after primary and booster immunizations with oral cholera vaccine in Swedish human volunteers. Large numbers of IgA-antibody-secreting cells (ASC) (detected by ELISPOT on cells isolated from small intestinal biopsies) were observed after two oral immunizations and a third single dose given 5 months (or in another study 5 years) later evoked strong immunologic memory. Adapted from Quiding et al. (1991)

at least 5 years in Swedish volunteers after oral cholera vaccination (Jertborn et al. 1994). In experimental studies in humans, Quiding et al. (1991) examined the kinetics of the antibody-secreting cell (ASC) response to the cholera B subunit (CTB) in the small intestine after single and booster oral cholera vaccinations. They found that duodenal IgA ASC responses to CTB peaked 1 week after immunization and decreased markedly over a 5-month period, but these responses could be quickly recalled by a booster administration of vaccine (Fig. 3).

Rudin et al. (1998) compared the kinetics and organ distribution of the antibody response after nasal and oral vaccination. They immunized Swedish female volunteers nasally or orally with CTB and measured specific antibody in serum and in nasal and vaginal secretions at different times after immunization. Strong systemic antibody responses to CTB were induced by both routes of vaccination. Nasal vaccination strongly increased CTB-specific IgA in nasal secretions, whereas no significant nasal IgA response was seen after oral vaccination. A striking difference between nasal and oral vaccination was that the nasal route elicited an antibody response with a later onset but of much longer duration than the oral route in both serum and at the mucosal expression sites (Fig. 4).

4.2 Sublingual Vaccination

The above considerations have prompted efforts to identify alternative routes of vaccine delivery. In this respect, the potential of the sublingual ("under the tongue") route for administration of vaccines is gaining increased interest due to recent studies indicating that this route may in fact induce broadly disseminated mucosal and systemic immune responses. Over the past few years, we and others have shown that sublingual administration of a variety of soluble, as well as

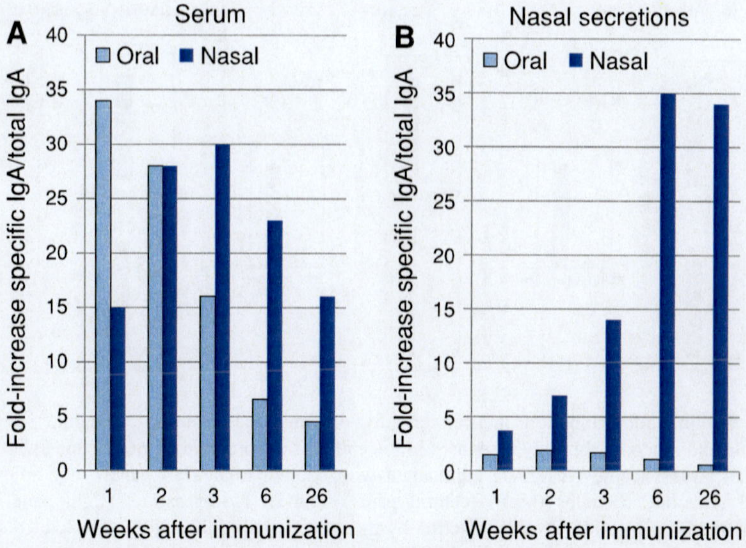

Fig. 4 Different kinetics of the mucosal and serum antibody response after mucosal immunizations by the oral as compared to the nasal routes. (B, C) Adapted from Rudin et al. (1998): The kinetics of both serum and mucosal antibody responses differ after oral (A) and nasal (B) immunization; nasal immunization gives rise to a less rapid but longer-lasting response than oral immunization.

particulate antigens, including live and killed bacteria and viruses, can evoke a broad spectrum of immune responses in mucosal and extra-mucosal tissues, ranging from secretory and systemic antibody responses to mucosal and systemic cytotoxic T lymphocyte (CTL) responses (Cuburu et al. 2007). Although only studied in animals so far, in all instances where this route of administration has been compared to the classical orogastric route, sublingually induced responses have been far more pronounced and required 10- to 50-fold lower amounts of antigen (Cuburu et al. 2007). Moreover, sublingual, but not oral administration of killed or live-attenuated influenza vaccine induced antiviral responses in the lungs of mice, and protected mice against lethal respiratory challenge with infectious virions (Song et al. 2008) (Fig. 5).

Importantly, antigens and adjuvants that have been administered sublingually are not redirected to the olfactory bulb epithelium; thus sublingual vaccines are less likely to have the same safety issues as nasal vaccines. More recently, we have documented that similar to nasal immunization, but at variance with orogastric immunization, sublingual administration of non-replicating antigens can also induce secretory antibody responses, and depending on the adjuvant used, CTL responses in the female reproductive tract (Cuburu et al. 2009). Another significant finding is that sublingual administration of a non-adjuvant vaccine consisting of human papillomavirus virus-like particles (VLPs) evoked virus-neutralizing antibody responses in serum and genital secretions, and provided protection against

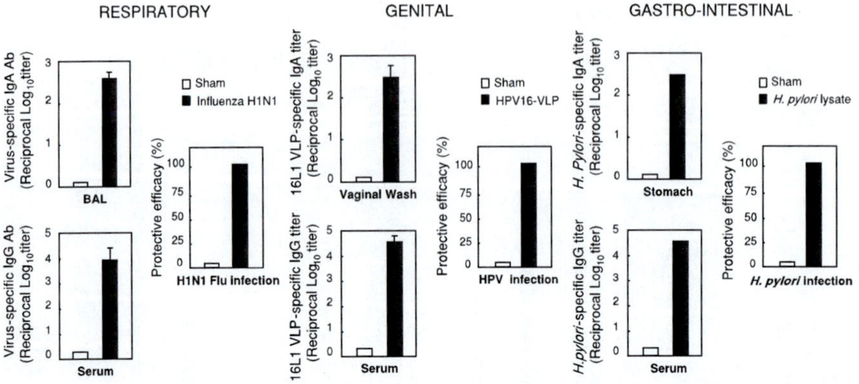

Fig. 5 Sublingual vaccination induces broadly disseminated protective immune responses. Systemic and mucosal antibody responses in mice after 2 consecutive immunizations with killed influenza virus vaccine (A/H1N1) adjuvanted with cholera toxin (left panel), non-adjuvanted HPV16 virus-like particles (VLP) (central panel), and H. pylori extract (right panel) were associated with protection against infection by the corresponding pathogen. Adapted from Song et al. (2008), Cuburu et al. (2009), and Rhagavan et al (2010)

genital challenge with HPV (Cuburu et al. 2009) (Fig. 5). Other recent experiments have shown that sublingual administration of an experimental *Helicobacter pylori* vaccine can effectively induce B and T cell responses in the stomach mucosa and protect mice against infection with *H. pylori* with an efficacy exceeding that achieved by orogastric immunization (Raghavan et al. 2010) (Fig. 5). Finally, sublingual immunization with experimental ETEC and *V. cholerae* whole cell vaccines, as well as purified fimbrial antigens, has proved efficient in giving rise to strong IgA antibody responses in the intestine, suggesting that this route may even be used as an alternative to the oral route for vaccination against enteric infections (Holmgren, unpublished data).

The exceptional ability of the murine sublingual mucosa to disseminate effector B and T cell responses to various mucosal tissues appears to be contributed by specialized dendritic cells residing in the sublingual epithelial and draining submaxillary (cervical) lymph nodes. These CCR7+ dendritic cells appear to respond to the chemokines CCL19 and CCL21 (Song et al. 2009) produced in the local microenvironment and to imprint B and T cells (including CTL precursors) to migrate to CCL28 that is expressed by epithelial cells in a variety of tissues, including the salivary glands, mammary glands, small and large intestines, respiratory tract and genital tract (Kunkel et al. 2003; Pan et al. 2000; Wang et al. 2000).

Controlled clinical trials are now being conducted to determine the safety and efficiency of this novel route of administration. The development of mucoadhesive formulations with enhanced permeabilizing properties to facilitate and prolong contact of vaccine antigens with the sublingual epithelium is likely to become a major milestone for the future emergence of sublingual vaccines.

4.3 Transcutaneous Vaccination

Another interesting route of vaccine administration relates to the use of skin-adhesive patches containing antigen and adjuvant (Glenn et al. 1998). This approach, called "transcutaneous immunization" has been shown to induce both systemic, intestinal and respiratory antibody responses in mice. The results of a clinical trial involving administration of *E. coli* heat-labile enterotoxin (LT) appear to be promising, and suggest that transcutaneous immunization with potent adjuvant-active antigens, such as LT, may also evoke both intestinal and systemic antibody responses in humans (Glenn et al. 2000). The ability of transcutaneous immunization to elicit intestinal antibody responses is intriguing and may relate to the observation that transcutaneous antigens co-administered with CT-like adjuvants induce IgA Ab-secreting cells that express CCR9 and CCR10 and can migrate to the small intestine (Chang et al. 2008).

4.4 Parenteral Vaccination

Finally, as discussed above (Fig. 1), parenteral vaccination routes may be effective for immunization against mucosal infections caused by pathogens which are taken up or penetrate the epithelium. For instance, parenteral vaccine-induced serum IgG antibodies can protect against intestinal pathogens either by preventing subepithelial microbial spread (e.g. shigellosis) or invasion through draining vessels (e.g. typhoid). In addition, parenteral administration might be used in tandem with mucosal vaccines, whether the latter are given by oral, nasal or sublingual route. Parenteral polio or cholera vaccines given as a booster have been found to stimulate antigen-specific S-IgA responses in naturally primed individuals although they did not induce any such response when given to immunologically naïve individuals. Thus, injectable and mucosal vaccines might synergize with each other in their protective profiles if given in tandem.

5 "Tropical Barriers" to Mucosal Vaccines

The oral polio vaccine (OPV), which was licensed more than 50 years ago, is a classic mucosal vaccine. In addition to its enormous impact in eradicating polio in most countries, this vaccine has served as a useful tool in elucidating the fundamental aspects of mucosal immunity in humans (Ogra and Karzon 1969; Ogra and Ogra 1973). Similar to the injectable, inactivated polio vaccine (IPV) but five times cheaper, OPV produces antibodies in the blood that prevent dissemination of poliovirus to the nervous system. However, unlike IPV, OPV also produces a local S-IgA immune response in the intestinal mucosa—the primary site of poliovirus entry. This intestinal immune response is the most critical property of the OPV, since it can rapidly stop person-to-person transmission of wild poliovirus ("herd protection"), making mass campaigns with OPV a most powerful strategy for the global eradication of polio. This would not be feasible with the injectable IPV. However, at the same time, concerns have been raised after reports of low or no response to OPV in children from certain developing countries, even after giving as many as 10 OPV doses. Like the OPV situation, several live oral vaccines have performed poorly in developing countries compared with industrialized countries. This is attributed mainly to chronic environmental enteropathy (CEE), also called tropical enteropathy, which is characterized by disturbances in digestive and absorptive functions. Factors that may contribute to CEE include poor sanitation, overgrowth of intestinal flora, and histological changes characterized by inflammation and blunting of small intestinal villi leading to malabsorption. Children living under extreme poverty are especially sensitive.

Other factors that might hurt the performance of oral vaccines in developing countries include: deficiencies in nutrients such as vitamin A (retinol) and zinc, which can influence the response to oral adjuvants and vaccines by affecting discrete subpopulations of intestinal dendritic cells and T cells; persistent activation of the gut innate immune system by infectious agents, such as helminths and concomitant viral and bacterial infections; and interferences by maternal breast milk (breast milk from mothers of low socioeconomic status in developing countries contains high titers of antibodies to enteric pathogens that can interfere with oral vaccine "take").

Strategies for coping with the different causes of immune hyporesponsiveness to oral vaccines in developing countries include the co-administration of vaccines with agents that improve gut integrity, such as zinc, vitamin A, and possibly probiotics; withdrawal of breast milk shortly before oral vaccination; and treatment of helminths prior to oral immunization. It would be interesting to determine if vaccines administered by a non-intestinal route could overcome these gut barriers.

6 Surrogates of Mucosal Vaccine-Induced Immunity

As of today, there is no method that has been qualified by regulatory bodies for analysis of mucosal immune responses to vaccines. Traditional approaches, such as measurement of secretory antibodies in external secretions or in organ lavages using immunoassays have not gained general acceptance, having either met with problems of reproducibility (even for a given individual tested on several occasions in a single day) or their impracticality on a large scale (e.g. gut and bronchoalveolar lavages), especially in young infants and children.

Probably, the most challenging problem that these methods will continue to face is the inherent compartmentalization of immune responses induced by mucosal immunization. Thus, immune responses measured in one mucosal tissue do not faithfully reflect responses induced in another.

Several approaches are now being developed based on the improved knowledge of mechanisms governing dissemination of mucosal immune responses and especially of mucosal plasmablasts. One such approach utilizes the known ability of recently activated antibody-secreting plasmablasts to circulate in blood after antigen/vaccine exposure, regardless of where these cells were activated. Combined immunomagnetic cell-sorting and ELISPOT assay can now be performed on small samples of whole blood (without gradient enrichment for mononuclear cells) and allows for partitioned measurement of systemic and mucosal antibody responses to vaccines by detecting antigen-specific plasmablasts with a specific mucosal pedigree (e.g. $\alpha4\beta7$, CCR10). This approach may in the future be expanded to cells with defined mucosal tissue tropism, such as cells expressing markers specific for the small intestine, large intestine, lung, or genital tract.

7 Perspectives

Better knowledge of human mucosal immune responsiveness during early life is required to establish the usefulness of different routes of vaccine administration against pathogens encountered by neonates and young infants from developing and industrialized countries. To explore the impact of environmental factors (tropical enteropathy, malnutrition and maternal factors) on mucosal responses to vaccines administered by different routes in developing countries, studies should be conducted with licensed killed and live mucosal vaccines, and for comparison, also with live and killed parenteral vaccines. Animal models could also be helpful in exploring the influence of these factors on mucosal immune responsiveness to antigens and adjuvants administered by these different routes.

The choice of mucosal vaccination route will impact overall vaccine design, including the selection of appropriate adjuvants and formulations, and thus, manufacturing issues. When compared with most licensed injectable vaccines, it is interesting to note that currently, there are no pure subunit vaccines formulated and licensed for mucosal administration. Because most injectable subunit vaccines are given with an adjuvant, a further challenge in the field will be the development of adjuvants to enhance the potency of future subunit vaccines administered by different mucosal routes.

Dearly needed are standardized, validated assays that do not require large sample volumes (especially in young children), and reference reagents for large scale measurements of mucosal immune responses to vaccines. Further research is needed to understand the mechanisms contributing to the generation and maintenance of mucosal adaptive B cell and T cell memory responses.

However, these challenges could be met with expanded use of animal models, multi-disciplinary efforts between basic scientists and clinical vaccinologists, and, most importantly, by implementing experimental systems using both animal models and human clinical trials to address the gaps in our understanding of the human mucosal immune system.

Acknowledgments The authors express their gratitude to Dr. Mi-Na Kweon for her comments regarding the contents and design of this review. Ms. Deborah Jin Hong. Mrs. Hyunsong Lee, and Pilim Choi are thanked for their expert assistance in the preparation of this manuscript. The International Vaccine Institute is supported by the governments of the Republic of Korea, Sweden, the Netherlands and Kuwait.

References

Berg EL et al (1989) Homing receptors and vascular addressins: cell adhesion molecules that direct lymphocyte traffic. Immunol Rev 108:5–18

Bilsborough J, Viney JL (2004) Gastrointestinal dendritic cells play a role in immunity, tolerance, and disease. Gastroenterology 127:300–309

Brandtzaeg P, Pabst R (2004) Let's go mucosal: communication on slippery ground. Trends in immunology. *Trends Immunol* 25:570–577.

Chang SY et al (2008) Cutting edge: Langerin + dendritic cells in the mesenteric lymph node set the stage for skin and gut immune system cross-talk. J Immunol 180:4361–4365

Cuburu N et al (2007) Sublingual immunization induces broad-based systemic and mucosal immune responses in mice. Vaccine 25:8598–8610

Cuburu N et al (2009) Sublingual immunization with nonreplicating antigens induces antibody-forming cells and cytotoxic T cells in the female genital tract mucosa and protects against genital papillomavirus infection. J Immunol 183:7851–7859

Czerkinsky C et al (1991) Antibody-producing cells in peripheral blood and salivary glands after oral cholera vaccination of humans. Infect Immun 59:996–1001

Eriksson K et al (1998) Specific-antibody-secreting cells in the rectums and genital tracts of nonhuman primates following vaccination. Infect Immunol 66:5889–5896

Fahlen-Yrlid et al (2009) CD11c(high)dendritic cells are essential for activation of CD4+ T cells and generation of specific antibodies following mucosal immunization. J Immunol 183: 5032–5041

Glenn GM RM et al (1998) Skin immunization made possible by cholera toxin. Nature 391:851

Glenn GM TD et al (2000) Transcutaneous immunization: a human vaccine delivery strategy using a patch. Nat Med 6:1403–1406

Holmgren J, Czerkinsky C (2005) Mucosal immunity and vaccines. Nat Med 11:S45–S53

Ishikawa H et al (1999) New gut associated lymphoid tissue "cryptopatches" breed murine intestinal intraepithelial T cell precursors. Immunol Res 20:243–250

Iwasaki A (2007) Mucosal dendritic cells. Annu Rev Immunol 25:381–418

Jang MH et al (2004) Intestinal villous M cells: an antigen entry site in the mucosal epithelium. Proc Natl Acad Sci USA 101:6110–6115

Jertborn M et al (1994) Immunological memory after immunization with oral cholera B subunit-whole-cell vaccine in Swedish volunteers. Vaccine 12:1078–1082

Jertborn M et al (2001) Local and systemic immune responses to rectal administration of recombinant cholera toxin B subunit in humans. Infect Immunol 69:4125–4128

Johansson EL et al (2001) Nasal and vaginal vaccinations have differential effects on antibody responses in vaginal and cervical secretions in humans. Infect Immun 69:7481–7486

Johansson EL et al (2004) Comparison of different routes of vaccination for eliciting antibody responses in the human stomach. Vaccine 22:984–990

Johansson-Lindbom B et al (2005) Functional specialization of gut CD103+ dendritic cells in the regulation of tissue-selective T cell homing. J Exp Med 202:1063–1073

Kiyono H, Fukuyama S (2004) NALT—versus Peyer's-patch-mediated mucosal immunity. Nat Rev Immunol 4:699–710

Kozlowski PA et al (1997) Comparison of the oral, rectal, and vaginal immunization routes for induction of antibodies in rectal and genital tract secretions of women. Infect Immun 65:1387–1394

Kozlowski PA et al (2002) Differential induction of mucosal and systemic antibody responses in women after nasal, rectal, or vaginal immunization: influence of the menstrual cycle. J Immunol 169:566–574

Kraehenbuhl JP, Neutra MR (2000) Epithelial M cells: differentiation and function. Annu Rev Cell Dev Biol 16:301–332

Kunkel EJ, Butcher EC (2003) Plasma-cell homing. Nat Rev Immunol 3:822–829

Kunkel EJ et al (2003) Chemokines in lymphocyte trafficking and intestinal immunity. Microcirculation 10:313–323

Kunkel EJ et al (2003) CCR10 expression is a common feature of circulating and mucosal epithelial tissue IgA Ab-secreting cells. J Clin Invest 111:1001–1010

Mora JR et al (2003) Selective imprinting of gut-homing T cells by Peyer's patch dendritic cells. Nature 424:88–93

Mora JR et al (2006) Generation of gut-homing IgA-secreting B cells by intestinal dendritic cells. Science 314:1157–1160

Mowat AM (2003) Anatomical basis of tolerance and immunity to intestinal antigens. Nat Rev Immunol 3:331–341

Nardelli-Haefliger D et al (2003) Specific antibody levels at the cervix during the menstrual cycle of women vaccinated with human papillomavirus 16 virus-like particles. J Natl Cancer Inst 95:1128–1137

Ogra PL, Karzon DT (1969) Poliovirus antibody response in serum and nasal secretions following intranasal inoculation with inactivated poliovaccine. J Immunol 102:15–23

Ogra PL, Karzon DT (1969) Distribution of poliovirus antibody in serum, nasopharynx and alimentary tract following segmental immunization of lower alimentary tract with poliovaccine. J Immunol 102:1423–1430

Ogra PL, Ogra SS (1973) Local antibody response to poliovaccine in the human female genital tract. J Immunol 110:1307–1311

Ogra PL (1999) Mucosal immunology. Academic Press, San Diego, pp xliii, 1628

Pan J et al (2000) A novel chemokine ligand for CCR10 and CCR3 expressed by epithelial cells in mucosal tissues. J Immunol 165:2943–2949

Quiding M et al (1991) Intestinal immune responses in humans. Oral cholera vaccination induces strong intestinal antibody responses and interferon-gamma production and evokes local immunological memory. J Clin Invest 88:143–148

Quiding-Järbrink M et al (1995) Induction of compartmentalized B-cell responses in human tonsils. Infect Immun 63:853–857

Quiding-Järbrink M et al (1997) Differential expression of tissue-specific adhesion molecules on human circulating antibody-forming cells after systemic, enteric, and nasal immunizations. A molecular basis for the compartmentalization of effector B cell responses. J Clin Invest 99:1281–1286

Raghavan S et al (2010) Sublingual protects against Heliocopeter pylori infection and induces T and B cell responses in the stomach. Infect Immun 78:4251–4260

Rakoff-Nahoum S et al (2004) Recognition of commensal microflora by toll-like receptors is required for intestinal homeostasis. Cell 118:229–241

Rescigno M, Di Sabatino A (2009) Dendritic cells in intestinal homeostasis and disease. J Clin Invest 119:2441–2450

Rudin A et al (1998) Differential kinetics and distribution of antibodies in serum and nasal and vaginal secretions after nasal and oral vaccination of humans. Infect Immun 66:3390–3396

Song JH et al (2008) Sublingual vaccination with influenza virus protects mice against lethal viral infection. Proc Natl Acad Sci USA 105:1644–1649

Song JH et al (2009) CCR7-CCL19/CCL21-regulated dendritic cells are responsible for effectiveness of sublingual vaccination. J Immunol 182(11):6851–6860

Stagg AJ et al (2002) Intestinal dendritic cells increase T cell expression of alpha4beta7 integrin. Eur J Immunol 32:1445–1454

Wang W et al (2000) Identification of a novel CC chemokine (CCL28) which binds CCR10 (GPR2). J Biol Chem 275:22313–22323

Wassén L et al (1996) Local intravaginal vaccination of the female genital tract. Scand J Immunol 44(4):408–414

Mucosal Immune Responses Induced by Transcutaneous Vaccines

L. B. Lawson, J. D. Clements and L. C. Freytag

Abstract The skin has been investigated as a site for vaccine delivery only since the late 1990s. However, much has been discovered about the cell populations that reside in the skin, their active role in immune responses, and the fate of transcutaneously applied antigens. Transcutaneous immunization (TCI) is a safe, effective means of inducing immune responses against a number of pathogens. One of the most notable benefits of TCI is the induction of immune responses in both systemic and mucosal compartments. This chapter focuses on the transport of antigen into and beyond intact skin, the cutaneous sentinel cell populations that play a role in TCI, and the types of mucosal immune responses that have been generated. A number of in vivo studies in murine models have provided information about the broad responses induced by TCI. Cellular and humoral responses and protection against challenge have been noted in the gastrointestinal, reproductive, and respiratory tracts. Clinical trials have demonstrated the benefits of this vaccine delivery route in humans. As with other routes of immunization, the type of vaccine formulation and choice of adjuvant may be critical for achieving appropriate responses and can be tailored to activate specific immune-responsive cells in the skin to increase the efficacy of TCI against mucosal pathogens.

Contents

L. B. Lawson, J. D. Clements and L. C. Freytag (✉)
Department of Microbiology and Immunology, Tulane University School of Medicine,
1430 Tulane Avenue, New Orleans, LA 70112, USA
e-mail: lfreyta@tulane.edu

Current Topics in Microbiology and Immunology (2012) 354: 19–37

DOI: 10.1007/82_2010_113

Published Online: 9 November 2010

1 Introduction

Transcutaneous immunization (TCI) also known as transdermal vaccine delivery (TVD) is a novel, safe, non-invasive method of inducing antigen-specific cellular and humoral immune responses via direct application of a vaccine antigen onto the skin. The advantages of needle-free immunization include easier and faster vaccine administration, increased safety, elimination of pain at the injection site, reduction of trained healthcare personnel, and improved compliance with vaccination schedules. The skin, like other epithelial surfaces, serves a crucial function in regulating exchange of matter between the body and the outside environment. The skin's role as a barrier against moisture loss, chemical or physical injury and pathogen entry has been extensively studied. However, only in the past few decades, the active role of immune-responsive cells of the skin has been noted (Silberberg-Sinakin et al. 1976; Sauder 1983; Streilin 1985). More recently, the concept of using the skin as a site of vaccine administration has been explored; the first investigation of topical vaccination was reported in 1997 (Tang et al. 1997). Since then, a substantial number of published reports have demonstrated the feasibility of TCI as an effective vaccine delivery method in animals and humans. It has also become evident that a key player in the outcome of TCI is the choice of adjuvant employed. The induction of humoral and cellular responses in both systemic and mucosal compartments, first reported in 1998 (Glenn et al. 1998b), is one of the most notable benefits of this technique over traditional parenteral vaccine administration.

2 Transport of Antigen Through the Skin

The skin is composed of three major layers: the epidermis, dermis, and hypodermis or subcutis (Young et al. 2006). Figure 1 displays a micrograph of the structure of the outermost layers of the skin; cells that are most involved in transcutaneous

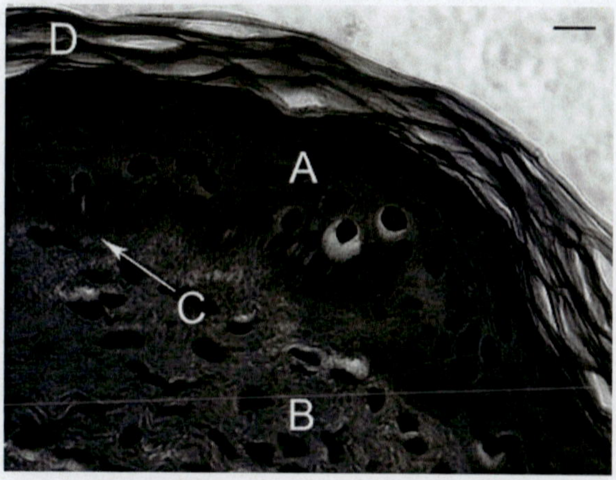

Fig. 1 Hematoxylin and eosin stain of porcine skin section showing the major tissue layers, the epidermis (*A*) and dermis (*B*), with the basement membrane (*C*) located at the junction between the two. The outermost region of the epidermis is the stratum corneum (*D*). *Bar* = 10 μm. Reprinted with permission from Macmillan Publishers Ltd: Clinical Pharmacology & Therapeutics (Lawson et al. 2007)

immune response are located within the epidermal and dermal layers. To achieve an efficacious immune response, antigens applied to the skin must traverse the topmost keratinized layers of the skin to reach the immune-responsive cells. The outer portion of the epidermis, the stratum corneum, is composed of non-nucleated highly keratinized cells surrounded by densely packed lipid molecules. This layer provides a barrier to moisture loss and pathogen entry, and also limits the permeation of large molecular-weight antigens. Various techniques have been considered to circumvent this limitation for TCI, including the use of adjuvants, disrupting the integrity of the stratum corneum by tape stripping, swabbing with alcohol or other solvents, hydration, ultrasound, microneedles, and other physical or chemical permeation enhancers. Tape stripping and solvent application not only abrogate the skin barrier but also activate resident cells to augment expression of cytokine and co-stimulatory molecules and to enhance antigen presentation (Nickoloff and Naidu 1994; Nishijima et al. 1997). While such methods can increase antigen permeation and typically improve immune response, transport of highly immunogenic antigens and adjuvants across intact skin with induction of protective immunity has also been demonstrated (Glenn et al. 1998a, b).

Another consideration for TCI is the anatomical site of antigen application. It is known that variations in the thickness and composition of the skin exist at different sites of the human body, indicating potential differences in permeability of applied antigens. A few studies have compared the efficacy of TCI at different anatomical sites in mice. Although there were differences in the role of skin-resident dendritic cells (DCs) following TCI on the ear versus the flank, no differences in T cell proliferation in the draining lymph nodes were observed (Wang et al. 2008). There were also no significant differences in serum antibody levels following ear or back TCI (Scharton-Kersten et al. 1999). However, there were greater serum antibody responses with administration of an HIV peptide and cholera toxin (CT) adjuvant on the back and abdomen compared to administration on the ear (Belyakov et al. 2004). Antigen-specific $CD8^+$ cytotoxic T lymphocytes (CTLs) in the gut mucosa were also lower with immunization on the ear than on the back or abdomen (Belyakov et al. 2004). In clinical trials, transcutaneous vaccines have been administered on the upper arm (Glenn et al. 2000; Frech et al. 2008) and forearm (Etchart et al. 2007) of volunteers.

3 Immune-Responsive Cells in the Skin

The skin is more than a passive barrier protecting the host against physical or chemical damage. We now know that non-inflamed skin is an immunologically active site that contains numerous cell populations of immune-responsive cells. The presence and function of these cells determines the response to antigens that permeate across the stratum corneum. Figure 2 is a schematic representation of the stratified layers of the epidermis, dermis and the main cell types involved in immune surveillance, antigen uptake, and initiation of immune responses. Contributors to the cutaneous immune response include keratinocytes, epidermal and

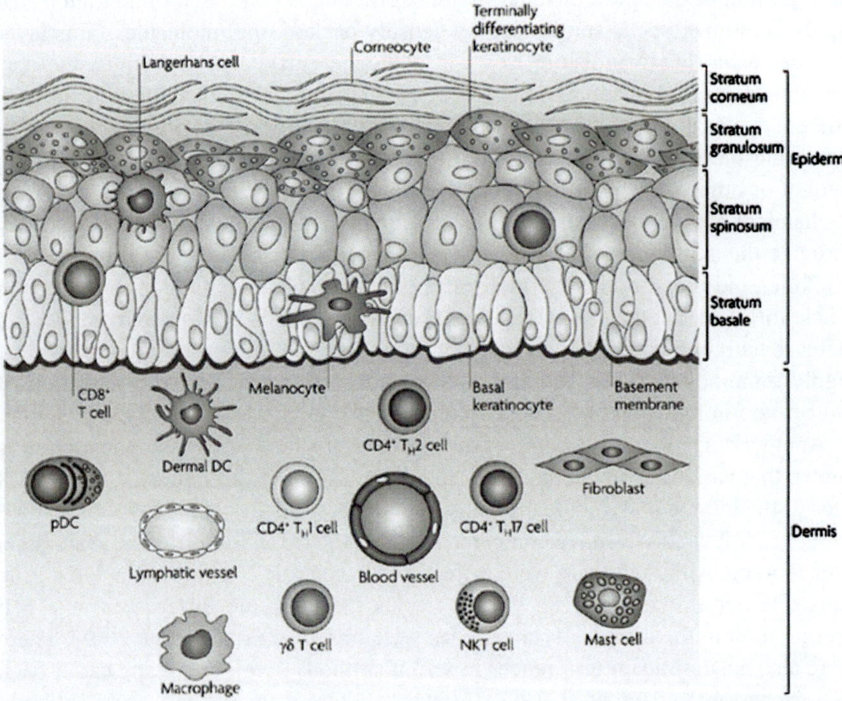

Fig. 2 Schematic representation of the skin anatomy and the cellular effectors involved in the generation of immune responses. Reprinted with permission from Macmillan Publishers Ltd: Nature Reviews Immunology (Nestle et al. 2009)

dermal DCs (dDCs), T lymphocytes, Natural Killer (NK)-T cells, mast cells and macrophages, among others. Curiously, the presence of B cells, B cell follicles, or germinal centers seen in some mucosal tissues has not been noted in the skin (Kapsenberg and Bos 1998).

3.1 Keratinocytes

Comprising 95% of epidermal cells (Wood et al. 1992), keratinocytes are epithelial cells that are predominant in the epidermis and are responsible for the production of keratin, a fibrous protein that contributes to the skin's protective barrier by providing structural support (Young et al. 2006). Through their production of various cytokines and chemokines, keratinocytes have a crucial role in maintaining the skin's physical barrier structure as well as in contributing to local innate and acquired immune responses. Cytokine and chemokine production by keratinocytes occurs both constitutively and in response to various stimuli. Disruption of the epidermal barrier can induce cytokine production by keratinocytes (Wood et al. 1992). Activation is also triggered by proinflammatory cytokines produced by other cells (Williams and Kupper 1996). Early in the immune response, cytokine production by keratinocytes induces motility of antigen presenting cells (APCs) in the skin (Kissenpfennig and Malissen 2006). Indicating their role in innate immune response, human keratinocytes express functional Toll-like receptors (TLRs) which contribute to the immune response against viral and bacterial pathogens (Köllisch et al. 2005; Kalali et al. 2008). TLR activation of keratinocytes has been shown to enhance DC activation in vitro (Sugita et al. 2007). Recent publications suggest that keratinocytes may also play a role as non-professional APCs because they express MHC class II molecules and can present peptide antigens to $CD4^+$ and $CD8^+$ T cells (Black et al. 2007). Keratinocytes play a role in directing the cutaneous immune response toward a cellular or humoral response, in the regulation of the thickness of the epidermis, and in promoting growth, maturation, and mobilization of leukocytes from the blood (Williams and Kupper 1996).

3.2 Dendritic Cells

The skin is rich in APCs such as macrophages and DCs, which act as sentinels patrolling the skin and are an essential component of innate defense against pathogens. While macrophages mostly function in pathogen clearance, DCs specialize in linking innate and adaptive immune responses and their primary role is antigen presentation rather than pathogen elimination. DCs are professional APCs, capable of efficiently capturing, processing, and presenting antigens on their surfaces in MHC molecules in close proximity to co-stimulatory molecules. DCs are especially potent at priming naive T cells to initiate antigen-specific immune responses.

Two types of DCs—dDCs and Langerhans cells (LCs)—are abundant in the skin of humans and animals. Upon stimulation, dDCs and LCs initiate antigen uptake, differentiate, become more mature, and migrate via afferent lymphatics to the draining lymph nodes, where they contact naive T and B cells. Within the epidermis, LCs play a critical role in antigen presentation. LCs comprise approximately 2% of the total epidermal cell population; however, these cells cover over 25% of the total surface area of the skin, as illustrated in Fig. 3. Their orientation parallel to the skin and dendrites maximizes exposure to foreign antigens that enter the skin (Yu et al. 1994). LCs typically localize within the upper level of the viable epidermis, although some are found deeper toward the basement membrane (Hauser et al. 1991). Most early studies of LC were focused on their role in contact hypersensitivity (Silberberg-Sinakin et al. 1976). Their role in systemic immune responses is now becoming more clearly understood.

A distinguishing characteristic of LCs is the presence of cytoplasmic Birbeck granules. The development of these tennis racket-shaped organelles is dependent on the expression of the endocytic receptor langerin/CD207. Once thought to be another defining characteristic of LC, langerin expression was recently shown not only in LCs but also in other distinct DC populations of the dermis (Bursch et al. 2007). Bone marrow-derived circulating DC can also express langerin (Chang et al. 2008). Another distinguishing molecule expressed by LCs is CD1a. This molecule is associated with the ability of LCs to present certain bacterial lipids and glycolipids as well as peptide antigen to T cells (Kapsenberg and Bos 1998).

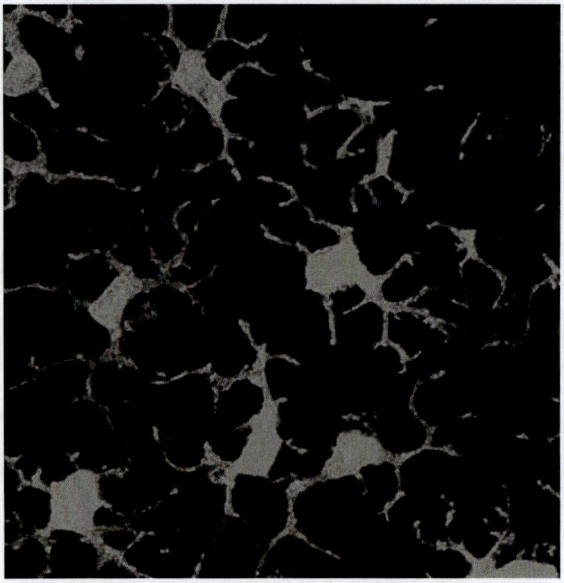

Fig. 3 Confocal micrograph showing the dense network of epidermal Langerhans cells in the ear of mice expressing enhanced green fluorescence protein under control of the *langerin* gene. Reprinted from Trends in Immunology (Kissenpfennig and Malissen 2006) with permission from Elsevier

Langerhans cells upregulate MHC class II molecules, co-stimulatory molecule CD40, and lymph node homing molecule CCR7 during migration from the skin to draining lymph nodes (Merad et al. 2008).

Like LCs, dDCs are active immune responders. dDCs were identified much more recently than their epidermal counterparts and are not as well characterized as LCs (Romani et al. 2006). dDCs are more abundant than LCs, and they have a distinct role in immune responses (Nestle et al. 1998). Expression of CD11c distinguishes dDCs from LCs. The CD1c (blood DC antigen-1) molecule is also expressed by dDCs but not LCs (Zaba et al. 2007). dDCs are typically localized in the perivascular region of the dermis (Nestle et al. 1998).

dDCs and LCs are comparable in their ability to present soluble antigen to T cells in vitro (Nestle et al. 1998). However, these two cell populations have distinguishing TLR expression profiles, indicating differences in their role in immune responses. dDCs express TLRs 1–8, while LCs have impaired expression of TLR2, TLR4, TLR5, and TLR8. As a result, LCs are less reactive to Gram-negative and Gram-positive bacteria, which likely prevents LCs from initiating an inflammatory response against commensal bacteria colonizing the skin. Langerhans cells and dDCs do react comparably to viral antigens (van der Aar et al. 2007). The TLR expression profile of LCs and dDCs is an important consideration in designing vaccine formulations for TCI.

3.3 T Cells

Substantial numbers of T lymphocytes exist in the human skin with limited distribution in the epidermis and a more prevalent population in the dermal perivascular region (Spetz et al. 1996; Clark et al. 2006). The T cells in non-inflamed skin express cutaneous-lymphocyte-associated antigen (CLA), which is a ligand for E-selectin. Interaction of CLA+ T cells with E-selectin in the cutaneous endothelium facilitates selective migration of lymphocytes to the skin. Various adhesion molecules, leukocyte chemoattractants and cell surface markers have also been implicated in the homing of T cells to the skin. In this context, an interesting recent observation indicates that Vitamin D_3, generated in the skin upon exposure to sunlight, can be converted to its active form ($1,25(OH)_2D_3$) by subsets of DC, macrophages and keratinocytes. This activated form has been shown to induce T cell expression of CCR10 chemokine receptor and migration toward keratinocyte-produced CCL27 in vitro (Sigmundsdottir et al. 2007). Regardless of the mechanisms governing T cell homing to the skin, it is evident that large pools of T cells are continuously present in the cutaneous environment, where they can immediately contact antigen-capturing DCs.

Although resident skin T cells are phenotypically diverse, most are Th1 effector memory cells, with lesser numbers of Th2 cells, central memory cells and regulatory T cells. Epidermal T cells are found in close proximity to LCs in the basal keratinocyte layer. The majority of epidermal T lymphocytes are $CD8^+$ $\alpha\beta$. In contrast, $CD4^+$ memory T cells predominate in the perivascular dermis (Kapsenberg and Bos 1998; Clark et al. 2006). Dermal T cells localize close to postcapillary venules in the epidermal–dermal junction (Fig. 2). Several subsets of $CD4^+$ Th1, Th2 and Th17 are found in the dermis. These have been associated with inflammatory skin diseases, but it is likely that they also participate in immune surveillance and immune responses to antigens encountered by APCs in the skin.

3.4 Other Immune-Responsive Cells

Other cell populations in the skin contribute to the outcome of TCI. Heib et al. 2007 demonstrated a role for dermal mast cells in LC migration, inflammation, and in the induction of CTL responses following TCI. A population of macrophages has been identified in the dermis of normal human skin based on expression of CD163, a scavenger receptor selectively expressed on monocytes and macrophages. These cells appear to be weak stimulators of T cell proliferation (Zaba et al. 2007). The roles of macrophages, granulocytes, NK cells, and $\gamma\delta$ T cells in skin immune responses have not been elucidated, but this information would be helpful for designing and formulating transcutaneous vaccines such that they generate desired immune responses (Warger et al. 2007).

4 Antigen Migration from the Skin

Running parallel to the skin surface, a network of lymphatic vessels exists just below the epidermis. These vessels form an interconnected mesh-like network (see Fig. 4) and drain through slightly larger ducts to collecting vessels in the deeper regions of the dermis. The collecting vessels actively propel lymphatic fluid from

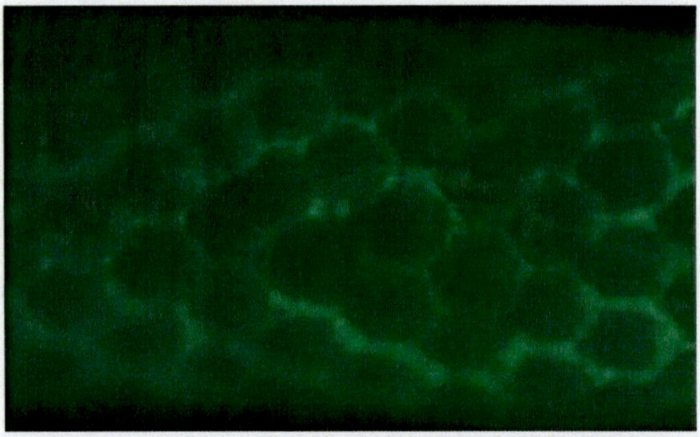

Fig. 4 Fluorescence micrograph showing the regular polygonal pattern of skin lymphatic vessels using fluorescent lymphatic tracers. Microscopic view is through the epidermis of a mouse tail. Reprinted by permission from Macmillan Publishers Ltd: Nature Reviews Immunology (Randolph et al. 2005)

the tissue to the lymph nodes. Flow in these vessels is unidirectional such that cells and molecules downstream in the lymph nodes do not return to or directly influence cells in the periphery (Randolph et al. 2005).

The migration of transcutaneously applied material has been studied using fluorescent dyes, fluorescently labeled proteins, and electron microscopy to better understand the responses induced by this immunization route. Fluorescent dye applied to the skin with or without protein immunogen was found in the regional draining, but not distal, lymph nodes of mice 24 h after administration. In the presence of protein immunogen, an increase in DC activation markers in the lymph nodes most proximal to the site of transcutaneous application was noted (Guebre-Xabier et al. 2003). In early investigations, ferritin-bearing LCs in draining lymph nodes were observed as soon as 4 h after the application of this protein on skin (Silberberg-Sinakin et al. 1976).

The use of knock-in mice expressing green fluorescent protein (GFP) under the control of the *langerin* gene has allowed researchers to distinguish trafficking of LC and other langerin$^+$ cells from that of dDC. dDC arrived in the lymph nodes 24 h post-treatment, while GFP-laden LCs were not detected until later time points (Kissenpfennig et al. 2005). Using similar techniques, the relative migration of LCs versus other APCs was shown to vary depending on the site (e.g. ear or flank) of TCI in mice (Wang et al. 2008). Together, these studies have demonstrated an active role for LC and other cell populations in the transport of antigens to draining lymph nodes following TCI.

When fluorescently labeled *E. coli* heat labile enterotoxin (LT) was applied to the skin of mice, the fluorescent label was detected in APCs in intestinal Peyer's patches but not in the spleen or non-draining lymph nodes at 24 and 48 h, suggesting that APCs migrate from the skin to directly present antigen to intestinal lymphocytes (Belyakov et al. 2004). Whether these skin-derived APCs reach other mucosal locations has not yet been determined.

5 Adjuvants for Transcutaneous Vaccines

A critical element in enhancing antigen-specific responses by TCI is the choice of method used to activate APCs in the skin. Different strategies have been employed to enhance the immune response, including disruption of the stratum corneum (by tape stripping, microneedles, electrical impulses, prolonged hydration), micro- or nanocarriers, and the use of adjuvants such as imiquimod, CpG, or bacterial enterotoxins (Partidos et al. 2004; Glenn and Kenney 2006).

The bacterial ADP-ribosylating enterotoxins (BARE)—CT, produced by various strains of *Vibrio cholerae*, and the closely related LT, produced by some enterotoxigenic strains of *Escherichia coli*—are effective adjuvants for systemic, mucosal and transdermal vaccines (Clements et al. 1988; Dickinson and Clements 1996; Glenn et al. 1998a; Freytag and Clements 1999, 2005). Both CT and LT are synthesized as multisubunit toxins with A and B components. The A-subunit is the enzymatically active moiety and consists of two chains, A1 and A2, joined by a proteolytically sensitive link (Arg192) subtended by a disulfide loop. Like other A–B toxins, CT and LT require nicking and disulfide reduction to be fully biologically active. When CT or LT first encounter a mammalian cell, they bind to the surface through interaction of the B-subunit pentamer. The A2 peptide of CT or LT facilitates association of A1 with the B-pentamer and helps direct retrograde transport of these molecules through the Golgi cisternae to the ER. Once in the ER, the A1 chain is transported across the membrane into the cytosol where it binds NAD^+ and transfers the ADP-ribose moiety from NAD^+ to the α subunit of one member of the heterotrimeric GTP-binding protein family. As a consequence, adenylate cyclase is irreversibly activated, leading to elevation in intracellular cyclic AMP (cAMP). Increased levels of cAMP activate protein kinase A which phosphorylates and opens the cystic fibrosis transmembrane conductance regulator chloride channel. Chloride efflux results in the concomitant osmotic movement of water into the gut lumen and the profuse watery diarrhea characteristic of cholera or enterotoxigenic *E. coli* infection in humans.

It has been reported that CT upregulates expression of co-stimulatory molecules on DC and promotes DC mobility, maturation and activation (Gagliardi et al. 2000). However, the exact mechanisms responsible for the adjuvant effects of BARE on DC have not been identified. The BARE can elicit mixed Th1/Th2 or Th2-biased immune responses, which may depend on the levels of cAMP induced in cells as cAMP ultimately suppresses DC production of IL-12 by inhibiting activity of the interferon regulatory factor 8 transcription factor (la Sala et al. 2010). Only a few studies have addressed the effects that CT and LT exert on skin-derived APCs. One suggested that CT adjuvant activity after skin immunization may be due to the secretion of proinflammatory cytokines from activated epidermal LCs and keratinocytes (Partidos et al. 2004). It has also been proposed that apoptosis of keratinocytes creates intercellular spaces resulting in more efficient diffusion of adjuvant and antigen molecules (Partidos et al. 2004).

Non-methylated CpG oligodeoxynucleotides (CpG ODNs) are TLR9 agonists. The adjuvant activity of CpG ODN has been attributed to several different effects on innate and adaptive immune responses. First, CpG ODNs cause B cells to proliferate and secrete immunoglobulin, synergizing strongly with antigen-specific effects mediated through B cells. In addition, CpG ODNs upregulates expression of co-stimulatory molecules and MHC class II molecules, improving antigen presentation. CpG ODNs also directly activate monocytes, macrophages and DC to secrete IFN-α/β, IL-6, IL-12, GM-CSF, chemokines, and TNF-α, which in turn stimulate T cells to secrete additional cytokines and NK cells to secrete IFN-γ. A T-helper function is provided by the strong Th1-like pattern of cytokine production that is dominated by IL-12 and IFN-γ, with little secretion of Th2 cytokines. The exact mechanisms responsible for the immunostimulatory action of CpG ODN are only now being resolved. One hypothesis is that CpG-DNA (either as a free molecule or encapsulated in whole bacteria) is taken up by an APC. After processing through a chloroquine-sensitive pathway, signaling is triggered by engagement of TLR9. The proteins myeloid differentiation factor 88 (MyD88), interleukin-1 receptor-associated kinase and tumor necrosis factor receptor-associated factor 6 activate cellular kinases such as IkB kinase and mitogen-activated protein kinase. Signal transduction through these well-known pathways leads to gene induction and evokes effector functions, such as cytokine secretion. CpG ODNs have been shown to function as effective adjuvants for transdermally delivered vaccines (Klimuk et al. 2004; Sugita et al. 2007).

Imiquimod (1-(2-methylpropyl)-1H-imidazo[4,5-c]quinolin-4-amine) is a synthetic derivative of imidazoquinoline, which is a ligand for TLR7. Imiquimod (marketed as Aldara^{TM}) is an FDA-approved therapy for the treatment of human external genital warts, actinic keratosis, and basal cell carcinoma. This compound acts as an immune modifier and activates DCs in vitro by inducing MyD88-dependent DC maturation and release of inflammatory cytokines. Rechtsteiner et al. (2005) recently described a study in which skin application of a CTL epitope in combination with imiquimod induced a robust CTL response against the target characterized by T cell proliferation, cytolytic activity and IFN-γ production. Topical imiquimod application to mouse skin induces migration of LCs from the epidermis to the local lymph nodes. It has been demonstrated that imiquimod also induces maturation of human epidermal LCs, enhances IL-12 production, and increases IFN-α production by $CD4^+$ T cells (Burns et al. 2000). It is thought that the effects of imiquimod on epidermal LCs are an important mechanism of action by which imiquimod induces Th1-dominant cellular responses in situ during the treatment of certain malignancies. Although it is known that dDCs, LCs and keratinocytes express intracytoplasmic TLR7, the exact effects of imiquimod on the activation of skin-derived APCs have not been defined.

Various nanocarriers and specifically tailored formulations show promise for TCI either by enhancing permeation through the stratum corneum or by increasing antigen uptake by APCs and other cells. The use of a lipid matrix for transcutaneous delivery of a *Helicobacter pylori* vaccine in mice induced protection against gastric challenge in the absence of co-administered adjuvants, although the addition of CT and CpG to the lipid formulation further enhanced protection (Hickey et al. 2009b). The use of particulate micro- and nanocarriers with encapsulated or adsorbed antigen can influence antigen uptake in the skin. The particle composition (lipid, polymer, virus-like particles, etc.), size, charge and degradability are important factors for interaction with DC, T cells, B cells and other components of the immune response. Mishra et al. (2006) demonstrated increased ex vivo macrophage uptake and in vivo lymphatic accumulation, follicular enlargement and both serum and salivary IgA responses with elastic liposomes applied transcutaneously. This supports the role of these and other carriers in modulating the immune response upon TCI.

Overall, it is clear that adjuvants play a fundamental role in the activation of skin DC upon transcutaneous delivery of vaccines. It is critical to design studies to understand how different adjuvants act upon skin APCs to influence the ultimate outcome of T cell activation. Deciphering the effects of adjuvants on skin APC maturation and activation can lead to the development of tailored vaccines for specific pathogens and specific immune responses.

6 Mucosal Immune Responses to Transcutaneous Antigens in Murine Models

TCI achieved by direct topical application of a vaccine preparation is thought to work because the vaccine components permeate the skin and interact directly with APC in the epidermis and dermis, which then migrate and interact with naive T cells in the lymph nodes to initiate adaptive immune responses (Kripke et al. 1990). Many published reports and results of clinical trials have demonstrated that TCI can induce robust systemic and mucosal immune responses in animals and humans (Yu et al. 2002; Glenn et al. 2007; Uddowla et al. 2007; Vogt et al. 2008).

6.1 Mucosal Antibody Responses in Mice Following TCI

Induction of antigen-specific antibody responses in mucosal tissues after TCI has been amply documented in animal models, particularly in mice. IgG and IgA antibodies against the immunizing antigen have been observed in the gastrointestinal, respiratory and genitourinary tracts. The mechanisms involved in the regulation of these responses are not well understood, but recent studies have documented the migration of activated DCs from the skin to the gut mucosa. Chang et al. 2008 found antigen-specific IgG and IgA antibody-secreting cells (ASC) in the small and large intestine after TCI with tetanus toxoid (TT) and CT but not after subcutaneous or intraperitoneal immunization. Others have also reported induction of specific antibodies in the intestine after TCI with various combinations of antigen and adjuvant. Among these studies, some significant observations include the generation of fecal anti-OVA IgA and IgG (Naito et al. 2007), anti-*E. coli* CS6 IgA and IgG (Yu et al. 2002) and anti-*H. pylori* IgA (Hickey et al. 2009b).

The use of TCI to protect against pathogens associated with periodontitis has been demonstrated. TCI of mice with a *Porphyromonas gingivalis* protein immunogen and CT adjuvant induced antigen-specific IgA and IgG ASC in spleens. However, ASC were present in much lower numbers in the salivary glands (Maeba et al. 2005). In long-term studies, serum IgG and IgA and salivary IgG levels remained elevated 1-year post-immunization, and oral challenge with *P. gingivalis* resulted in significantly less bone loss (Ishikura et al. 2009).

The ability to induce antigen-specific ASC in the female reproductive tract of mice using TCI has also been demonstrated. In one study (Gockel et al. 2000), the numbers of ASC detected in the uterus and vagina of mice given TCI with TT and CT were found to exceed the numbers of ASC in the small intestine and salivary glands. IgG and IgA antibodies were also detected in feces, vaginal lavage, saliva, and sera of these mice. There were no mucosal or systemic IgA responses in the absence of CT adjuvant (Gockel et al. 2000). In mice immunized transcutaneously with the major outer membrane protein (MOMP) of *Chlamydia muridarum*, the number of antigen-specific ASC in vaginal tissue was increased to a greater extent by co-delivery with CpG ODN when compared to CT (Berry et al. 2004). In another study (Skelding et al. 2006), TCI with MOMP and a mixture of CpG and CT induced antigen-specific ASC in lung tissue and protection against respiratory chlamydial challenge (Skelding et al. 2006). More recently, Hickey et al. 2009a reported that TCI with *C. muridarum* MOMP and Lipid C (a lipid-based adjuvant) or CT plus CpG was able to elicit MOMP-specific pulmonary IgG and vaginal IgG and IgA and to partially protect against chlamydia infection following vaginal or nasal challenge.

6.2 Cell-Mediated Immune Responses in Mice Following TCI

While induction of mucosal antibodies in response to TCI has been extensively documented, fewer studies have examined the antigen-specific cellular mucosal responses induced by this immunization strategy. Proliferation by $CD8^+$ T cells is one cellular response that has been demonstrated in in vivo murine studies (Stoitzner et al. 2006). Skin-derived DCs have been shown to play a direct role in antigen presentation after TCI with recombinant viral vectors and in the induction of $CD8^+$ T cell responses (He et al. 2006). TCI with imiquimod plus a peptide containing a T cell epitope has generated antigen-specific CTL in the spleen (Rechtsteiner et al. 2005).

Cell-mediated responses in the murine mucosa have also been noted after TCI with an HIV peptide. Following transdermal delivery of the vaccine, antigen-specific $CD8^+$ CTLs were observed in the Peyer's patches of the small intestine and in the spleen. The vaccine was adjuvanted by CT, LT or a combination of CT and CpG. This immunization strategy resulted in reduction of viral loads after intrarectal challenge of mice with recombinant vaccinia virus encoding HIV gp160 (Belyakov et al. 2004).

In mice transcutaneously immunized with *C. muridarum* MOMP and a mixture of CT and CpG, a balanced Th1/Th2 cytokine response was noted, and clearance of chlamydia infection was enhanced following intravaginal challenge (Berry et al. 2004).

With most antigens applied transcutaneously, the use of appropriate adjuvant is essential for inducing spleen and skin-draining lymph node lymphoproliferative or cytokine responses to antigen. Interestingly, TCI with CT as an adjuvant for TT induced a mixed Th1/Th2 response in contrast to the predominant Th2-type response elicited by oral or nasal immunization with CT and TT (Hammond et al. 2001). Transcutaneous application of LT adjuvant and a mutant of this protein (LT-R192G) has also induced a balanced Th1/Th2 response with robust antibody production, lymphocyte proliferation, and cytokine production in the lymph nodes (Hammond et al. 2001).

An interesting approach for increasing the efficacy of transcutaneous vaccines has been to immunize with whole organisms instead of purified subunit antigens. TCI against influenza, using formalin-inactivated influenza virus in the presence or absence of CT, induced systemic and mucosal antibody responses as well as cytokines. Titers of hemagglutination inhibition (HAI) and neutralizing antibody were enhanced when CT was included in the vaccine preparation (Skountzou et al. 2006; Skountzou and Kang 2009). This study also revealed that TCI with inactivated influenza virus induced secretion of IL-4 and IFN-γ by $CD4^+$ and $CD8^+$ T cells, which was stronger in the presence of CT or two other immunostimulants—oleic acid or retinoic acid.

Together, these studies illustrate three important concepts of TCI: (1) Murine models are useful for evaluating the immunogenicity of transcutaneous antigen/adjuvant combinations. (2) Antigen-specific antibody and T cells can be generated in mucosal tissues of the oral cavity, large and small intestines, respiratory tract, and female reproductive tract using TCI. (3) As with other immunization routes, the magnitude and quality of the immune responses elicited by TCI is heavily influenced by adjuvant.

7 Mucosal Immune Responses After TCI in Humans

Obtaining approvals to evaluate new immunization strategies in humans is a difficult and lengthy process with ethical and safety considerations limiting the number of permutations that can be tested in individual studies. However, the striking advantages and safety profiles of TCI predicted from animal studies have paved the way to initiate a number of clinical trials. The safety of TCI in humans has been demonstrated in studies with live-attenuated virus (Etchart et al. 2007) and bacterial toxins (Glenn et al. 2000; Guerena-Burgueno et al. 2002; Frech et al. 2008). No severe adverse reactions were noted in three separate TCI studies. Vaccine recipients also rated the transcutaneous route as being more acceptable than the subcutaneous route (Etchart et al. 2007).

Etchart et al. (2007) performed TCI with a live-attenuated measles virus. Adults in this study had been immunized as infants with live-attenuated measles vaccine. While subcutaneous but not TCI enhanced serum IgG antibodies when compared to levels present before the trial, salivary IgA levels were elevated after transcutaneous but not subcutaneous immunization. TCI also induced virus-specific IFN-γ production by peripheral blood mononuclear cells, suggesting a Th1-type response following the transcutaneous boost with measles vaccine.

TCI with *E. coli* LT, which simultaneously acts as antigen and adjuvant, induced LT-specific serum antibody that was enhanced by boosting at 12 weeks and further increased with a second boost at 35 weeks. Urine and fecal IgG and IgA were also detected (Glenn et al. 2000). When compared to placebo, the transcutaneous LT vaccine was effective for reducing the occurrence and severity of travelers' diarrhea caused by enterotoxigenic *E. coli*, indicating that TCI is safe and can impart protection against enteric disease (Frech et al. 2008).

In another study, adult volunteers received a dermal patch containing LT and the *E. coli* colonization factor CS6. The majority of vaccinees developed anti-CS6 serum IgG and IgA as well as delayed-type hypersensitivity responses. Modest immunogenicity was detected in people who received CS6 without the LT adjuvant (Guerena-Burgueno et al. 2002).

Transdermal vaccines against influenza virus infections would be very desirable, as these vaccines are intended for yearly mass administration to humans. Several studies have demonstrated the feasibility of TCI against influenza. Frech et al. (2005) demonstrated that rates of seroconversion against influenza antigens were increased after an LT-containing patch was applied on top of an injection site where a traditional influenza vaccine had been injected. This effect was particularly noticeable in elderly volunteers. A more recent study (Vogt et al. 2008) reported induction of effector CD4 and CD8 T cell responses as well as influenza-specific IFN-γ-producing T cells after transcutaneous administration of a commercially available influenza vaccine. Although no adjuvant was given in this study, the skin was treated with superglue (cyanoacrylate glue) followed by tape stripping (Vogt et al. 2008).

Although safety and efficacy are still a concern for the development of transcutaneously delivered vaccines in humans, the studies presented here provide a solid foundation to support the advancement of promising TCI vaccines from the bench to the bedside.

8 Conclusion

The skin serves a critical protective role for the detection of and responding to invading pathogens. Immunization through cutaneous surfaces takes advantage of the assortment of immune-responsive cells in the skin to initiate an adaptive immune response. The past few decades have brought about a deeper understanding of the cutaneous cells involved in TCI and the important antibody and cell-mediated responses. Both human and murine studies support the use of TCI for induction of protective systemic and mucosal immune responses. There are many variables to consider with this route of immunization, such as site of administration, type of pretreatment if any, dosing, and the selection of appropriate adjuvant(s). Immune responses have been generated in multiple mucosal compartments (respiratory, digestive, and female genitourinary tract), making this non-invasive immunization route a promising vaccine delivery strategy for protection against a variety of pathogens.

References

Belyakov IM, Hammond SA, Ahlers JD et al (2004) Transcutaneous immunization induces mucosal CTLs and protective immunity by migration of primed skin dendritic cells. J Clin Invest 113:998–1007

Berry LJ, Hickey DK, Skelding KA et al (2004) Transcutaneous immunization with combined cholera toxin and CpG adjuvant protects against *Chlamydia muridarum* genital tract infection. Infect Immun 72:1019–1028

Black AP, Ardern-Jones MR, Kasprowicz V et al (2007) Human keratinocyte induction of rapid effector function in antigen-specific memory CD4$^+$ and CD8$^+$ T cells. Eur J Immunol 37:1485–1493

Burns RP Jr, Ferbel B, Tomai M et al (2000) The imidazoquinolines, imiquimod and R-848, induce functional, but not phenotypic, maturation of human epidermal Langerhans' cells. Clin Immunol 94:13–23

Bursch L, Wang L, Igyarto B et al (2007) Identification of a novel population of Langerin$^+$ dendritic cells. J Exp Med 204:3147–3156

Chang S-Y, Cha H-R, Igarashi O et al (2008) Langerin$^+$ dendritic cells in the mesenteric lymph node set the stage for skin and gut immune system cross-talk. J Immunol 180:4361–4365

Clark RA, Chong B, Mirchandani N et al (2006) The vast majority of CLA+ T cells are resident in normal skin. J Immunol 176:4431–4439

Clements JD, Hartzog NM, Lyon FL (1988) Adjuvant activity of *Escherichia coli* heat-labile enterotoxin and effect on the induction of oral tolerance in mice to unrelated protein antigens. Vaccine 6:269–277

Dickinson BL, Clements JD (1996) Use of *Escherichia coli* heat-labile enterotoxin as an oral adjuvant. In: Kiyono H, Ogra PL, McGhee JR (eds) Mucosal vaccines. Academic Press, San Diego, CA

Etchart N, Hennino A, Friede M et al (2007) Safety and efficacy of transcutaneous vaccination using a patch with the live-attenuated measles vaccine in humans. Vaccine 25:6891–6899

Frech SA, DuPont HL, Bourgeois AL et al (2008) Use of a patch containing heat-labile toxin from *Escherichia coli* against traveller' diarrhoea: a phase II, randomised, double-blind, placebo-controlled field trial. Lancet 371:2019–2025

Frech SA, Kenney RT, Spyr CA et al (2005) Improved immune responses to influenza vaccination in the elderly using an immunostimulant patch. Vaccine 23:946–950

Freytag LC, Clements JD (2005) Mucosal adjuvants. Vaccine 23:1804–1813

Freytag LC, Clements JD (1999) Bacterial toxins as mucosal adjuvants. Curr Top Microbiol Immunol 236:215–236

Gagliardi MC, Sallusto F, Marinaro M et al (2000) Cholera toxin induces maturation of human dendritic cells and licences them for Th2 priming. Eur J Immunol 30:2394–2403

Glenn GM, Flyer DC, Ellingsworth LR et al (2007) Transcutaneous immunization with heat-labile enterotoxin: development of a needle-free vaccine patch. Expert Rev Vaccines 6:809–819

Glenn GM, Kenney RT (2006) Mass vaccination: solutions in the skin. Curr Top Microbiol Immunol 304:247–268

Glenn GM, Rao M, Matyas GR et al (1998a) Skin immunization made possible by cholera toxin. Nature 391:851–852

Glenn GM, Scharton-Kersten T, Vassell R et al (1998b) Transcutaneous immunization with cholera toxin protects mice against lethal mucosal toxin challenge. J Immunol 161:3211–3214

Glenn GM, Taylor DN, Li X et al (2000) Transcutaneous immunization: a human vaccine delivery strategy using a patch. Nat Med 6:1403–1406

Gockel CM, Bao S, Beagley KW (2000) Transcutaneous immunization induces mucosal and systemic immunity: a potent method for targeting immunity to the female reproductive tract. Mol Immunol 37:537–544

Guebre-Xabier M, Hammond SA, Epperson DE et al (2003) Immunostimulant patch containing heat-labile enterotoxin from *Escherichia coli* enhances immune responses to injected influenza virus vaccine through activation of skin dendritic cells. J Virol 77:5218–5225

Guerena-Burgueno F, Hall ER, Taylor DN et al (2002) Safety and immunogenicity of a prototype enterotoxigenic *Escherichia coli* vaccine administered transcutaneously. Infect Immun 70:1874–1880

Hammond SA, Walwender D, Alving CR et al (2001) Transcutaneous immunization: T cell responses and boosting of existing immunity. Vaccine 19:2701–2707

Hauser C, Elbe A, Stingl G (1991) The Langerhans cell. In: Goldsmith LA (ed) Physiology, biochemistry, and molecular biology of the skin, vol 2. Oxford University Press, New York

He Y, Zhang J, Donahue C et al (2006) Skin-derived dendritic cells induce potent CD8$^+$ T cell immunity in recombinant lentivector-mediated genetic immunization. Immunity 24:643–56

Heib V, Becker M, Warger T et al (2007) Mast cells are crucial for early inflammation, migration of Langerhans cells, and CTL responses following topical application of TLR7 ligand in mice. Blood 110:946–953

Hickey DK, Aldwell FE, Beagley KW (2009a) Transcutaneous immunization with a novel lipid-based adjuvant protects against Chlamydia genital and respiratory infections. Vaccine 27:6217–6225

Hickey DK, Aldwell FE, Tan ZY et al (2009b) Transcutaneous immunization with novel lipid-based adjuvants induces protection against gastric *Helicobacter pylori* infection. Vaccine 27:6983–6990

Ishikura K, Hashizume T, Kurita-Ochiai T et al (2009) Transcutaneous immunization with the outer membrane protein of *P. gingivalis* elicits long-term protective immunity in the oral cavity. J Oral Biosci 51:1 10

Kalali BN, Köllisch G, Mages J et al (2008) Double-stranded RNS induces an antiviral defense status in epidermal keratinocytes through TLR3-, PKR-, and MDA5/RIG-I-mediated differential signaling. J Immunol 181:2964–2074

Kapsenberg ML, Bos JD (1998) Skin, contribution to immunity. In: Delves PJ, Roitt IM (eds) Encyclopedia of immunology. Academic Press, New York

Kissenpfennig A, Henri S, Dubois B et al (2005) Dynamics and function of Langerhans cells in vivo: dermal dendritic cells colonize lymph node areas distinct from slower migrating Langerhans cells. Immunity 22:643–654

Kissenpfennig A, Malissen B (2006) Langerhans cells—revisiting the paradigm using genetically engineered mice. Trends Immunol 27:132–139

Klimuk SK, Najar HM, Semple SC et al (2004) Epicutaneous application of CpG oligodeoxy-nucleotides with peptide or protein antigen promotes the generation of CTL. J Invest Dermatol 122:1042–1049

Köllisch G, Kalali BN, Voelcker V et al (2005) Various members of the Toll-like receptor family contribute to the innate immune response of human epidermal keratinocytes. Immunology 114:531–541

Kripke ML, Munn CG, Jeevan A et al (1990) Evidence that cutaneous antigen-presenting cells migrate to regional lymph nodes during contact sensitization. J Immunol 145:2833–2838

la Sala A, He J, Laricchia-Robbio L et al (2010) Cholera toxin inhibits IL-12 production and CD8a+ dendritic cell differentiation by cAMP-mediated inhibition of IRF8 function. J Exp Med 206:1227–1235

Lawson LB, Freytag LC, Clements JD (2007) Use of nanocarriers for transdermal vaccine delivery. Clin Pharmacol Ther 82:641–643

Maeba S, Otake S, Namikoshi J et al (2005) Transcutaneous immunization with a 40-kDa outer membrane protein of *Porphyromonas gingivalis* induces specific antibodies which inhibit coaggregation by *P. gingivalis*. Vaccine 23:2513–2521

Merad M, Ginhoux F, Collin M (2008) Origin, homeostasis and function of Langerhans cells and other langerin-expressing dendritic cells. Nat Rev Immunol 8:935–946

Mishra D, Dubey V, Asthana A et al (2006) Elastic liposomes mediated transcutaneous immunization against Hepatitis B. Vaccine 24:4847–4855

Naito S, Maeyama J, Mizukami T et al (2007) Transcutaneous immunization by merely prolonging the duration of antigen presence on the skin of mice induces a potent antigen-specific antibody response even in the absence of an adjuvant. Vaccine 25:8762–8770

Nestle FO, Di Meglio P, Qin JZ et al (2009) Skin immune sentinels in health and disease. Nat Rev Immunol 9:679–691

Nestle FO, Filgueira L, Nickoloff NO et al (1998) Human dermal dendritic cells process and present soluble protein antigens. J Invest Dermatol 110:762–766

Nickoloff BJ, Naidu Y (1994) Perturbation of epidermal barrier function correlates with initiation of cytokine cascade in human skin. J Am Acad Dermatol 30:535–546

Nishijima T, Tokura Y, Imokawa G et al (1997) Altered permeability and disordered cutaneous immunoregulatory function in mice with acute barrier disruption. J Invest Dermatol 109:175–182

Partidos CD, Beignon AS, Briand JP et al (2004) Modulation of immune responses with transcutaneously deliverable adjuvants. Vaccine 22:2385–2390

Randolph GJ, Angeli V, Swartz MA (2005) Dendritic-cell trafficking to lymph nodes through lymphatic vessels. Nat Rev Immunol 5:617–628

Rechtsteiner G, Warger T, Osterloch P et al (2005) Priming of CTL by transcutaneous peptide immunization with imiquimod. J Immunol 174:2476–2480

Romani N, Ebner S, Tripp CH et al (2006) Epidermal Langerhans cells—changing views on their function in vivo. Immunol Lett 106:119–125

Sauder DN (1983) Immunology of the epidermis: changing perspectives. J Invest Dermatol 81:185–186

Scharton-Kersten T, Glenn GM, Vassell R et al (1999) Principles of transcutaneous immunization using cholera toxin as an adjuvant. Vaccine 17:S37–S43

Sigmundsdottir H, Pan J, Debes GF et al (2007) DCs metabolize sunlight-induced vitamin D3 to 'program' T cell attraction to the epidermal chemokine CCL27. Nat Immunol 8:285–293

Silberberg-Sinakin I, Thorbecke GJ, Baer RL et al (1976) Antigen-bearing Langerhans cells in skin, dermal lymphatics and in lymph nodes. Cell Immunol 25:137–151

Skelding KA, Hickey DK, Horvat JC et al (2006) Comparison of intranasal and transcutaneous immunization for induction of protective immunity against *Chlamydia muridarum* respiratory tract infection. Vaccine 24:355–366

Skountzou I, Kang SM (2009) Transcutaneous immunization with influenza vaccines. Curr Top Microbiol Immunol 333:347–368

Skountzou I, Quan FS, Jacob J et al (2006) Transcutaneous immunization with inactivated influenza virus induces protective immune responses. Vaccine 24:6110–6119

Spetz A-L, Strominger J, Groh-Spies V (1996) T Cell subsets in normal human epidermis. Am J Pathol 149:665–674

Stoitzner P, Tripp CH, Eberhart A et al (2006) Langerhans cells cross-present antigen derived from skin. Proc Natl Acad Sci 103:7783–7788

Streilin JW (1985) Circuits and signals of the skin-associated lymphoid tissues (SALT). J Invest Dermatol 85:10s–13s

Sugita K, Kabashima K, Atarashi K (2007) Innate immunity mediated by epidermal keratinocytes promotes acquired immunity involving Langerhans cells and T cells in the skin. Clin Exp Immunol 147:176–183

Tang D-C, Shi Z, Curiel DT (1997) Vaccination onto bare skin. Nature 388:729–730

Uddowla S, Freytag LC, Clements JD (2007) Effect of adjuvants and route of immunizations on the immune response to recombinant plague antigens. Vaccine 25:7984–7993

van der Aar AMG, Sylva-Steenland RMR, Bos JD et al (2007) Loss of TLR2, TLR4, and TLR5 on Langerhans cells abolishes bacterial recognition. J Immunol 178:1986–1990

Vogt A, Mahe B, Costagliola D et al (2008) Transcutaneous anti-influenza vaccination promotes both CD4 and CD8 T cell immune responses in humans. J Immunol 180:1482–1489

Wang L, Bursch LS, Kissenpfennig A et al (2008) Langerin expressing cells promote skin immune responses under defined conditions. J Immunol 180:4722–4727

Warger T, Schild H, Rechsteiner G (2007) Initiation of adaptive immune responses by transcutaneous immunization. Immunol Lett 109:13–20

Williams IR, Kupper TS (1996) Immunity at the surface: homeostatic mechanisms of the skin immune system. Life Sci 58:1485–1507

Wood LC, Jackson SM, Elias PM et al (1992) Cutaneous barrier perturbation stimulates cytokine production in the epidermis of mice. J Clin Invest 90:482–487

Young B, Lowe JS, Stevens A et al (2006) Wheater's functional histology. Elsevier, Philadelphia, PA

Yu J, Cassels F, Scharton-Kersten T et al (2002) Transcutaneous immunization using colonization factor and heat-labile enterotoxin induces correlates of protective immunity for enterotoxigenic *Escherichia coli*. Infect Immun 70:1056–1068

Yu RC, Abrams DC, Alaibac M et al (1994) Morphological and quantitative analyses of normal epidermal Langerhans cells using confocal scanning laser microscopy. Br J Dermatol 131:843–848

Zaba LC, Fuentes-Duculan J, Steinman RM et al (2007) Normal human dermis contains distinct populations of $CD11c^{+}BDCA\text{-}1^{+}$ dendritic cells and $CD163^{+}FXIIIA^{+}$ macrophages. J Clin Invest 117:2517–2525

M Cell-Targeted Mucosal Vaccine Strategies

M. Yamamoto, D. W. Pascual and H. Kiyono

Abstract Immune responses in the aerodigestive tract are characterized by production and transport of specific IgA antibodies across the epithelium to act as a first line of defense against pathogens in the external environment. To sample antigens on mucosal surfaces in the intestine and upper respiratory tract, the immune system relies on a close collaboration between specialized antigen-sampling epithelial M cells and lymphoid cells. Depending on various factors, local antigen presentation in the mucosal tissue leads to tolerance or initiation of an active immune response. Recently, molecules that could be used to target vaccine antigens to apical M cell surfaces have been identified. Here we review the M cell-targeted vaccine strategy, an approach that could be used to enhance uptake and efficacy of vaccines delivered in the nasal cavity or intestine.

M. Yamamoto (✉)
Department of Oral Immunology,
Nihon University School of Dentistry at Matsudo,
Matsudo, Chiba 271-8587, Japan
e-mail: yamamoto.masafumi@nihon-u.ac.jp

D. W. Pascual
Department of Immunology and Infectious Diseases,
Montana State University, Bozeman, MT 59717, USA

H. Kiyono
Division of Mucosal Immunology,
Department of Microbiology and Immunology,
The Institute of Medical Science, The University of Tokyo,
Minato-ku, Tokyo 108-8639, Japan

Current Topics in Microbiology and Immunology (2012) 354: 39–52
DOI: 10.1007/82_2011_134

Published Online: 19 June 2011

Contents

1 Introduction

Mucosal surfaces provide a first line of defense against the plethora of potential pathogens and nonself antigens that perturb the host. Since mucosal tissues normally harbor a vast variety of commensal microorganisms, the mucosa is a site of continuous stimulation requiring tolerance to the normal flora, but immune reactions to pathogens (Kiyono et al. 2008). These tissues are protected by secretory IgA (*S*IgA) antibodies which constitute greater than 80% of all antibodies produced in mucosa-associated tissues of humans. Mucosal IgA antibodies are induced, transported, and regulated by mechanisms that are completely different from those used to generate systemic antibody responses (Craig and Cebra 1971). The mucosal immune system can be subdivided into two primary components: the organized mucosa-associated lympho-reticular tissues (MALTs), where antigen-specific T and B cells are activated and imprinted with mucosal homing molecules for direct migration to specific effector sites, and the diffuse lamina propria regions or glandular tissues, which serve as the effector sites for synthesis of polymeric IgA and the execution of T cell responses (Kiyono and Fukuyama 2004; Kunisawa et al. 2005).

MALTs are situated along the surfaces of various mucosal tissues and include the nasopharynx-associated lymphoid tissue (NALT), bronchus-associated lymphoid tissue (BALT), and the gut-associated lymphoid tissue (GALT) such as Peyer's patches (PP), isolated lymphoid follicles, and colonic patches. The most extensively studied MALTs are PP and NALT in the digestive and airway tissues, respectively (Kiyono and Fukuyama 2004). Peyer's Patches usually number 8 to 10 in the small intestine of mice and hundreds in humans. In rodents, NALT is found on both sides of the nasopharyngeal duct dorsal to the cartilaginous soft palate. Humans generally do not share the same anatomical features of NALT, except possibly at an early age (Debertin et al. 2003), but they do possess oropharyngeal lymphoid tissues, including unpaired nasopharyngeal tonsils (adenoids), bilateral tubular palatines, and the lingual tonsil, which together are known as Waldeyer's ring and appear to be functionally equivalent to murine NALT (Kiyono and Fukuyama 2004).

The induction of SIgA responses is known to be generally dependent on cognate help provided by $CD4^+$ T helper (Th) cells in MALT. The antigen-specific lymphocytes in MALT are programmed to home primarily local effector tissues using a mucosal imprinting system which bridges mucosal inductive and effector sites, whereas lymphocytes activated in peripheral lymph nodes have a distinct systemic homing program (Kiyono and Fukuyama 2004; Kunisawa et al. 2008). The MALT contains antigen-presenting cells (APC) of all major types, including several dendritic cell (DC) subsets, macrophages, and MHC class II^+ B cells for initiation of mucosal immune responses. In addition, germinal centers are present with a high frequency of surface IgA^+ B cells and inter-nodular zones predominantly populated by $CD4^+$ and $CD8^+$ T cell subsets (Kiyono et al. 2008). The MALT is the site for the induction of regulatory T cells (T_{reg} cells) in addition to Th1 and Th2 cells (Izcue et al. 2009; Lloyd and Hawrylowicz 2009; Murai et al. 2009; Unutmaz and Pulendran 2009). Recently, it has been shown that some of these T_{reg} cells differentiate into follicular helper T cells (T_{FH} cells) which support IgA B cell responses in MALT (Tsuji et al. 2009). The $CD4^+$ T cell axis between T_{reg} and T_{FH} cells would account for the simultaneous induction of tolerance and IgA responses in mucosal compartments. Another important trait of MALTs is that these lymphoid tissues are covered by a specialized epithelium, termed follicle-associated epithelium (FAE), which contains micro-fold or membranous (M) cells, a professional antigen-sampling epithelial cell specialized for the uptake of antigens from the lumen of the aerodigestive tract (Bockman and Cooper 1973; Owen and Jones 1974). M cells have also been identified in the crypt epithelium of human tonsils and adenoids (Karchev and Kabakchiev 1984).

The development of effective mucosal vaccines will require the precise characterization and understanding of the molecular and cellular mechanisms involved in the antigen-sampling, -processing and -presentation initially executed by M cells and APC in MALT for the induction of protective immunity. In this article, we will summarize the recent progress made in the characterization of airway and digestive tract M cells. In particular, we will focus on the development of M cell-targeted vaccines for prevention of diseases in the aerodigestive tract.

2 Characterization of M Cells in the Aerodigestive Tract

2.1 *Immunobiological Features of M Cells*

Originally described as part of the FAE associated with GALT and NALT, M cells have shared unique structural features in comparison with other mucosal epithelial cells. M cells have tight junctions and desmosomes in contact with adjacent columnar epithelial cells and interdigitating lateral membranes (Fig. 1). The processes on their luminal surfaces are spaced more widely and are often shorter and more irregular in shape than the microvilli of absorptive cells (Kraehenbuhl and Neutra 2000; Neutra et al. 1996; Niedergang and Kraehenbuhl 2000).

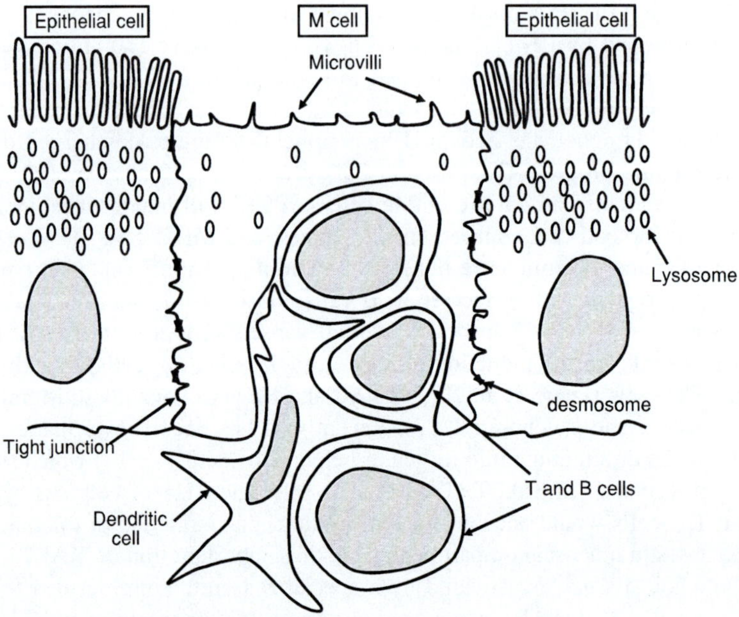

Fig. 1 Diagram of M cells in the follicle-associated epithelium. M cells have tight junctions and desmosomes in contact with adjacent columnar epithelial cells. Luminal surfaces of M cells are characterized by short microvilli, a thin mucus layer, small cytoplasmic vesicles, a reduced glycocalyx and sparse lysosomes. The basolateral surface of the M cells forms an intraepithelial pocket that contains DC, T cells or B cells

Furthermore, compared with adjacent columnar epithelial cells, they are characterized by short microvilli, a thin mucus layer, small cytoplasmic vesicles, a reduced glycocalyx, sparse lysosomes, and a deep invagination of their basolateral membrane which enfolds lymphoid cells (Frey et al. 1996; Kraehenbuhl and Neutra 2000; Neutra et al. 1996; Niedergang and Kraehenbuhl 2000). These unique features allow M cells to selectively and efficiently transfer inhaled or ingested luminal antigens to APC located in the M cell pocket or directly below in the FAE of MALT (Kraehenbuhl and Neutra 2000). M cells take up macromolecules, particles, and microorganisms by adsorptive endocytosis via clathrin-coated pits and vesicles (Neutra et al. 1987; Sicinski et al. 1990), fluid-phase endocytosis (Bockman and Cooper 1973; Owen 1977), and phagocytosis involving extension of cellular processes and reorganization of sub-membrane actin assemblies (Jones et al. 1994). All of these uptake mechanisms result in the transport of foreign material into endosomal tubules and vesicles and large multivesicular bodies that lie between the apical membrane and the intraepithelial pocket (Neutra et al. 1987). Immunocytochemical analysis has revealed the presence of an endosomal protease, cathepsin E, in rabbit M cells (Finzi et al. 1993), but the possible presence of other endosomal hydrolases in M cell transport vesicles has not yet been examined.

M cells are defined by a combination of the above described morphologic features and the presence of the fucose epitope recognized by the *Ulex europaeus* agglutinin-1 (UEA-1) lectin on mouse M cell membrane (Kraehenbuhl and Neutra 2000; Neutra et al. 1996). Recently, we generated a novel M cell-specific monoclonal antibody (NKM 16-2-4). This antibody reacts with murine M cells in FAE of PP, but not with epithelial cells or goblet cells (Nochi et al. 2007). M cells have been shown to develop in villous epithelium in addition to the FAE of organized lymphoid tissues in the intestine (Jang et al. 2004). These cells, termed villous M cells, take up bacteria, as well as bacterial antigens, for subsequent induction of antigen-specific immune responses (Jang et al. 2004), suggesting that villous M cells could be an alternative to the FAE-dependent antigen-sampling pathway. NKM 16-2-4 reacts with villous M cell. Thus, it is considered a pan-marker for murine PP and villous M cells (Nochi et al. 2007).

2.2 *Origin of M Cells*

The origin of M cells and the regulation of their development are still controversial. One study showed that intravenous injection of PP lymphocytes into severe combined immunodeficient mice resulted in the formation of new lymphoid follicles and FAE with typical M cells (Savidge and Smith 1995). A similar phenomenon was seen in vitro when co-culture of PP B cells with an enterocyte cell line triggered the conversion of enterocytes into M cell-like epithelial cells (Kerneis et al. 1997). Furthermore, B cells have been proposed to play a role in the organogenesis of the mucosal immune barrier system (Golovkina et al. 1999). Two different strains of B cell-null mice have exhibited drastic reductions in FAE size and M cell numbers (Golovkina et al. 1999). On the other hand, others have found that the absence of mature T and B cells does not prevent the formation of FAE and M cells, and instead suggest that signaling of lymphotoxin α/β from non-B and non-T cells plays a critical role in formation of M cells in FAE of PP (Debard et al. 2001).

2.3 *Role of DC in Aerodigestive Tract*

In addition to M cells, DC in the lamina propria extend their dendrites into the lumen and sample antigens (Chieppa et al. 2006; Niess et al. 2005; Rescigno et al. 2001). A recent study has suggested that these lamina propria DC are capable of initiating systemic IgG responses, whereas antigen transport by M cells into the PP is required for induction of intestinal IgA responses (Martinoli et al. 2007), a finding consistent with the report that DC in PP are responsible for intestinal IgA production (Fleeton et al. 2004). Villous M cells and intraepithelial DC have been reported in the respiratory tract (Jahnsen et al. 2006; Teitelbaum et al. 1999). Furthermore, we recently demonstrated the presence of M cells in the single layer of epithelium covering the nasal cavity turbinate in addition to the FAE in NALT

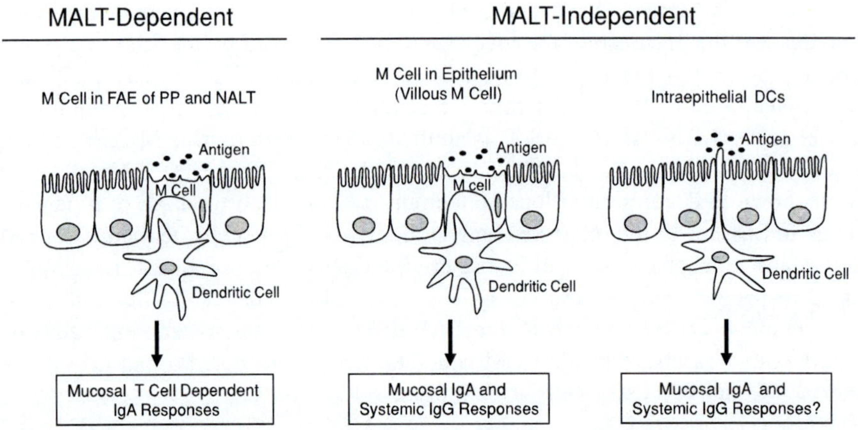

Fig. 2 MALT-dependent and -independent antigen-sampling system at aerodigestive surfaces. Antigens are captured by M cells located in follicle-associated epithelium (FAE) of lymphoid follicles, intestinal villi or the epithelial cell layer in the nasal cavity. The antigens are then transported to subepithelial DC for processing and presentation. Alternatively, lamina propia or intraepithelial DC extends their dendrites through the epithelial layer for direct capture of luminal antigens. Antigen uptake through M cells in FAE of MALT leads to the induction of mucosal IgA responses. On the other hand, M cells located in the intestinal villi or nasal epithelium as well as intraepithelial DC are thought to play a critical role in the induction of systemic IgG responses in addition to mucosal IgA

(submitted for publication). Taken together, these results suggest that tissue in the aerodigestive tracts is equipped with a diversified antigen-uptake and presenting system which consists of MALT M cells, villous M cells, lamina propria DC, and intraepithelial DC (Fig. 2).

3 Targeting Vaccines to Nasal M Cells for Induction of Specific IgA and CTL

Although most human pathogens infect the host by means of a mucosal surface, the majority of vaccines are administered intramuscularly, a route that poorly induces antigen-specific mucosal immune responses (Ogra et al. 2001). It is essential to select a mucosal route of vaccination to induce mucosal immune responses. Nasal administration of vaccines is preferred to oral administration because the former can be used to deliver vaccine without degradation by digestive enzymes and acids. Because M cells are extremely efficient in the uptake of luminal antigens, it is a logical strategy to target vaccines to these cells. In this regard, several approaches incorporating an M cell-specific lectin (Manocha et al. 2005; Wang et al. 2005), peptide (Higgins et al. 2004) or microbial invasion molecules of reovirus or Yersinia (Clark et al. 1998; Wang et al. 2003; Wu et al.

Table. 1 M cell-targeting molecules for development of mucosal vaccine

M cell ligands
Ulex europaeus agglutinin-1 (UEA-1)
Reovirus protein $\sigma 1$
Yersinia invasin
YQCSYTMPHPPV
M cell-specific molecules
NKM 16-2-4 (specific for $\alpha(1,2)$-fucose-containing carbohydrate moiety)
FimH of enterobacteria (specific for glycoprotein 2 expressed by M cells)

2001) have been tested as M cell-targeting delivery vehicles for nasal or oral vaccines (Table 1).

In our mucosal DNA vaccination studies, recombinant reovirus protein $\sigma 1$, which can bind NALT M cells, has proved effective as an antigen delivery molecule. It facilitated nasal immunization with luciferase and β-galactosidase plasmid reporter gene constructs (Wu et al. 2000, 2001). Furthermore, nasal delivery of a human immunodeficiency virus type 1 (HIV-1) envelope protein-encoding plasmid complexed to protein $\sigma 1$ via poly-L-lysine successfully induced potent and long-lived HIV-specific cytotoxic T lymphocytes (CTL) in both respiratory and systemic lymphoid tissues (Wang et al. 2003).

Alternative M cell ligands have also been tested, including UEA-1 (Table 1). When mice were nasally immunized with UEA-1-poly-L-lysine complexed to plasmid encoding HIV envelope, significant envelope-specific mucosal and systemic antibodies, as well as CTL, were induced (Wang et al. 2005). These findings suggest that targeted delivery of mucosal DNA vaccines to M cells could be highly effective for induction of cellular and humoral immunity against infectious diseases (Fig. 3).

4 Intestinal M Cell-Targeted Vaccine Strategies

Nasal immunization has proven to be an effective method for stimulating both mucosal and systemic immunity. However, nasal immunization can be problematic due to the possible migration of vaccine antigen, adjuvant, and/or delivery molecule into the central nervous system via the olfactory nerves. Nasally administered cholera toxin (CT) and adenovirus vectors have been shown to temporally accumulate in the olfactory nerves and epithelial regions of mice (Lemiale et al. 2003; van Ginkel et al. 2000). Clinical studies have also linked *Escherichia coli* heat-labile enterotoxin (LT)-based adjuvants with the development of Bell's palsy in nasal vaccine recipients (Lewis et al. 2009; Mutsch et al. 2004). This has raised concerns about potential health threats posed by nasal vaccines. It should be noted that the targeted delivery of vaccine to M cells in the respiratory tract could overcome this problem. Nevertheless, oral vaccine delivery may be safer in some cases, and oral immunization would be more effective for induction of immune responses in the intestine. A practical advantage of oral vaccination is the lack of necessity for

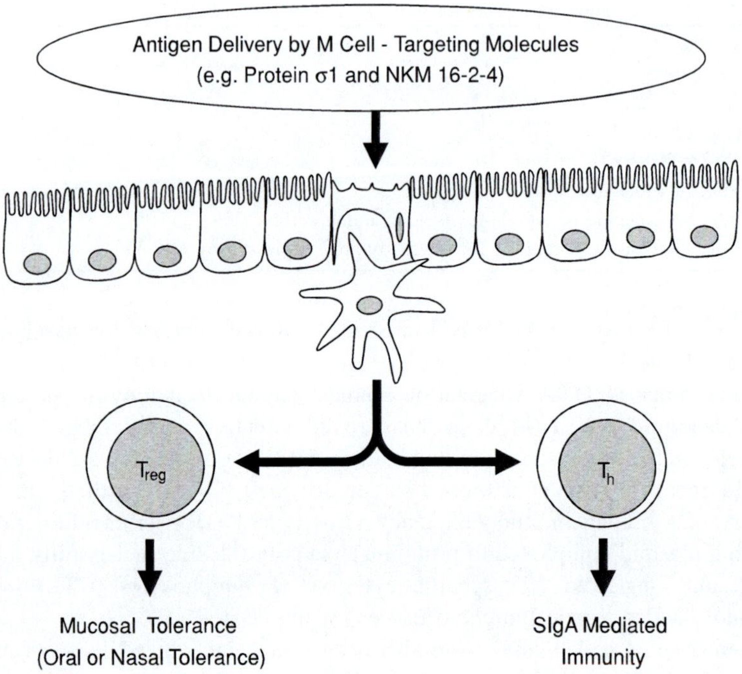

Fig. 3 FAE M cell-targeting antigen delivery system for induction of active or quiescent immunity. Different fusion molecules consisting of antigen and M cell-targeting molecules have been shown to effectively induce Th2 type cell-mediated protective immunity and/or T_{reg} cell-mediated mucosal tolerance

delivery devices (e.g. nebulizers, needles) but the obstacles are greater compared to other immunization routes because of the extremely large surface area and harsh degradative environment of the gastrointestinal tract.

Despite the hurdles, the success of oral poliovirus and rotavirus vaccines (Holmgren and Czerkinsky 2005) has encouraged many mucosal immunologists and vaccinologists to tackle the challenges associated with oral vaccine development. Oral administration of vaccine antigens in conjunction with enterotoxin adjuvants (CT, LT, or nontoxic mutant derivatives thereof) has been shown to effectively induce antigen-specific protective immune responses in both mucosal and systemic compartments (de Haan et al. 1996; Di Tommaso et al. 1996; Douce et al. 1997; Giuliani et al. 1998; Yamamoto et al. 1997, 1998). Moreover, the concept of M cell targeting has also been applied for the development of oral vaccines. For example, antigen expressed in attenuated *Salmonella* vectors, which can bind to M cells, has stimulated antigen-specific mucosal immune responses (Yamamoto et al. 2001). As described above, several M cell-specific molecules have been examined as M cell-targeted delivery vehicles for mucosal vaccines (Clark et al. 1998; Higgins et al. 2004; Manocha et al. 2005; Wang et al. 2003, 2005; Wu et al. 2001). However, some of these molecules are not solely

M cell-specific and bind to other neighboring cells. The murine M cell-specific UEA-1 lectin also reacts strongly with goblet cells and the mucus layer covering the intestinal epithelium (Kandori et al. 1996). Since the NKM 16-2-4 M cell-specific monoclonal antibody has been shown to be solely specific (Nochi et al. 2007), an obvious experiment was to test whether NKM 16-2-4 could be used as a carrier for M cell-targeted oral vaccines (Table 1). Indeed, oral administration of CT adjuvant with a chimeric vaccine consisting of botulinum toxoid (BT) and NKM 16-2-4 induced strong antigen-specific IgG and mucosal IgA responses, as well as protective immunity against lethal challenge with botulinum toxin (Nochi et al. 2007). Considering the anatomical and physiological conditions of the gastrointestinal tract, the selective targeting of vaccine to M cells should allow for lowering of vaccine dosage since the antigen can be specifically delivered to the inductive tissue. In this regard, it should be noted that because of the M cell targeting ability of NKM 16-2-4, as little as 50 μg BT was sufficient for the induction of protective immunity in this murine model. An epitope analysis indicated that NKM 16-2-4 distinguishes $\alpha(1,2)$-fucosylated M cells from goblet cells containing abundant sialic acids neighboring the $\alpha(1,2)$ fucose moiety and from non-$\alpha(1,2)$-fucosylated epithelial cells (Nochi et al. 2007). These results suggest that the use of monoclonal antibody NKM 16-2-4 to target vaccine antigens to the M cell-specific carbohydrate moiety could be highly effective for delivery of vaccines into the intestinal mucosa (Fig. 3).

In addition to NKM 16-2-4, glycoprotein 2 (GP2) has been found to be specifically expressed in the apical plasma membrane of PP M cells (Terahara et al. 2008). A recent study has shown that GP2 selectively binds a subset of commensal and pathogenic enterobacteria, including *E. coli* and *Salmonella typhimurium*, by recognizing FimH, a component of type I pili on the bacterial outer membrane (Hase et al. 2009). Interestingly, deficiency of bacterial FimH or host GP2 leads to defects in transcytosis of type-I-piliated bacteria through M cells, resulting in an attenuation of PP-mediated antigen-specific immune responses (Hase et al. 2009). These findings suggest that the GP2-dependent transcytotic pathway could provide another target for delivery of mucosal vaccines to M cells.

5 Targeting M Cells for Induction of Tolerance

Oral administration of a single high dose or repeated low doses of protein has been shown to induce mucosal tolerance (Mowat 2003; Weiner 2000; Xiao and Link 1997). The former mode induces tolerance by clonal anergy/deletion of effector cells, whereas the latter, based on repeated low-dose administration, causes active suppression of effector cells (Faria and Weiner 1999; Fujihashi et al. 2001a, b; Jun et al. 2005; Xiao and Link 1997). Previous studies have demonstrated that PP (Fujihashi et al. 2001a, b; Mowat 2003) and NALT (Kiyono and Fukuyama 2004; Wu et al. 2001) actively facilitate immunity or unresponsiveness by luminal antigen sampling (Fleeton et al. 2004; Weiner 2000; Wu et al. 2001) via M cells, suggesting that M cells play a crucial role in the induction of mucosal tolerance. Previous studies have demonstrated that mucosal administration of ovalbumin fused to reovirus protein σ1 (OVA-pσ1) induces a state of unresponsiveness in both mucosal and systemic lymphoid tissues (Rynda et al. 2008; Suzuki et al. 2008). In fact, tolerance could be achieved even with a single low dose of OVA-pσ1 delivered either nasally (Rynda et al. 2008) or orally (Suzuki et al. 2008). In contrast, parenteral delivery of OVA-pσ1 failed to induce tolerance to OVA. Interestingly, the pσ1-induced mucosal tolerance resisted co-treatment with the potent mucosal adjuvants, CT and CpG oligodeoxynucleotides, and tolerance was not broken after peripheral challenge with OVA (Rynda et al. 2008). In contrast, mucosal tolerance established by OVA without an M cell targeting vehicle has typically been abrogated by the presence of mucosal adjuvants (Lycke 2005).

It is now generally agreed that mucosal tolerance is established and maintained at the levels of T cells. Such suppression occurs via activation of specific regulatory cells, among which $CD25^+$ $CD4^+$ T regulatory (T_{reg}) cells have been best described (Fujihashi et al. 2001a, b; Weiner 2000). Specific T_{reg} cells are known to express the nuclear forkhead box P3 (FoxP3) transcription factor and suppress the immune response in an IL-10- and/or TGF-β-dependent fashion (Faria et al. 2003; Sakaguchi et al. 2006, 2008). Interestingly, $FoxP3^+$ $CD25^+$ $CD4^+$ T cells secreting IL-10 and TGF-β were significantly increased in the mucosal compartment after nasal or oral administration of OVA-pσ1 (Rynda et al. 2008; Suzuki et al. 2008). Furthermore, adoptive transfer of OVA-pσ1-primed $CD25^+$ $CD4^+$ or $CD25^-$ $CD4^+$ T cells significantly inhibited antigen-specific proliferation of OVA-transgenic $CD4^+$ T cells. This suppression was due to increased production of IL-10 by OVA-pσ1-induced T_{reg} cells, as evidenced by the lack of OVA-specific tolerance in OVA-pσ1-dosed IL-$10^{-/-}$ mice (Rynda et al. 2008). Mucosal administration of OVA-pσ1 also induced clonal deletion of OVA-specific $CD4^+$ T cells (Rynda et al. 2008; Suzuki et al. 2008), offering an additional suppressive mechanism for protein σ1 if it can survive delivery beyond the initial cell binding to mucosal epithelium or M cells. Taken together, these findings suggest that reovirus protein σ1-mediated targeting of protein antigen to M cells could be an effective strategy for establishing tolerance (Fig. 3). Because the nasal and oral routes provide an easy way to administer antigens, vaccines, or drugs, the M cell-targeting protein antigen delivery system for induction of mucosal and systemic unresponsiveness could provide important advantages for the development of therapeutic approaches to treat diseases.

6 Conclusion and Future Directions

Recent progress in our understanding of the molecular and cellular characteristics of M cells in the aerodigestive tract has allowed testing the possibility of M cell-targeted vaccines. The mucosal immune system is a remarkable defense mechanism that provides the means to generate highly specific responses against a myriad of potentially pathogenic microorganisms that invade via mucosal surfaces. The mucosal immune system consists of several distinct but harmonized antigen-sampling and presentation mechanisms for MALT-dependent and -independent induction of inhaled and/or ingested antigen-specific immune responses. Of course, one of the major portals of antigen entry is M cells. Despite the recent advances in our knowledge, we still lack a global view of how M cells develop and orchestrate mucosal immune responses after sampling antigens in the lumen of the aerodigestive tract. The orientation towards tolerance or active immune responses is also a critical issue to clarify. Finally, the development of vaccines that trigger mucosal as well as systemic immune responses is of global importance, and the M cell-targeted vaccine strategy offers the potential for safe and effective delivery of mucosal vaccines.

Acknowledgments This work was supported by grants from the Ministry of Education, Culture, Sports, Science, and Technology of Japan, and the Ministry of Health and Labor of Japan; the Global Center of Excellence Program "Center of Education and Research for Advanced Genome-Based Medicine—For Personalized Medicine and the Control of Worldwide Infectious Diseases"; the "Development of Fundamental Technologies for Production of High-Value Materials Using Transgenic Plants" project of the Ministry of Economy, Trade and Industry and GATES Grand Challenges Explorations; an "Academic Frontier" Project for Private Universities matching fund subsidy from the Ministry of Education, Culture, Sports, Science and Technology, 2007–2011. This work was supported in part by the National Institutes of Health grants R01 AI078938 and P01 AT004986, and by Montana Agricultural Station and US Department of Agriculture Formula Funds.

References

Bockman DE, Cooper MD (1973) Pinocytosis by epithelium associated with lymphoid follicles in the bursa of Fabricius, appendix, and Peyer's patches. An electron microscopic study. Am J Anat 136:455–477

Chieppa M, Rescigno M, Huang AY et al (2006) Dynamic imaging of dendritic cell extension into the small bowel lumen in response to epithelial cell TLR engagement. J Exp Med 203:2841–2852

Clark MA, Hirst BH, Jepson MA (1998) M-cell surface beta 1 integrin expression and invasin-mediated targeting of *Yersinia pseudotuberculosis* to mouse Peyer's patch M cells. Infect Immun 66:1237–1243

Craig SW, Cebra JJ (1971) Peyer's patches: an enriched source of precursors for IgA-producing immunocytes in the rabbit. J Exp Med 134:188–200

de Haan L, Verweij WR, Feil IK et al (1996) Mutants of the *Escherichia coli* heat-labile enterotoxin with reduced ADP-ribosylation activity or no activity retain the immunogenic properties of the native holotoxin. Infect Immun 64:5413–5416

Debard N, Sierro F, Browning J et al (2001) Effect of mature lymphocytes and lymphotoxin on the development of the follicle-associated epithelium and M cells in mouse Peyer's patches. Gastroenterology 120:1173–1182

Debertin AS, Tschernig T, Tonjes H et al (2003) Nasal-associated lymphoid tissue (NALT): frequency and localization in young children. Clin Exp Immunol 134:503–507

Di Tommaso A, Saletti G, Pizza M et al (1996) Induction of antigen-specific antibodies in vaginal secretions by using a nontoxic mutant of heat-labile enterotoxin as a mucosal adjuvant. Infect Immun 64:974–979

Douce G, Fontana M, Pizza M et al (1997) Intranasal immunogenicity and adjuvanticity of site-directed mutant derivatives of cholera toxin. Infect Immun 65:2821–2828

Faria AM, Weiner HL (1999) Oral tolerance: mechanisms and therapeutic applications. Adv Immunol 73:153–264

Faria AM, Maron R, Ficker SM et al (2003) Oral tolerance induced by continuous feeding: enhanced up-regulation of transforming growth factor-beta/interleukin-10 and suppression of experimental autoimmune encephalomyelitis. J Autoimmun 20:135–145

Finzi G, Cornaggia M, Capella C et al (1993) Cathepsin E in follicle associated epithelium of intestine and tonsils: localization to M cells and possible role in antigen processing. Histochemistry 99:201–211

Fleeton MN, Contractor N, Leon F et al (2004) Peyer's patch dendritic cells process viral antigen from apoptotic epithelial cells in the intestine of reovirus-infected mice. J Exp Med 200:235–245

Frey A, Giannasca KT, Weltzin R et al (1996) Role of the glycocalyx in regulating access of microparticles to apical plasma membranes of intestinal epithelial cells: implications for microbial attachment and oral vaccine targeting. J Exp Med 184:1045–1059

Fujihashi K, Dohi T, Rennert PD et al (2001a) Peyer's patches are required for oral tolerance to proteins. Proc Natl Acad Sci USA 98:3310–3315

Fujihashi K, Kato H, van Ginkel FW et al (2001b) A revisit of mucosal IgA immunity and oral tolerance. Acta Odontol Scand 59:301–308

Giuliani MM, Del Giudice G, Giannelli V et al (1998) Mucosal adjuvanticity and immunogenicity of LTR72, a novel mutant of *Escherichia coli* heat-labile enterotoxin with partial knockout of ADP-ribosyltransferase activity. J Exp Med 187:1123–1132

Golovkina TV, Shlomchik M, Hannum L et al (1999) Organogenic role of B lymphocytes in mucosal immunity. Science 286:1965–1968

Hase K, Kawano K, Nochi T et al (2009) Uptake through glycoprotein 2 of FimH(+) bacteria by M cells initiates mucosal immune response. Nature 462:226-230

Higgins LM, Lambkin I, Donnelly G et al (2004) In vivo phage display to identify M cell-targeting ligands. Pharm Res 21:695–705

Holmgren J, Czerkinsky C (2005) Mucosal immunity and vaccines. Nat Med 11:S45–S53

Izcue A, Coombes JL, Powrie F (2009) Regulatory lymphocytes and intestinal inflammation. Annu Rev Immunol 27:313–338

Jahnsen FL, Strickland DH, Thomas JA et al (2006) Accelerated antigen sampling and transport by airway mucosal dendritic cells following inhalation of a bacterial stimulus. J Immunol 177:5861–5867

Jang MH, Kweon MN, Iwatani K et al (2004) Intestinal villous M cells: an antigen entry site in the mucosal epithelium. Proc Natl Acad Sci USA 101:6110–6115

Jones BD, Ghori N, Falkow S (1994) Salmonella typhimurium initiates murine infection by penetrating and destroying the specialized epithelial M cells of the Peyer's patches. J Exp Med 180:15–23

Jun S, Gilmore W, Callis G et al (2005) A live diarrheal vaccine imprints a Th2 cell bias and acts as an anti-inflammatory vaccine. J Immunol 175:6733–6740

Kandori H, Hirayama K, Takeda M et al (1996) Histochemical, lectin-histochemical and morphometrical characteristics of intestinal goblet cells of germfree and conventional mice. Exp Anim 45:155–160

Karchev T, Kabakchiev P (1984) M-cells in the epithelium of the nasopharyngeal tonsil. Rhinology 22:201–210

Kerneis S, Bogdanova A, Kraehenbuhl JP et al (1997) Conversion by Peyer's patch lymphocytes of human enterocytes into M cells that transport bacteria. Science 277:949–952

Kiyono H, Fukuyama S (2004) NALT- versus Peyer's-patch-mediated mucosal immunity. Nat Rev Immunol 4:699–710

Kiyono H, Kunisawa J, McGhee J et al (2008) The mucosal immune system. In: Paul WE (ed) Fundamental immunology. Lippincott-Raven, Philadelphia

Kraehenbuhl JP, Neutra MR (2000) Epithelial M cells: differentiation and function. Annu Rev Cell Dev Biol 16:301–332

Kunisawa J, Fukuyama S, Kiyono H (2005) Mucosa-associated lymphoid tissues in the aerodigestive tract: their shared and divergent traits and their importance to the orchestration of the mucosal immune system. Curr Mol Med 5:557–572

Kunisawa J, Nochi T, Kiyono H (2008) Immunological commonalities and distinctions between airway and digestive immunity. Trends Immunol 29:505–513

Lemiale F, Kong WP, Akyurek LM et al (2003) Enhanced mucosal immunoglobulin A response of intranasal adenoviral vector human immunodeficiency virus vaccine and localization in the central nervous system. J Virol 77:10078–10087

Lewis DJ, Huo Z, Barnett S et al (2009) Transient facial nerve paralysis (Bell's palsy) following intranasal delivery of a genetically detoxified mutant of *Escherichia coli* heat labile toxin. PLoS One 4:e6999

Lloyd CM, Hawrylowicz CM (2009) Regulatory T cells in asthma. Immunity 31:438–449

Lycke N (2005) From toxin to adjuvant: basic mechanisms for the control of mucosal IgA immunity and tolerance. Immunol Lett 97:193–198

Manocha M, Pal PC, Chitralekha KT et al (2005) Enhanced mucosal and systemic immune response with intranasal immunization of mice with HIV peptides entrapped in PLG microparticles in combination with *Ulex europaeus*-I lectin as M cell target. Vaccine 23:5599–5617

Martinoli C, Chiavelli A, Rescigno M (2007) Entry route of *Salmonella typhimurium* directs the type of induced immune response. Immunity 27:975–984

Mowat AM (2003) Anatomical basis of tolerance and immunity to intestinal antigens. Nat Rev Immunol 3:331–341

Murai M, Turovskaya O, Kim G et al (2009) Interleukin 10 acts on regulatory T cells to maintain expression of the transcription factor Foxp3 and suppressive function in mice with colitis. Nat Immunol 10:1178–1184

Mutsch M, Zhou W, Rhodes P et al (2004) Use of the inactivated intranasal influenza vaccine and the risk of Bell's palsy in Switzerland. N Engl J Med 350:896–903

Neutra MR, Frey A, Kraehenbuhl JP (1996) Epithelial M cells: gateways for mucosal infection and immunization. Cell 86:345–348

Neutra MR, Phillips TL, Mayer EL et al (1987) Transport of membrane-bound macromolecules by M cells in follicle- associated epithelium of rabbit Peyer's patch. Cell Tissue Res 247: 537–546

Niedergang F, Kraehenbuhl JP (2000) Much ado about M cells. Trends Cell Biol 10:137–146

Niess JH, Brand S, Gu X et al (2005) CX3CR1-mediated dendritic cell access to the intestinal lumen and bacterial clearance. Science 307:254–258

Nochi T, Yuki Y, Matsumura A et al (2007) A novel M cell-specific carbohydrate-targeted mucosal vaccine effectively induces antigen-specific immune responses. J Exp Med 204:2789–2796

Ogra PL, Faden H, Welliver RC (2001) Vaccination strategies for mucosal immune responses. Clin Microbiol Rev 14:430–445

Owen RL (1977) Sequential uptake of horseradish peroxidase by lymphoid follicle epithelium of Peyer's patches in the normal unobstructed mouse intestine: an ultrastructural study. Gastroenterology 72:440–451

Owen RL, Jones AL (1974) Epithelial cell specialization within human Peyer's patches: an ultrastructural study of intestinal lymphoid follicles. Gastroenterology 66:189–203

Rescigno M, Urbano M, Valzasina B et al (2001) Dendritic cells express tight junction proteins and penetrate gut epithelial monolayers to sample bacteria. Nat Immunol 2:361–367

Rynda A, Maddaloni M, Mierzejewska D et al (2008) Low-dose tolerance is mediated by the microfold cell ligand, reovirus protein sigma1. J Immunol 180:5187–5200

Sakaguchi S, Ono M, Setoguchi R et al (2006) Foxp3+ CD25+ CD4+ natural regulatory T cells in dominant self-tolerance and autoimmune disease. Immunol Rev 212:8–27

Sakaguchi S, Yamaguchi T, Nomura T et al (2008) Regulatory T cells and immune tolerance. Cell 133:775–787

Savidge TC, Smith MW (1995) Evidence that membranous (M) cell genesis is immunoregulated. Adv Exp Med Biol:239–241

Sicinski P, Rowinski J, Warchol JB et al (1990) Poliovirus type 1 enters the human host through intestinal M cells. Gastroenterology 98:56–58

Suzuki H, Sekine S, Kataoka K et al (2008) Ovalbumin-protein sigma 1 M-cell targeting facilitates oral tolerance with reduction of antigen-specific CD4+ T cells. Gastroenterology 135:917–925

Teitelbaum R, Schubert W, Gunther L et al (1999) The M cell as a portal of entry to the lung for the bacterial pathogen *Mycobacterium tuberculosis*. Immunity 10:641–650

Terahara K, Yoshida M, Igarashi O et al (2008) Comprehensive gene expression profiling of Peyer's patch M cells, villous M-like cells, and intestinal epithelial cells. J Immunol 180:7840–7846

Tsuji M, Komatsu N, Kawamoto S et al (2009) Preferential generation of follicular B helper T cells from Foxp3+ T cells in gut Peyer's patches. Science 323:1488–1492

Unutmaz D, Pulendran B (2009) The gut feeling of T_{reg} cells: IL-10 is the silver lining during colitis. Nat Immunol 10:1141–1143

van Ginkel FW, Jackson RJ, Yuki Y et al (2000) Cutting edge: the mucosal adjuvant cholera toxin redirects vaccine proteins into olfactory tissues. J Immunol 165:4778–4782

Wang X, Hone DM, Haddad A et al (2003) M cell DNA vaccination for CTL immunity to HIV. J Immunol 171:4717–4725

Wang X, Kochetkova I, Haddad A et al (2005) Transgene vaccination using *Ulex europaeus* agglutinin I (UEA-1) for targeted mucosal immunization against HIV-1 envelope. Vaccine 23:3836–3842

Weiner HL (2000) Oral tolerance, an active immunologic process mediated by multiple mechanisms. J Clin Invest 106:935–937

Wu Y, Boysun MJ, Csencsits KL et al (2000) Gene transfer facilitated by a cellular targeting molecule, reovirus protein sigma1. Gene Ther 7:61–69

Wu Y, Wang X, Csencsits KL et al (2001) M cell-targeted DNA vaccination. Proc Natl Acad Sci USA 98:9318–9323

Xiao BG, Link H (1997) Mucosal tolerance: a two-edged sword to prevent and treat autoimmune diseases. Clin Immunol Immunopathol 85:119–128

Yamamoto M, Briles DE, Yamamoto S et al (1998) A nontoxic adjuvant for mucosal immunity to pneumococcal surface protein A. J Immunol 161:4115–4121

Yamamoto M, McGhee JR, Hagiwara Y et al (2001) Genetically manipulated bacterial toxin as a new generation mucosal adjuvant. Scand J Immunol 53:211–217

Yamamoto S, Kiyono H, Yamamoto M et al (1997) A nontoxic mutant of cholera toxin elicits Th2-type responses for enhanced mucosal immunity. Proc Natl Acad Sci USA 94:5267–5272

Virus-Like Particles for Antigen Delivery at Mucosal Surfaces

K. Schneider-Ohrum and T. M. Ross

Abstract Virus-like particles are a new type of vaccine platform that presents an attractive alternative to more traditional live-attenuated or inactivated/subunit vaccines. Virus-like particles (VLP) are composed of viral structural proteins that assemble spontaneously in cells, mimicking the live virus without the possibility of replication. They are readily recognized by the immune system, inducing both humoral and cellular immune responses. Here we review the development of VLP as vaccine delivery systems at mucosal surfaces. We first summarize the current status of VLP vaccines in general, and then discuss their use in mucosal vaccination approaches for several viruses that enter the host via the urogenital, respiratory or gastrointestinal tract.

Contents

K. Schneider-Ohrum · T. M. Ross (✉)
Center for Vaccine Research, Department of Microbiology and Molecular Genetics,
University of Pittsburgh, Pittsburgh, PA, USA
e-mail: tmr15@pitt.edu

Current Topics in Microbiology and Immunology (2012) 354: 53–73
DOI: 10.1007/82_2011_135

Published Online: 10 July 2011

1 Introduction

Vaccination is the most effective way to combat diseases caused by infectious agents. Most vaccines, such as the smallpox vaccine, have been derived empirically, and many modern vaccines still follow these principles, developed decades ago. Despite success in the eradication of smallpox and in the control of infectious diseases such as polio or measles, development of vaccines against more complex viral pathogens has proved more challenging. Infectious diseases such as malaria, tuberculosis, human immunodeficiency virus (HIV) and dengue hemorrhagic fever result in a large number of deaths, especially in developing countries. New and emerging diseases, such as Nipah virus and the looming avian influenza pandemic, represent additional challenges for the vaccine development community.

Advances in recombinant genetics have facilitated the development of new vaccine technology platforms, such as virus-like particle (VLP) vaccines, which present a promising alternative to more traditional vaccination approaches. In this chapter, an update will be given on VLP as vaccine candidates, with emphasis on the use of VLP vaccines for generation of mucosal immunity.

2 Characteristics of VLP

Virus-like particles are composed of multiple copies of viral structural proteins, which upon expression, spontaneously assemble into structures resembling native virus. In contrast to the virus of origin, VLP generally do not contain the viral genome and are therefore replication-incompetent and non-pathogenic. They range in size from 25 to 120 nm, depending on the viral background, and they structurally and morphologically resemble the virus from which they are derived (Fig. 1) (Johnson and Chiu 2000; Ellenberger et al. 2004).

Virus-like particles have been generated from non-enveloped and enveloped viruses belonging to various virus families (Table 1). Administration of VLP as vaccines can protect the host against the specific viral infection (e.g. HIV VLP and influenza VLP) or they can be used as antigen presentation platforms, in the form of chimeric VLP, which present foreign antigens (e.g. phage Qbeta VLP) (Grgacic and Anderson 2006; McBurney et al. 2006; Bessa et al. 2008). Several different expression systems are currently used to derive VLP. The viral structural proteins can be produced in bacterial, yeast, plant, insect or mammalian cell

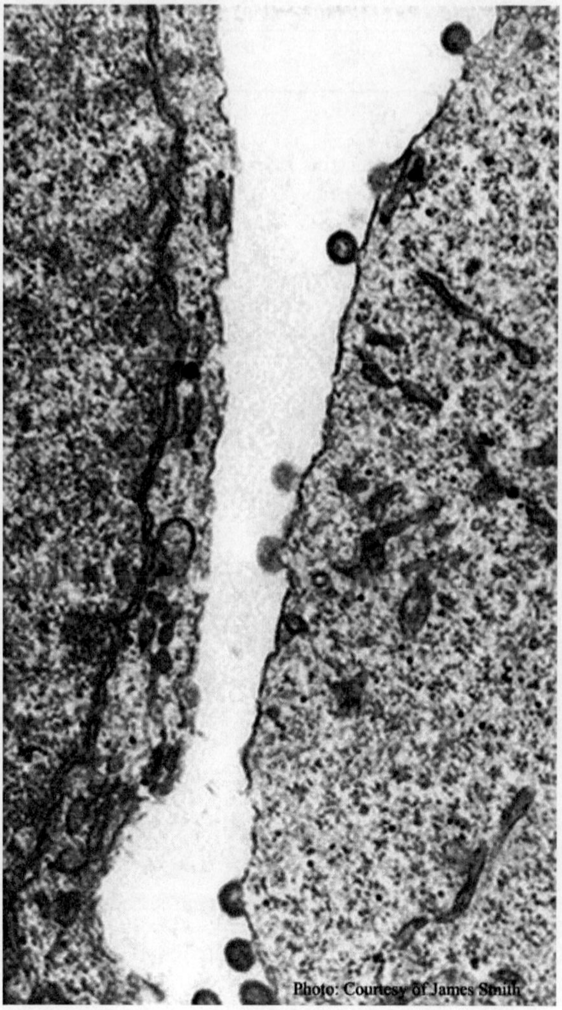

Fig. 1 *HIV-1 virus-like particles*. Transmission electron microscopy of HIV virus-like particles budding from 293T cells transfected with vaccine constructs expressing HIV-1 genes (photo kindly provided by James Smith, Centers for Disease Control and Prevention)

expression systems. What makes VLP good vaccine candidates? In order to answer this question, it is important to briefly review more traditional vaccine approaches.

3 Vaccination Strategies

3.1 Traditional Vaccines

Currently, two vaccine approaches are widely used by manufacturers: live-attenuated or inactivated/subunit vaccines. The advantage of live-attenuated vaccines is the ability to elicit robust immune responses, leading to life-long

Table 1 Examples of current VLP vaccine strategies

Family	Virus	Genome	Envelope	Particle composition	Expression systems	Vaccine status
Caliciviridae	Noro	ssRNA	no	Capsid	Baculovirus yeast	Phase I preclinical
Hepeviridae	Hepatitis E	ssRNA	no	Capsid	Baculovirus	Preclinical
Flaviviridae	Hepatitis C	ssRNA	yes	Core E1, E2	Baculovirus	Preclinical
Retroviridae	HIV, SIV	ssRNA	yes	Gag, env	Baculovirus mammalian cells yeast	Preclinical Phase I
Bunyaviridae	Rift Valley Fever	seg. ssRNA	yes	Capsid, G_N, G_C	Mammalian cells	Preclinical
Orthomyxoviridae	Influenza	seg. ssRNA	yes	HA, (NA), M1/gag	Baculovirus mammalian cells tobacco	Phase I preclinical preclinical
Reoviridae	Bluetongue	seg. ssDNA	no	VP3, VP7	Baculovirus	Preclinical
	Rota		no	VP2, VP6, VP7	Baculovirus	Preclinical
Papilloviridae	Papilloma	dsDNA	no	L1	Baculovirus Yeast	Licensed Licensed
Hepadnaviridae	Hepatitis B	dsDNA	yes	HBsAg	Yeast Potato Native subviral Envelope particles (plasma-derived) Mammalian cells	Licensed Preclinical Licensed (Developing countries) Licensed

immunity. Attenuated vaccines are capable of inducing highly durable T and B cell responses and often require only a single immunization. Examples of live-attenuated vaccines are measles, yellow fever and oral polio vaccines (Ravanfar et al. 2009). However, live-attenuated vaccines harbor safety risks since the pathogen can revert to a wild-type phenotype with potentially devastating outcomes. Furthermore, there is a risk of transmission of the attenuated pathogen from vaccinated individuals to others, including newborns, who lack a mature immune system and hence, may not be able to control the infection. Not surprisingly, live-attenuated vaccines are contra-indicated for use in immune-compromised individuals. Due to the potential safety risks associated with live-attenuated vaccines, there has been a trend toward development of safer inactivated or subunit vaccines, such as those for influenza, rabies and hepatitis B. But safety comes at a price. Inactivated or subunit vaccines are less immunogenic than live vaccines. They therefore require multiple booster immunizations and/or supplementation with adjuvants.

3.2 *Virus-Like Particles as a Vaccine Platform*

The mammalian immune system is designed to optimally respond to microbial invaders, such as viruses. Viruses are highly immunogenic due to their (a) repetitive, ordered structure; (b) particulate nature; and (c) expression of pathogen-associated molecular patterns (PAMP) which activate the host innate immune system via Toll-like receptors (TLR) and other intracellular pattern recognition receptors (PRR) (Takeuchi and Akira 2009). Virus-like particles mimic native virus in structure and size, but lack the genetic information required for replication, making them safer than live-attenuated vaccines. Although VLP induce less robust immune responses than live-attenuated vaccines, they are more immunogenic than subunit vaccines. In the context of a VLP, antigens are presented in a highly repetitive and ordered fashion, leading to the induction of a robust humoral immune response (Bright et al. 2008). The particulate nature of VLP makes them prime targets for uptake and presentation by antigen-presenting cells (APC) to the adaptive arm of the immune system (Yan et al. 2004). In contrast to native virus, the genome-less VLP does not contain nucleic acid-derived pathogen-associated molecular patterns recognized by TLR or the Rig-1-like receptors (RLR). Not present in the VLP is double stranded RNA (dsRNA, TLR3 and RIG-I/MDA-5 agonist), single stranded RNA (ssRNA, TLR7/8 agonist) or DNA enriched in unmethylated cytosine-guanine motifs (CpG, TLR9 agonist), all of which are potent activators of the innate immune system (Akira 2006). Nevertheless, VLP do trigger innate responses. The mechanisms responsible are poorly understood but may be due in part to incorporation of proteins from the VLP expression system (e.g. yeast or baculovirus) into the particle (Demi et al. 2005). It is also possible to attach or package immune stimulatory molecules onto or into the VLP for stronger activation of innate immune responses (Jegerlehner et al. 2007).

4 Mucosal Immunity, an Overview

The principal mucosal site used by pathogens to enter mammalian hosts is the digestive, respiratory or urogenital tract (Lavelle 2005). Therefore, an effective and specialized innate and adaptive immune system protecting these surfaces has evolved. Local lymphoid tissues associated with the mucosae are the mucosa-associated lymphoid tissues (MALT) that include the Peyer's patches (PP) and smaller lymphoid follicles in the intestine and the oro-pharyngeal tonsils in Waldeyer's ring, forming together a large lymphoid organ system (Holmgren and Czerkinsky 2005; Brandtzaeg 2007). In order for the mucosal immune system to respond to a pathogen, the antigen must traverse or be transported across the mucosal epithelium. The M cell plays an important role in luminal antigen uptake in the intestine and adenoids (Niedergang and Kweon 2005). M cells are specialized epithelial cells that have a characteristic invagination of their basolateral plasma membrane (a "pocket") that harbors lymphocytes, macrophages and dendritic cells (DC) (Kraehenbuhl and Neutra 2000). M cells bind and transcytose luminal particles or protein antigens into the pocket where they are taken up by the resident phagocytic cells. The main APC in the M cell pocket is the DC (Kelsall and Strober 1996a, b). In addition to the DC residing underneath M cells, another population of DC in the gut lamina propria plays a role in antigen sampling. These DC send dendrites through the epithelium to sample antigens in the lumen (Rescigno et al. 2001). The formation of the dendrites is dependent on the chemokine receptor CX3CR1 whose ligand is the epithelial cell-derived chemokine fractalkine (Niedergang and Kweon 2005). Recognition of conserved molecular patterns such as lipopolysaccharide (LPS) via PRR sends a "danger signal" to the DC, leading to maturation, upregulation of MHC class II and co-stimulatory molecules (CD80, CD86 and CD40) and secretion of pro-inflammatory cytokines such as type I IFN and IL-12. After antigen presentation and priming of naive B and T cells by the APC, the activated lymphocytes travel through the lymph into blood and then migrate to specific mucosal effector sites, a process dictated by specific homing receptors (Campbell et al. 2003; Kunkel and Butcher 2003).

A hallmark and main adaptive humoral effector function of the mucosal immune system is the synthesis of polymeric IgA antibodies which are transported across columnar epithelial cells and into luminal secretions via the polymeric Ig receptor (Brandtzaeg 2007). T cell and epithelial cell-derived cytokines such as transforming growth factor (TGF-β), IL-10 and IL-6 play an important role in the development of IgA-secreting B cells (Goodrich and McGee 1998; Asano et al. 2004). In addition to IgA, smaller amounts of locally synthesized IgG and IgM, as well as serum IgG transudated into tissues, also contribute to mucosal immune defense (Czerkinsky and Holmgren 2010). Cytotoxic T cell responses are also elicited and are critical for the control of certain types of gastrointestinal and respiratory infections (Belyakov and Ahlers 2011).

5 Examples of VLP Vaccines

Virus-like particles are ideal mucosal vaccine candidates because their particulate nature and size promotes uptake by M cells and DC, they closely mimic the natural pathogen, and they are good activators of the innate immune system (Demi et al. 2005), leading in turn to activation of the humoral and cellular arms of the adaptive immune response. Virus-like particles can be used as viral vaccines or in the form of chimeric VLP as antigen and/or adjuvant delivery systems (Jennings and Bachmann 2008). Various examples of VLP vaccines will be discussed, with emphasis on VLP vaccines in the context of mucosal immunity.

5.1 Human Papilloma Virus

Human papilloma virus (HPV) is one of the most common sexually transmitted infectious agents worldwide and specific types of HPV have been linked to the development of cervical cancer (HPV strains 16 and 18, which cause 70% of cervical cancers) and other types of cancer (zur Hausen 1996, 2009). The first HPV vaccines to be licensed for use in humans are Gardasil®, a quadrivalent HPV VLP vaccine developed by Merck to prevent infection by HPV types 6, 11, 16 and 18 (types 6 and 11 cause 90% of genital warts), and Cervarix™, a bivalent HPV-16/18 VLP vaccine developed by GlaxoSmithKline (Schiller et al. 2008). Both vaccines are composed of the HPV L1 major capsid protein, which can self-assemble into VLP that are structurally and antigenically similar to the HPV virion (Kirnbauer et al. 1992). Both vaccines are also administered parenterally via three injections into the deltoid muscle. The vaccines differ in their valencies, the cell types employed for recombinant expression of the L1 protein, and in the adjuvant used. The L1 proteins for Gardasil are expressed in yeast (*Saccharomyces cervisiae*) whereas Cervarix™ VLP are produced in the *Trichoplusia ni* insect-cell-line infected with recombinant baculovirus expressing the L1 protein (Schiller et al. 2008). Gardasil® contains the classical alum adjuvant (aluminum hydroxy-phosphate sulfate). Cervarix contains AS04 adjuvant, a combination of mono-phosphoryl lipid A (detoxified *Salmonella minnesota* LPS) and aluminum hydroxide (Wang 2007; Schwarz and Leo 2008). Aluminum compounds are the most widely used adjuvants in human vaccines and induce primarily a Th2 type immune response (Lindblad 2004). Recently, the mechanism of alum-based adjuvants has been described. Alum leads to an increase in antigen-specific T cell proliferation via the induction of IL-1, which it does by activating caspase-1 to produce active IL-1β and IL-18. This caspase-1 activation is dependent on the activation of NOD-like (NLR) intracellular microbial sensors, which form cytoplasmic complexes, called inflammasomes (Martinon et al. 2009). Monophosphoryl lipid A not only efficiently promotes antibody responses, but also induces cellular immune responses through activation of the innate arm of the immune system, particularly DC (Ulrich and Myers 1995).

Both HPV VLP vaccines performed well in clinical trials with higher than 95% prophylactic efficacy in preventing infection and lesions related to the targeted HPV strains in young women (Schiller et al. 2008). More results can be expected soon from trials currently underway in men and older women.

HPV has a specific tropism for the squamous epithelium of the skin or mucosal sites and after establishing infection the virus remains localized in the epithelial cells of the mucosa. The viral replication cycle is exclusively intraepithelial and there is no viremia, allowing the virus to evade the immune system. Despite this, 90% of all primary infections with HPV are cleared by the immune system, with innate, cellular and humoral responses all playing a role (Passmore et al. 2006; Stanley et al. 2006). Several months after natural HPV infection, low levels of virus-specific IgG in serum and IgA in cervical secretions are detected

(Passmore et al. 2007). The HPV VLP vaccines, which are not delivered via a mucosal route, elicit their protection primarily by inducing high levels of antiviral neutralizing IgG in serum, which transudates into reproductive tract tissues and secretions (Nardelli-Haefliger et al. 2003; Schiller and Davies 2004). Time will tell whether the current HPV vaccines are effective for providing long-term protection, or whether booster immunizations will be necessary. Issues that will need to be addressed in future generations of HPV vaccines for developing countries, which have the highest rates of cervical cancer, will be the current (a) high costs of production; (b) requirement for three immunizations; (c) need for a cold chain; (d) limited number of oncogenic HPV strains; and (e) the requirement for needle-based intramuscular administration. In a pilot study comparing two different mucosal administration routes for HPV16L1 VLP in humans, bronchial vaccination with aerosolized VLP produced similar neutralizing antibody titers when compared to intramuscular VLP injection, but nasal vaccination with aerosol was poorly immunogenic (Nardelli-Haefliger et al. 2005). A more recent study in mice found that co-administration of the HPV16L1 VLP with *E.coli* heat-labile enterotoxin (LT) adjuvant significantly improved the titers of specific serum IgG and vaginal IgA after nasal or bronchial immunization (Revaz et al. 2007). These results will aid the development of a mucosally administered HPV VLP vaccine formulation with appropriate mucosal adjuvants for human use.

5.2 *Influenza*

Influenza, a member of the *Orthomyxoviridae* family, is an enveloped virus that contains a segmented RNA genome (eight segments encoding for at least 11 proteins) of negative polarity. The segmented nature of the genome allows for the generation of viral diversity (Lamb 2001). Influenza can be subdivided into three types: A, B and C. Influenza epidemics occur almost every winter around the globe, caused by circulating influenza A subtypes (H3N2 and H1N1) and influenza B. The annual influenza epidemics lead to approximately 300,000 hospitalizations and 36,000 deaths in the US alone (Simonsen et al. 2007). About 90% of all influenza-related deaths occur in the elderly (Simonsen et al. 1998). However, the H1N1 "Spanish" influenza pandemic of 1918 resulted in the deaths of >50 million people worldwide, and the recent H1N1 swine flu outbreak, originating in Mexico, illustrates how fast a virus with pandemic potential can spread across the globe (Johnson and Mueller 2002; Charatan 2009; Fraser et al. 2009). In 1997, and again in 2004, the highly pathogenic avian influenza (HPAI) of the H5N1 subtype emerged as an extremely pathogenic virus in poultry and humans (Subbarao and Luke 2007). H5N1 has the potential to evolve into a virus that could cause a new pandemic. It therefore represents a serious threat for global health.

The immune control of influenza involves a combination of cellular and humoral responses (Doherty et al. 1997; Gerhard et al. 1997). The viral antigens, hemagglutinin (HA) and neuraminidase (NA), are the major surface glycoproteins of the virus and thus important targets for the host immune response (Wilson and Cox 1990). The goal of the influenza vaccine is to induce antigen-specific memory T and B cells. The memory B cells secrete high avidity neutralizing antibodies to HA and NA (Lamb 2001). The memory CD8+ T cells quickly acquire effector functions which include cytolytic killing of infected cells and secretion of proinflammatory cytokines that inhibit virus replication. Activated memory CD4+ T helper cells support these B cell and CD8+ T cell functions (Doherty et al. 1997). The efficacy of a vaccine is, like the control of an infection, dependent on the fitness of the immune system of the immunized individual. The immunization of immunocompromised people, very young children, and the elderly is therefore less effective and more challenging.

Current vaccine strategies against influenza infection are inactivated virus, either administered as whole or split vaccines via intramuscular injection. The vaccines are effective in protecting healthy adults from infection with antigenically matched influenza viruses, but perform relatively poorly in the elderly. Due to antigenic drift, the vaccine formulations must be updated and administered every year. The correlate of protection with the conventional influenza vaccines is primarily the induction of neutralizing antibodies against the viral HA envelope protein. The licensed trivalent inactivated vaccines (TIV) contain 15 μg of each of the three HA, derived from the influenza A subtypes H1N1 and H3N2 and influenza B virus of the specific season (Bridges et al. 2002). The conventional inactivated influenza vaccines induce virtually no cross-protection against unmatched strains. Currently, there is only one licensed influenza vaccine given via a mucosal route. This is the intranasal FluMist® vaccine, developed by MedImmune (Belshe 2004). The vaccine is based on cold-adapted, live-attenuated influenza master strains. In contrast to TIV, the live-attenuated vaccine induces some degree of heterotypic immunity and can therefore protect against drifted strains (Belshe 2004). In addition to induction of CTL and serum IgG antibodies, the live-attenuated FluMist vaccine elicits significantly higher levels of nasal S-IgA compared to the inactivated intramuscular vaccine (Cox et al. 2004). Manufacture of both vaccines requires the growth of live virus in chicken eggs and has long production times.

Virus-like particle vaccines represent an attractive alternative to inactivated and live-attenuated influenza vaccines for several reasons: (a) there is no live virus involved in the production process which makes them extremely safe; (b) development and production time are relatively short; and (c) there are a variety of egg-free expression systems available. The VLP vaccines can be made without the need to grow up large stocks of live virus, which is especially important due to the emergence of avian influenza A H5N1 viruses with the capacity to infect humans (Claas et al. 1998; Subbarao et al. 1998). Handling H5N1 viruses requires Biosafety Level 3 facilities that hinder practical large scale growth of these viruses in eggs or tissue culture. Particular effort has therefore been put into the development of VLP vaccines for pandemic influenza strains.

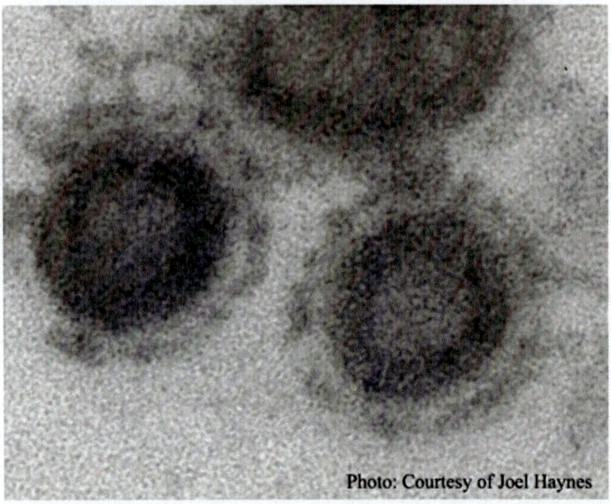

Fig. 2 *Influenza virus-like particles*. Thin section electron microscopy of H1N1-pseudotyped Gag-VLPs produced in insect cells. The globular heads of the HA protein are visible (photo kindly provided by Joel Haynes, Ligocyte Pharmaceuticals, Inc.)

There are several VLP-based influenza vaccine candidates under development and some are currently in clinical trials. Influenza VLP vaccines have recently been reviewed in great detail (Haynes 2009; Kang et al. 2009a) and here we will focus mainly on results obtained with mucosally administered influenza VLP. The majority of influenza VLP contain the viral HA and NA envelope proteins and the M1 matrix protein (Latham and Galarza 2001; Galarza et al. 2005; Bright et al. 2007; Quan et al. 2007). Expression or exogenous addition of recombinant NA is required in mammalian cell expression systems for cleavage of HA terminal sialic acids by NA (Ali et al. 2000). In insect cells, N-glycans are not modified after translation by the addition of sialic acid, which eliminates the requirement for NA in insect-cell-based expression systems (Galarza et al. 2005; Quan et al. 2007). Another approach (Fig. 2) is to produce influenza-pseudotyped Gag virus-like particles via the expression of influenza-HA, NA and a lentiviral Gag protein (Haynes et al. 2009). Currently, the expression system of choice for influenza and other VLP is the recombinant baculovirus/insect-cell expression system. The advantages of this system are (a) the large amounts of recombinant protein that can be produced in this high-density culture system; (b) the absence of mammalian cell-derived tissue culture supplements, reducing the risk of opportunistic pathogen introduction; (c) the insect cells have the capacity to perform post-translational modifications such as glycosylation and phosphorylation; and (d) the baculovirus can be inactivated by chemical treatment (Noad and Roy 2003; Cox 2008). One drawback of the system is that influenza VLP and baculovirus are of similar size (80–120 nm). Thus, it is difficult to remove all traces of the baculovirus from the influenza vaccine formulation (Pushko et al. 2005).

Recently, H5N1 influenza VLP have been successfully produced in a plant-based transient expression system using *Nicotiana benthamiana* tobacco plants (D'Aoust et al. 2008). Advantages of a plant-based expression system are safety and the capacity to produce VLP in large scale. Intramuscular immunization of mice with tobacco plant-derived VLP has protected against lethal challenge with a heterologous H5N1 influenza strain (D'Aoust et al. 2008).

Parenteral or mucosal (intranasal) immunization with seasonal and pandemic influenza VLP has been quite successful. Galarza et al. (2005) immunized mice via both routes with two doses of influenza A/Udorn H3N2 baculovirus-derived VLP (composed of HA and M1) with or without IL-12 as adjuvant. The mice that received the vaccine by the intranasal route developed higher antibody titers to HA than the animals that received the vaccine by the intramuscular route or mice that were given two sub-lethal doses of live virus (Galarza et al. 2005). In regard to cross-protection, influenza-HA-M1 VLP derived from the mouse-adapted A/PR/8/34 H1N1 virus given via the intranasal route conferred cross-protection against a lethal challenge with the A/WSN/33 H1N1 influenza strain (Quan et al. 2007). These results suggest that mucosally administered influenza vaccine may provide better protection against antigenic variants within a subtype than parenterally administered vaccines. Furthermore, the induction of anti-HA IgG in the nasal mucosa and the priming of virus-specific cellular responses, which were readily recalled after virus challenge, were observed in mice intranasally immunized with HA-M1 VLP (Quan et al. 2007).

H5N1 influenza VLP protect against drifted strains, which is of particular interest, since the subtype or clade that may emerge and cause a pandemic is difficult to predict. To date, 10 different clades of highly pathogenic avian influenza viruses (HPAI) with the potential to develop into human-to-human transmissible strains have been identified. In addition to H5N1, HPAI strains from subtypes H7N7 and H9N2 have also infected people in the last decade. Intramuscular immunization of mice with a baculovirus-derived influenza VLP containing HA and NA from the clade 2 virus A/Indonesia/05/2005 has proved successful for eliciting protection against the heterologous clade 1 strain A/Vietnam/1203/2004 (Bright et al. 2008). Cross-clade protection by the same VLP was confirmed in the more suitable ferret model (Mahmood et al. 2008). Another important consideration in vaccine development is the longevity of the induced immune responses. Intranasal immunization with a clade 1 H5N1 VLP induced high levels of long-lived H5N1-specific antibodies which were still 100% protective 7 months after vaccination (Kang et al. 2009b). The intransally administered VLP induced virus-specific systemic IgG and mucosal IgG and IgA responses (Kang et al. 2009a).

An alternative approach to these influenza VLP vaccines is the use of a chimeric VLP displaying influenza antigens. Bessa et al. (2008) generated VLP derived from the RNA bacteriophage Qβ on which the influenza M2 protein was subsequently covalently attached. A single intranasal immunization with M2-Qb-VLP induced M2-specific IgG and IgA in serum and broncheoalveolar fluid and protected against a lethal challenge with influenza virus (Bessa et al. 2008). Current and future human trials with influenza VLP vaccines will reveal whether the promising results obtained in animal models can be translated to humans.

5.3 Norovirus

Norovirus (or Norwalk virus), belonging to the *Caliciviridae* virus family, is one of the leading causes of nonbacterial gastroenteritis in humans (Fankhauser et al. 1998). Noroviruses are classified into 5 genogroups (I–V) and 32 genotypes based on the sequence diversity in the complete capsid protein VP1. The human norovirus strains are clustered within the genogroups I, II and III (Patel et al. 2009). Norovirus outbreaks peak in the winter months. Fecal-oral transmission is the most prevalent way of viral spread, which is often very fast and extensive, especially in densely populated areas such as hospitals, hotels, schools, nursing homes, cruise ships and military vessels (Estes et al. 2000; Patel et al. 2009). Clinical symptoms of a norovirus infection include nausea, vomiting and a non-bloody diarrhea. These usually last anywhere between 2 and 6 days, depending on the patient (Rockx et al. 2002; Patel et al. 2009). Even though the symptoms subside relatively quickly, infected patients can still shed virus for up to 14 days, which makes it especially important to monitor people working in the food industry to avoid spreading of the disease (Graham et al. 1994). Norovirus research has been hampered by the inability to grow norovirus in tissue culture. There are currently no suitable small animal models for studies of human norovirus, but the discovery of murine norovirus (MNV) strains, which are capable of replicating in vitro and in vivo, has opened new doors in norovirus research (Karst et al. 2003; Wobus et al. 2004). In addition, the finding that recombinant norovirus capsid protein self-assembles into VLP has provided a tool to study serum antibody responses to infection, to generate antisera, and to identify a cellular receptor for norovirus (Jiang et al. 1992; Green et al. 1993). The human histo-blood group antigens (HBGA) may act as receptors for norovirus and play a role in a subject's susceptibility to norovirus infection (Hutson et al. 2003; Lindesmith et al. 2003). Norovirus VLP produced in either the baculovirus system, yeast or plants are the premier candidates for vaccine development (Green et al. 1993; Xia et al. 2007; Santi et al. 2008). Several studies in small animals and human volunteers showed that the VLP are highly immunogenic after parenteral injection or oral administration (Green et al. 1993; Ball et al. 1998, 1999; Tacket et al. 2003). Obstacles in the development of a norovirus vaccine are (a) the lack of known correlates of immune protection; (b) the existence of several norovirus types within the three genogroups that infect humans; and (c) the lack of long-term and cross-protective immunity (Patel et al. 2009). A recent study employing an alphavirus-adjuvanted murine norovirus-like particle vaccine showed that passive transfer of sera from mice immunized with the MNV VLP protected naive mice against MNV challenge, whereas adoptive transfer of purified CD4+ or CD8+ T cells did not (LoBue et al. 2009). These results suggest that humoral immunity induced by the VLP vaccine is likely to be the main correlate of protection. In the same study, multi-valent human norovirus VLP vaccines were generated employing the same Venezuelan Equine Encephalitis virus replicon system (Baric et al. 2002; LoBue et al. 2009). The VLP were co-administered to mice via footpad injection with alphavirus adjuvant particles. The homotypic and heterotypic immunity to human and murine norovirus strains was then evaluated (LoBue et al. 2009). These vaccines induced antibody responses that cross-reacted against norovirus VLP that were not present in the vaccine formulation. Furthermore, immunization of mice with multi-valent human norovirus VLP vaccines resulted in reduced viral loads after MNV challenge (LoBue et al. 2009).

In addition to the mouse/MNV model, the gnotobiotic pig represents an animal model that can be used to study human norovirus infections and vaccine approaches. Pigs with the ABO histo-blood group phenotype A + and/or H + are especially susceptible to infection with a GII.4 human norovirus strain (Cheetham et al. 2007; Souza et al. 2007a). Oral immunization of A/H gnotobiotic pigs with baculovirus-derived human norovirus VLP (HS66 strain) and an attenuated LT mucosal adjuvant, LTR192G, protected pigs from developing diarrhea after challenge with the homologous HS66 strain (Souza et al. 2007b). A second group of pigs received a VLP-immune stimulatory complexes (ISCOM) vaccine, which conferred only 75% protection, despite the induction of higher intestinal IgM and IgA and systemic IgG antibody titers compared to the VLP + LTR192G group, suggesting that factors other than antibody are important for protection (Souza et al. 2007a). This study and others show that norovirus VLP vaccines successfully induce a protective immune response in two different animal models. Follow-up studies in human volunteers may lead to a successful norovirus VLP vaccine.

5.4 Human Immunodeficiency Virus

Human immunodeficiency virus (HIV) type 1, the infectious agent causing the acquired immunodeficiency syndrome (AIDS), has claimed millions of lives since its introduction into the human population and approximately 40 million people are now living with HIV/AIDS (Gallo et al. 1983; Robinson 2007). Most of the HIV-infected people live in Sub-Saharan Africa and have limited access to life-saving antiretroviral drugs. Even in more developed parts of the world, HIV is still a major health concern. Antiretroviral medications are expensive, require strict compliance to prevent the emergence of drug-resistant strains, have adverse side effects, and need to be taken for the rest of the life. Therefore, a primary goal in HIV research is the development of a vaccine that will contain the HIV pandemic by eliciting neutralizing antibodies and robust cell-mediated immune responses. However, HIV presents unique challenges for vaccine development. Circulating strains are extremely diverse due to the high mutation rate that is characteristic of lentiviruses (Karlsson Hedestam et al. 2008). The gp120 viral envelope (Env) glycoprotein is the most variable gene and rapidly evolves under immune pressure to evade the host neutralizing antibody response (Burton et al. 2004).

Traditional vaccine approaches have focused on the elicitation of neutralizing antibodies, and this has proved successful in protection against many infectious agents. However, in the case of HIV, vaccine strategies that elicit both humoral and cell-mediated immune responses will be required for preventing infection. HIV is spread mainly via sexual contact, entering the host at a mucosal surface. Thus, vaccines must elicit mucosal immune responses in order to prevent infection (Lehner 2003; Letvin 2005). Virus-like particle-based HIV vaccines are a multiple protein approach that enhances both humoral and cell-mediated immune responses. An advantage of VLP-based HIV vaccines is the presentation of the Env glycoprotein in its natural form on the particle surface. The oligomeric Env protein on the VLP is biologically active and mediates binding to CD4 and chemokine co-receptors (CCR5 or CXCR4), allowing for VLP uptake and antigen processing by DC or macrophages (Young et al. 2006). Virus-like particles as HIV vaccines have been reviewed previously (Young et al. 2006). We will, therefore, focus on their application as mucosally delivered HIV vaccines.

As a member of the *Retroviridae* family, HIV contains two positive-sense RNA strands, which are converted by the viral reverse transcriptase (RT) into dsDNA (provirus), which integrates into the host genome. The proviral genome consists of nine open reading frames, encoding for 15 viral proteins (Gotte et al. 1999). The three major genes are the group-associated antigen (*gag*) genes which encode structural core proteins, the polymerase (*pol*) genes that encode viral enzymes and the envelope (*env*) gene which encodes the gp120 receptor binding protein and the gp41 fusion protein. The viral genome also encodes two regulatory proteins (Tat and Rev) and four accessory proteins (Nef, Vif, Vpu and Vpr) (Gotte et al. 1999). Expression of Gag alone leads to spontaneous formation of lentiviral VLP. However, normally the virus also contains Matrix, Nucleocapsid and Env proteins. In order to mimic the virus and to present as many antigenic sites as possible, HIV VLP for vaccination are composed of multiple proteins. Most VLP are generated by expressing the Gag-Pol polypeptide precursor and some form of the Env protein. Integration and recombination is prevented by removing the viral integrase and specific nucleotide sequence elements in the long terminal repeats (Young et al. 2006).

Lentivirus-like particles can be delivered in the form of DNA plasmids or viral vectors, resulting in the expression of the VLP in vivo. Alternatively, the VLP can be produced and purified in vitro using an insect or mammalian cell-based expression system (Wagner et al. 1992; Gay et al. 1998; Montefiori et al. 2001; Smith et al. 2004; Young et al. 2004; Ellenberger et al. 2005).

Several nonhuman primate models have been developed to assess HIV vaccine strategies. Simian immunodeficiency virus (SIV) obtained from African monkeys is genetically similar to HIV and causes immunodeficiency in Asian macaques (Letvin and King 1990). Additionally, chimeric simian immunodeficiency viruses (SHIV) composed of the SIV backbone expressing HIV envelopes have been created in the laboratory (Reimann et al. 1996). Both SHIV and SIV VLP containing Gag and truncated Env proteins have been produced in a baculovirus expression system (Yao et al. 2003). Expression of truncated Env resulted in higher expression levels. Intranasal administration of the SIV VLP in BALB/c mice elicited a systemic and mucosal antibody response that was further enhanced when cholera toxin (CT) was co-administered as adjuvant (Yao et al. 2003). Importantly, the SIV VLP generated neutralizing antibodies against the SIV_{1A11}

and SIV_{mac239} strains, which was tested by immunizing mice and New Zealand rabbits, respectively. SIV Env-specific cellular responses were also elicited by the SIV VLP, as shown by antigen-specific IFN-γ and IL-4 production in an ELISPOT assay (Yao et al. 2003).

Another interesting approach is the use of baculovirus-derived SHIV VLP in combination with inactivated influenza vaccine as the adjuvant (Kang et al. 2004). In contrast to cholera toxin, influenza vaccine is safe and accepted for human use, even for HIV positive subjects. These VLP were administered intranasally to mice in combination with influenza-HA, inactivated influenza or CpG oligodeoxynucleotides (ODN) as adjuvant. The combination with inactivated influenza virus or influenza-HA protein-enhanced systemic IgG and mucosal IgA antibody responses to the HIV Env protein, increased neutralizing antibody titers to HIV, and increased numbers of IFN-γ- and IL-4-producing T cells when compared to SHIV VLP alone. Addition of inactivated influenza virus induced a mixed T helper (Th) type 1 and 2 response, whereas the combination of VLP and CpG produced mainly a Th1-type response. Furthermore, CTL activity was enhanced in the mice that received the SHIV VLP in combination with the influenza virus or CpG ODN (Kang et al. 2004). Using a combination of two vaccines against distinctive pathogens in one immunization would be highly desirable, especially if one vaccine can function as the adjuvant for the other.

A major obstacle in the development of an AIDS vaccine is the high diversity between HIV strains. Mainly based on the genetic sequence variations of the surface envelope proteins, HIV-1 isolates can be divided into three groups: M (Major), N (Non-M, Non-O) and O (Outlier). Group M is the most common and subdivides into several clades (A–D, F–H, J and K). B is the most prevalent clade in the United States and Europe, whereas clade C is mainly found in India, China and Sub-Saharan Africa (Thomson et al. 2002). The high diversity between the strains will require that a vaccine elicit a broadly reactive immune response. There are different approaches to address this issue. One is the generation of a polyvalent vaccine, which consists of a mixture of the different envelope antigens derived from several strains, administered at the same time (McBurney and Ross 2007). An alternative strategy is the generation of a consensus sequence vaccine, which is based on a computational analysis of the amino acid sequences of the various envelope proteins and the generation of a consensus sequence based on the most common amino acid in each position (McBurney and Ross 2007). In a recent study, monovalent, polyvalent and consensus Env-VLP vaccines were directly compared for their ability to elicit a broadly reactive cell-mediated immune response (McBurney and Ross 2009). The vaccines were based on clade B or clade C envelope sequences. The VLP were produced in mammalian cells and were administered via the intranasal route to BALB/c mice, employing CpG ODN as the adjuvant. Both the polyvalent and consensus clade B VLP vaccines were determined to have elicited a broader cell-mediated immune response than the monovalent clade B vaccine using an IFN-γ ELISPOT assay. The number of specific T cell epitopes recognized after immunization with the consensus and polyvalent B Env-VLP vaccines was significantly higher than the monovalent Env-VLP.

Importantly, vaccination with the consensus VLP vaccines (both clade B and C) resulted in a broader mucosal cell-mediated immune response than the polyvalent and the monovalent vaccine (McBurney and Ross 2009). A consensus based vaccine might therefore protect a vaccinated person from a wider range of isolates compared to a polyvalent vaccine.

In animals, VLP-based HIV vaccines have successfully elicited humoral and cellular immune responses systemically and at the mucosal sites relevant to HIV transmission. Results from ongoing preclinical studies in nonhuman primates and future clinical trials will ultimately determine whether VLP are a promising vaccine platform for a HIV vaccine.

6 Conclusion

Virus-like particles represent an attractive platform for vaccine design for a variety of pathogens. They are easy to produce, non-infectious, closely mimic the native virus, can be administered via parenteral or mucosal routes and they successfully induce cellular and humoral immune responses. Future studies will show the potential of VLP-based vaccine strategies, leading to licensing, and aiding in the eradication of infectious diseases.

References

Akira S (2006) TLR signaling. Curr Top Microbiol Immunol 311:1–16

Ali A, Avalos RT, Ponimaskin E et al (2000) Influenza virus assembly: effect of influenza virus glycoproteins on the membrane association of M1 protein. J Virol 74:8709–8719

Asano T, Kaneko H, Terada T et al (2004) Molecular analysis of B-cell differentiation in selective or partial IgA deficiency. Clin Exp Immunol 136:284–290

Ball JM, Hardy ME, Atmar RL et al (1998) Oral immunization with recombinant Norwalk virus-like particles induces a systemic and mucosal immune response in mice. J Virol 72:1345–1353

Ball JM, Graham DY, Opekun AR et al (1999) Recombinant Norwalk virus-like particles given orally to volunteers: phase I study. Gastroenterology 117:40–48

Baric RS, Yount B, Lindesmith L et al (2002) Expression and self-assembly of Norwalk virus capsid protein from venezuelan equine encephalitis virus replicons. J Virol 76:3023–3030

Belshe RB (2004) Current status of live attenuated influenza virus vaccine in the US. Virus Res 103:177–185

Belyakov IM, Ahlers JD (2011) Mucosal immunity and HIV-1 infection: applications for mucosal AIDS vaccine development. Curr Top Microbiol (in press)

Bessa J, Schmitz N, Hinton HJ et al (2008) Efficient induction of mucosal and systemic immune responses by virus-like particles administered intranasally: implications for vaccine design. Eur J Immunol 38:114–126

Brandtzaeg P (2007) Induction of secretory immunity and memory at mucosal surfaces. Vaccine 25:5467–5484

Bridges CB, Fukuda K, Uyeki TM et al (2002) Prevention and control of influenza. Recommendations of the advisory committee on immunization practices (ACIP). MMWR Recomm Rep 51:1–31

Bright RA, Carter DM, Daniluk S et al (2007) Influenza virus-like particles elicit broader immune responses than whole virion inactivated influenza virus or recombinant hemagglutinin. Vaccine 25:3871–3878

Bright RA, Carter DM, Crevar CJ et al (2008) Cross-clade protective immune responses to influenza viruses with H5N1 HA and NA elicited by an influenza virus-like particle. PLoS ONE 3:e1501

Burton DR, Desrosiers RC, Doms RW et al (2004) HIV vaccine design and the neutralizing antibody problem. Nat Immunol 5:233–236

Campbell DJ, Debes GF, Johnston B et al (2003) Targeting T cell responses by selective chemokine receptor expression. Semin Immunol 15:277–286

Charatan F (2009) UN warns that swine flu outbreak could turn into pandemic. BMJ 338:b1751

Cheetham S, Souza M, McGregor R et al (2007) Binding patterns of human norovirus-like particles to buccal and intestinal tissues of gnotobiotic pigs in relation to A/H histo-blood group antigen expression. J Virol 81:3535–3544

Claas EC, Osterhaus AD, van Beek R et al (1998) Human influenza A H5N1 virus related to a highly pathogenic avian influenza virus. Lancet 351:472–477

Cox MM (2008) Progress on baculovirus-derived influenza vaccines. Curr Opin Mol Ther 10:56–61

Cox RJ, Brokstad KA, Ogra P (2004) Influenza virus: immunity and vaccination strategies. Comparison of the immune response to inactivated and live, attenuated influenza vaccines. Scand J Immunol 59:1–15

Czerkinsky C, Holmgren J (2010) Mucosal delivery routes for optimal immunization: targeting immunity to the right tissues. Curr Top Microbiol Immunol (in press)

D'Aoust MA, Lavoie PO, Couture MM et al (2008) Influenza virus-like particles produced by transient expression in Nicotiana benthamiana induce a protective immune response against a lethal viral challenge in mice. Plant Biotechnol J 6:930–940

Demi L, Speth C, Dierich MP et al (2005) Recombinant HIV-1 Pr55^{gag} virus-like particles: potent stimulators of innate and acquired immune responses. Mol Immunol 42:259–277

Doherty PC, Topham DJ, Tripp RA et al (1997) Effector CD4+ and CD8+ T-cell mechanisms in the control of respiratory virus infections. Immunol Rev 159:105–117

Ellenberger D, Li B, Smith J et al (2004) Optimization of a multi-gene HIV-1 recombinant subtype CRF02_AG DNA vaccine for expression of multiple immunogenic forms. Virology 319:118–130

Ellenberger D, Wyatt L, Li B et al (2005) Comparative immunogenicity in rhesus monkeys of multi-protein HIV-1 (CRF02_AG) DNA/MVA vaccines expressing mature and immature VLPs. Virology 340:21–32

Estes MK, Ball JM, Guerrero RA et al (2000) Norwalk virus vaccines: challenges and progress. J Infect Dis 181(Suppl 2):S367–S373

Fankhauser RL, Noel JS, Monroe SS et al (1998) Molecular epidemiology of "Norwalk-like viruses" in outbreaks of gastroenteritis in the United States. J Infect Dis 178:1571–1578

Fraser C, Donnelly CA, Cauchemez S et al (2009) Pandemic potential of a strain of influenza A (H1N1): Early Findings. Science 324:1557–1561

Galarza JM, Latham T, Cupo A (2005) Virus-like particle (VLP) vaccine conferred complete protection against a lethal influenza virus challenge. Viral Immunol 18:244–251, 365–372

Gallo RC, Sarin PS, Gelmann EP et al (1983) Isolation of human T-cell leukemia virus in acquired immune deficiency syndrome (AIDS). Science 220:865–867

Gay B, Tournier J, Chazal N et al (1998) Morphopoietic determinants of HIV-1 Gag particles assembled in baculovirus-infected cells. Virology 247:160–169

Gerhard W, Mozdzanowska K, Furchner M et al (1997) Role of the B-cell response in recovery of mice from primary influenza virus infection. Immunol Rev 159:95–103

Goodrich ME, McGee DW (1998) Regulation of mucosal B cell immunoglobulin secretion by intestinal epithelial cell-derived cytokines. Cytokine 10:948–955

Gotte M, Li X, Wainberg MA (1999) HIV-1 reverse transcription: a brief overview focused on structure-function relationships among molecules involved in initiation of the reaction. Arch Biochem Biophys 365:199–210

Graham DY, Jiang X, Tanaka T et al (1994) Norwalk virus infection of volunteers: new insights based on improved assays. J Infect Dis 170:34–43

Green KY, Lew JF, Jiang X et al (1993) Comparison of the reactivities of baculovirus-expressed recombinant Norwalk virus capsid antigen with those of the native Norwalk virus antigen in serologic assays and some epidemiologic observations. J Clin Microbiol 31:2185–2191

Grgacic EV, Anderson DA (2006) Virus-like particles: passport to immune recognition. Methods 40:60–65

Haynes JR (2009) Influenza virus-like particle vaccines. Expert Rev Vaccines 8:435–445

Haynes JR, Dokken L, Wiley JA et al (2009) Influenza-pseudotyped Gag virus-like particle vaccines provide broad protection against highly pathogenic avian influenza challenge. Vaccine 27:530–541

Holmgren J, Czerkinsky C (2005) Mucosal immunity and vaccines. Nat Med 11:S45–S53

Hutson AM, Atmar RL, Marcus DM et al (2003) Norwalk virus-like particle hemagglutination by binding to h histo-blood group antigens. J Virol 77:405–415

Jegerlehner A, Maurer P, Bessa J et al (2007) TLR9 signaling in B cells determines class switch recombination to IgG2a. J Immunol 178:2415–2420

Jennings GT, Bachmann MF (2008) The coming of age of virus-like particle vaccines. Biol Chem 389(5):521–536

Jiang X, Wang M, Graham DY et al (1992) Expression, self-assembly, and antigenicity of the Norwalk virus capsid protein. J Virol 66:6527–6532

Johnson JE, Chiu W (2000) Structures of virus and virus-like particles. Curr Opin Struct Biol 10:229–235

Johnson NP, Mueller J (2002) Updating the accounts: global mortality of the 1918–1920 "Spanish" influenza pandemic. Bull Hist Med 76:105–115

Kang SM, Guo L, Yao Q et al (2004) Intranasal immunization with inactivated influenza virus enhances immune responses to coadministered simian-human immunodeficiency virus-like particle antigens. J Virol 78:9624–9632

Kang SM, Yoo DG, Lipatov AS et al (2009a) Induction of long-term protective immune responses by influenza H5N1 virus-like particles. PLoS ONE 4:e4667

Kang SM, Song JM, Quan FS et al (2009b) Influenza vaccines based on virus-like particles. Virus Res 143(2):140–146

Karlsson Hedestam GB, Fouchier RA, Phogat S et al (2008) The challenges of eliciting neutralizing antibodies to HIV-1 and to influenza virus. Nat Rev Microbiol 6:143–155

Karst SM, Wobus CE, Lay M et al (2003) STAT1-dependent innate immunity to a Norwalk-like virus. Science 299:1575–1578

Kelsall BL, Strober W (1996a) Distinct populations of dendritic cells are present in the subepithelial dome and T cell regions of the murine Peyer's patch. J Exp Med 183:237–247

Kelsall BL, Strober W (1996b) The role of dendritic cells in antigen processing in the Peyer's patch. Ann N Y Acad Sci 778:47–54

Kirnbauer R, Booy F, Cheng N et al (1992) Papillomavirus L1 major capsid protein self-assembles into virus-like particles that are highly immunogenic. Proc Natl Acad Sci USA 89:12180–12184

Kraehenbuhl JP, Neutra MR (2000) Epithelial M cells: differentiation and function. Annu Rev Cell Dev Biol 16:301–332

Kunkel EJ, Butcher EC (2003) Plasma-cell homing. Nat Rev Immunol 3:822–829

Lamb RA (2001) Orthomyxoviridae: the viruses and their replication. In: Fields virology. Lippincott Williams and Wilkins, PA, USA, pp 1487–1531

Latham T, Galarza JM (2001) Formation of wild-type and chimeric influenza virus-like particles following simultaneous expression of only four structural proteins. J Virol 75:6154–6165

Lavelle EC (2005) Generation of improved mucosal vaccines by induction of innate immunity. Cell Mol Life Sci 62:2750–2770

Lehner T (2003) Innate and adaptive mucosal immunity in protection against HIV infection. Vaccine 21(Suppl 2):S68–S76

Letvin NL (2005) Progress toward an HIV vaccine. Annu Rev Med 56:213–223

Letvin NL, King NW (1990) Immunologic and pathologic manifestations of the infection of rhesus monkeys with simian immunodeficiency virus of macaques. J Acquir Immune Defic Syndr 3:1023–1040

Lindblad EB (2004) Aluminium compounds for use in vaccines. Immunol Cell Biol 82:497–505

Lindesmith L, Moe C, Marionneau S et al (2003) Human susceptibility and resistance to Norwalk virus infection. Nat Med 9:548–553

LoBue AD, Thompson JM, Lindesmith L et al (2009) Alphavirus-adjuvanted norovirus-like particle vaccines: heterologous, humoral, and mucosal immune responses protect against murine norovirus challenge. J Virol 83.3212–3227

Mahmood K, Bright RA, Mytle N et al (2008) H5N1 VLP vaccine induced protection in ferrets against lethal challenge with highly pathogenic H5N1 influenza viruses. Vaccine 26:5393–5399

Martinon F, Mayor A, Tschopp J (2009) The inflammasomes: guardians of the body. Annu Rev Immunol 27:229–265

McBurney SP, Ross TM (2007) Developing broadly reactive HIV-1/AIDS vaccines: a review of polyvalent and centralized HIV-1 vaccines. Curr Pharm Des 13:1957–1964

McBurney SP, Ross TM (2009) Human immunodeficiency virus-like particles with consensus envelopes elicited broader cell-mediated peripheral and mucosal immune responses than polyvalent and monovalent Env vaccines. Vaccine 27(32):4337–4349

McBurney SP, Young KR, Nwaigwe CI et al (2006) Lentivirus-like particles without reverse transcriptase elicit efficient immune responses. Curr HIV Res 4:475–484

Montefiori DC, Safrit JT, Lydy SL et al (2001) Induction of neutralizing antibodies and gag-specific cellular immune responses to an R5 primary isolate of human immunodeficiency virus type 1 in rhesus macaques. J Virol 75:5879–5890

Nardelli-Haefliger D, Wirthner D, Schiller JT et al (2003) Specific antibody levels at the cervix during the menstrual cycle of women vaccinated with human papillomavirus 16 virus-like particles. J Natl Cancer Inst 95:1128–1137

Nardelli-Haefliger D, Lurati F, Wirthner D et al (2005) Immune responses induced by lower airway mucosal immunisation with a human papillomavirus type 16 virus-like particle vaccine. Vaccine 23:3634–3641

Niedergang F, Kweon MN (2005) New trends in antigen uptake in the gut mucosa. Trends Microbiol 13:485–490

Noad R, Roy P (2003) Virus-like particles as immunogens. Trends Microbiol 11:438–444

Passmore JA, Milner M, Denny L et al (2006) Comparison of cervical and blood T-cell responses to human papillomavirus-16 in women with human papillomavirus-associated cervical intraepithelial neoplasia. Immunology 119:507–514

Passmore JA, Marais DJ, Sampson C et al (2007) Cervicovaginal, oral, and serum IgG and IgA responses to human papillomavirus type 16 in women with cervical intraepithelial neoplasia. J Med Virol 79:1375–1380

Patel MM, Hall AJ, Vinje J et al (2009) Noroviruses: a comprehensive review. J Clin Virol 44:1–8

Pushko P, Tumpey TM, Bu F et al (2005) Influenza virus-like particles comprised of the HA, NA, and M1 proteins of H9N2 influenza virus induce protective immune responses in BALB/c mice. Vaccine 23:5751–5759

Quan FS, Huang C, Compans RW et al (2007) Virus-like particle vaccine induces protective immunity against homologous and heterologous strains of influenza virus. J Virol 81:3514–3524

Ravanfar P, Satyaprakash A, Creed R et al (2009) Existing antiviral vaccines. Dermatol Ther 22:110–128

Reimann KA, Li JT, Veazey R et al (1996) A chimeric simian/human immunodeficiency virus expressing a primary patient human immunodeficiency virus type 1 isolate env causes an AIDS-like disease after in vivo passage in rhesus monkeys. J Virol 70:6922–6928

Rescigno M, Urbano M, Valzasina B et al (2001) Dendritic cells express tight junction proteins and penetrate gut epithelial monolayers to sample bacteria. Nat Immunol 2:361–367

Revaz V, Zurbriggen R, Moser C et al (2007) Humoral and cellular immune responses to airway immunization of mice with human papillomavirus type 16 virus-like particles and mucosal adjuvants. Antiviral Res 76:75–85

Robinson HL (2007) HIV/AIDS vaccines. Clin Pharmacol Ther 82:686–693

Rockx B, De Wit M, Vennema H et al (2002) Natural history of human calicivirus infection: a prospective cohort study. Clin Infect Dis 35:246–253

Santi L, Batchelor L, Huang Z et al (2008) An efficient plant viral expression system generating orally immunogenic Norwalk virus-like particles. Vaccine 26:1846–1854

Schiller JT, Davies P (2004) Delivering on the promise: HPV vaccines and cervical cancer. Nat Rev Microbiol 2:343–347

Schiller JT, Castellsague X, Villa LL et al (2008) An update of prophylactic human papillomavirus L1 virus-like particle vaccine clinical trial results. Vaccine 26(Suppl 10):K53–K61

Schwarz TF, Leo O (2008) Immune response to human papillomavirus after prophylactic vaccination with AS04-adjuvanted HPV-16/18 vaccine: improving upon nature. Gynecol Oncol 110:S1–S10

Simonsen L, Clarke MJ, Schonberger LB et al (1998) Pandemic versus epidemic influenza mortality: a pattern of changing age distribution. J Infect Dis 178:53–60

Simonsen L, Taylor RJ, Viboud C et al (2007) Mortality benefits of influenza vaccination in elderly people: an ongoing controversy. Lancet Infect Dis 7:658–666

Smith JM, Amara RR, Campbell D et al (2004) DNA/MVA vaccine for HIV type 1: effects of codon-optimization and the expression of aggregates or virus-like particles on the immunogenicity of the DNA prime. AIDS Res Hum Retroviruses 20:1335–1347

Souza M, Cheetham SM, Azevedo MS et al (2007a) Cytokine and antibody responses in gnotobiotic pigs after infection with human norovirus genogroup II.4 (HS66 strain). J Virol 81:9183–9192

Souza M, Costantini V, Azevedo MS et al (2007b) A human norovirus-like particle vaccine adjuvanted with ISCOM or mLT induces cytokine and antibody responses and protection to the homologous GII.4 human norovirus in a gnotobiotic pig disease model. Vaccine 25:8448–8459

Stanley M, Lowy DR, Frazer I (2006) Chapter 12: Prophylactic HPV vaccines: underlying mechanisms. Vaccine 24(Suppl 3):S3/106–S3/113

Subbarao K, Luke C (2007) H5N1 viruses and vaccines. PLoS Pathog 3:e40

Subbarao K, Klimov A, Katz J et al (1998) Characterization of an avian influenza A (H5N1) virus isolated from a child with a fatal respiratory illness. Science 279:393–396

Tacket CO, Sztein MB, Losonsky GA et al (2003) Humoral, mucosal, and cellular immune responses to oral Norwalk virus-like particles in volunteers. Clin Immunol 108:241–247

Takeuchi O, Akira S (2009) Innate immunity to virus infection. Immunol Rev 227:75–86

Thomson MM, Perez-Alvarez L, Najera R (2002) Molecular epidemiology of HIV-1 genetic forms and its significance for vaccine development and therapy. Lancet Infect Dis 2:461–471

Ulrich JT, Myers KR (1995) Monophosphoryl lipid A as an adjuvant. Past experiences and new directions. Pharm Biotechnol 6:495–524

Wagner R, Fliessbach H, Wanner G et al (1992) Studies on processing, particle formation, and immunogenicity of the HIV-1 gag gene product: a possible component of a HIV vaccine. Arch Virol 127:117–137

Wang KL (2007) Human papillomavirus and vaccination in cervical cancer. Taiwan J Obstet Gynecol 46:352–362

Wilson IA, Cox NJ (1990) Structural basis of immune recognition of influenza virus hemagglutinin. Annu Rev Immunol 8:737–771

Wobus CE, Karst SM, Thackray LB et al (2004) Replication of Norovirus in cell culture reveals a tropism for dendritic cells and macrophages. PLoS Biol 2:e432

Xia M, Farkas T, Jiang X (2007) Norovirus capsid protein expressed in yeast forms virus-like particles and stimulates systemic and mucosal immunity in mice following an oral administration of raw yeast extracts. J Med Virol 79:74–83

Yan M, Peng J, Jabbar IA et al (2004) Despite differences between dendritic cells and Langerhans cells in the mechanism of papillomavirus-like particle antigen uptake, both cells cross-prime T cells. Virology 324:297–310

Yao Q, Bu Z, Vzorov A et al (2003) Virus-like particle and DNA-based candidate AIDS vaccines. Vaccine 21:638–643

Young KR, Smith JM, Ross TM (2004) Characterization of a DNA vaccine expressing a human immunodeficiency virus-like particle. Virology 327:262–272

Young KR, McBurney SP, Karkhanis LU et al (2006) Virus-like particles: designing an effective AIDS vaccine. Methods 40:98–117

zur Hausen H (1996) Papillomavirus infections–a major cause of human cancers. Biochim Biophys Acta 1288:F55–F78

zur Hausen H (2009) Papillomaviruses in the causation of human cancers—a brief historical account. Virology 384:260–265

Recent Advances in Microparticle and Nanoparticle Delivery Vehicles for Mucosal Vaccination

E. A. McNeela and E. C. Lavelle

Abstract The great potential of mucosal vaccination is widely accepted but progress in the clinical development of subunit mucosal vaccines has been disappointing. Of the available approaches, the use of polymer-based microparticles is attractive because these delivery vehicles can be specifically tailored for vaccines and they offer the potential for integration of adjuvant. Here we address recent developments in the use of particulates as mucosal vaccines and the potential of novel targeting strategies, formulation approaches and adjuvant combinations to enhance the efficacy of particle-based mucosal vaccines. This review discusses the current status of mucosal vaccines based on particles and highlights several of the strategies that are currently under investigation for improving their immunogenicity. These include enhancing the stability of formulations in the luminal environment, increasing uptake by specifically targeting particles to mucosal inductive sites, and augmenting immunogenicity through co-formulation with immunostimulatory agents.

Contents

E. A. McNeela (✉) · E. C. Lavelle
Adjuvant Research Group, School of Biochemistry and Immunology,
Trinity College, Dublin 2, Ireland
e-mail: mcneele@tcd.ie

Current Topics in Microbiology and Immunology (2012) 354: 75–99
DOI: 10.1007/82_2011_140

Published Online: 9 September 2011

1 Introduction

The majority of human pathogens infect via the mucosae, including *Vibrio cholerae*, enterotoxigenic *Escherichia coli* (ETEC), influenza virus, human immunodeficiency virus type 1 (HIV-1), rotavirus and respiratory syncytial virus. Mucosal immunization is likely to induce greatest local immunity and prevent infection at sites of pathogen entry (Czerkinsky and Holmgren 2011). Mucosal immunization would obviate many of the problems associated with parenteral vaccination, such as the requirement for sterile needles and trained personnel, and it would improve patient compliance (Giudice and Campbell 2006; Lavelle 2001). Although most of the vaccines currently administered in humans are injected, there are several licensed mucosal vaccines, including oral vaccines against poliovirus, *Salmonella typhi* and *V. cholerae* and an intranasal (i.n.) vaccine for influenza virus (Brandtzaeg and Johansen 2008). These mucosal vaccines are based on killed or live-attenuated microorganisms, and their efficacy has highlighted the potential of mucosal vaccination. Much of the current vaccine research has focused on the development of subunit vaccines that are composed of purified native or recombinant components of microorganisms. Subunit vaccines are safer because they lack contaminants that are often present in whole-cell vaccines and they cannot revert to a virulent form, as reported for the live-attenuated oral polio vaccine (Minor 2009). However, most soluble subunit antigens are poorly immunogenic when administered at mucosal surfaces, and they require appropriate delivery systems and/or adjuvants in order to generate potent immune responses (Lavelle 2005; O'Hagan 1998).

A number of adjuvants and delivery systems have been evaluated for mucosal vaccines, including liposomes, immunostimulatory complexes, CpG oligodeoxynucleotides, bacterial toxins, nanoparticles and microparticles. Microparticles are attractive for mucosal vaccine delivery because they are similar in size to many pathogens that the host immune system has evolved to fight (O'Hagan et al. 2006). As a consequence, these particles and associated antigens may be rapidly taken up by antigen-presenting cells (APC) following immunization. The biodegradable and biocompatible polymers poly(lactide-co-glycolide) (PLG) and poly(lactic acid) (PLA) are the most widely used materials for the construction of microparticles (Cleland 1999). The US Food and Drug Administration (FDA) has approved the use of these materials for various clinical applications, including resorbable sutures and implants for controlled drug delivery. It has been suggested that the efficacy of microparticles is primarily related to their ability to protect encapsulated antigens, release antigen over extended time periods and to direct antigen to and retain it in local lymphoid tissues (Gupta et al. 1998; Vyas and Gupta 2007). However, recent findings suggest that these particulates can additionally enhance adaptive immunity by triggering innate responses (Sharp et al. 2009).

In the early 1990s, several groups reported the induction of mucosal and systemic immune responses to antigens entrapped in PLA/PLG microparticles after mucosal delivery in mice (Challacombe et al. 1992; Eldridge et al. 1989; Maloy et al. 1994; Moldoveanu et al. 1993). Furthermore, protective immunity against various pathogens, including *Streptococcus pneumoniae* (Fattal et al. 2002; Seong et al. 1999), *Bordetella pertussis* (Cahill et al. 1995; Conway et al. 2001) and *Salmonella typhimurium* (Allaoui-Attarki et al. 1997; Fattal et al. 2002) was generated in rodents by mucosal immunization with PLG microparticulate vaccines. However, despite these early encouraging results, studies in humans have been disappointing, and there are currently no licensed polymer-based microparticle mucosal vaccines (Katz et al. 2003; Lambert et al. 2001; Tacket et al. 1994). Significant improvements in the development of microparticles for human mucosal vaccination are needed, and recent studies have focused on strategies to enhance their efficacy. This review discusses the current status of mucosal vaccines based on particulates and highlights several of the strategies that are currently under investigation for improving their immunogenicity.

2 Mucosal Immunity to PLG/PLA Polymer-Formulated Microparticle Vaccines

The initiation of adaptive immunity following mucosal immunization occurs at specialized sites in the mucosae that contain organized mucosa-associated lymphoid tissue (MALT). Humoral immunity at these sites is mediated by secretory IgA (SIgA), which has been shown to neutralize toxins and to prevent the attachment and entry of pathogens at mucosal surfaces (Macpherson et al. 2008; Mestecky and Russell 2009). Serum IgG antibody responses may also be induced by mucosal immunization. Effectors of cellular immunity in mucosal tissues are $CD8^+$ cytotoxic T lymphocytes (CTL), $CD4^+$ T helper (Th) cells and Natural Killer (NK) cells. Cellular responses can be induced by mucosal immunization with vaccines, such as the oral typhoid vaccine (Salerno-Goncalves et al. 2002). Although vaccines can potentially be delivered via numerous mucosal routes, the majority of microparticle studies have focused on the oral and i.n. routes for vaccine administration.

Many investigators have shown that systemic antibody responses to antigens entrapped within or adsorbed onto PLG/PLA microparticles are greater than those produced in response to oral or i.n. immunization with soluble antigens (Carcaboso et al. 2003; Carcaboso et al. 2004; Challacombe et al. 1992; Florindo et al. 2009; Kende et al. 2002; Tabata et al. 1996; Vajdy and O'Hagan 2001; Yeh et al. 2002). Furthermore, several studies have reported the augmentation of antigen-specific IgA in mucosal secretions (Challacombe et al. 1992; Florindo et al. 2009; Tabata et al. 1996; Ugozzoli et al. 1998) and the induction of cell-mediated immune responses (Carpenter et al. 2005; Florindo et al. 2009; Moore et al. 1995; Vajdy and O'Hagan 2001) following mucosal delivery of microparticulate vaccines. More importantly, a number of vaccines utilizing PLG/PLA microparticles have elicited protective immunity in mice after oral delivery (Table 1).

From these studies (Table 1), it is apparent that oral immunization of mice with PLG/PLA-associated vaccines generally produces low titers of serum IgG antibodies but results in significant protection against mucosal microbial challenge, which in some studies was greater than that induced by systemic immunization. Therefore, it is important that additional immune parameters, including mucosal, humoral and cellular responses, and especially protective efficacy, be measured when evaluating mucosal vaccines in experimental animals.

One concern with oral vaccination studies is that contamination of the nasal cavity with antigen can occur when vaccine is given in a large volume. Douce et al. (1999) addressed this issue in a study examining the adjuvanticity of detoxified *E. coli* heat-labile toxin (LT) derivatives, and the authors stressed the importance of analyzing individual (rather than pooled) samples from immunized subjects. Furthermore, i.n. administration of vaccine to anaesthetized mice can result in antigen dissemination to the lungs when volumes >20 μl are administered in the naris (Minne et al. 2007; Thompson et al. 1999). These factors should be taken into consideration when designing oral or i.n. vaccination protocols in mice.

Despite encouraging results in mice, there are no studies showing consistent induction of protective immunity in humans following oral delivery of microparticulate vaccines. A study by Tacket et al. (1994) demonstrated antigen-specific jejunal IgA responses in some human subjects orally immunized with ETEC colonization factor antigen encapsulated in PLG microspheres, and one-third of the volunteers were protected against challenge. A subsequent Phase I trial using microencapsulated CS6 ETEC antigen reportedly increased antigen-specific serum IgA and IgG, but the benefits of microparticles over soluble antigen were not clear due to the small number of subjects (Katz et al. 2003). In a more recent study, oral immunization of human subjects with CRM197 diphtheria antigen conjugated to starch microparticles, given as a booster vaccination in previously immunized individuals, failed to significantly increase anti-diptheria toxin neutralizing antibody in serum (Rydell et al. 2006). Nevertheless, the ETEC study (Tacket et al. 1994) indicates that microparticle-based oral vaccines can induce protective immunity against a mucosal pathogen, and hence, support the development of improved microparticle systems.

Table 1 Protective immunity in mice following oral administration of vaccines in PLG/PLA particles

Antigen	Immunization protocol	Outcome	Reference
Pertussis toxoid and filamentous haemagglutinin	100 μg/dose of each orally (500 μl) on weeks 0, 4 and 8	Compared to antigens alone orally; similar or lower serum IgG antibody titers but greater protection post aerosol challenge with *B. pertussis*.	Conway et al. (2001)
DNA encoding HIV envelope glycoprotein	10 μg/dose (volume not specified) orally on days 0, 7 and 14	Compared to i.m. particulate DNA vaccine; similar serum IgG but higher fecal IgA antibody responses. Better protection after intrarectal challenge.	Kaneko et al. (2000)
DNA encoding rotavirus proteins	75 μg/dose (500 μl) orally once	Compared to naked DNA orally; serum IgG antibodies not significantly different. Significantly greater protection after oral challenge.	Herrmann et al. (1999)
Fimbrial protein of *B. pertussis*	10 μg/dose (500 μl) orally once	Compared to alum-formulated i.p. fimbriae; lower serum IgG antibody responses. Similar protection after intranasal challenge with *B. pertussis*.	Jones et al. (1996)
Phosphorylcholine	280 μg/dose (500 μl) orally on days 1, 2, 3, 28, 29 and 30	Compared to i.p. antigen (15 μg/dose); lower serum IgG antibodies. Significantly greater protection after oral challenge with *S. typhimurium*.	Allaoui-Attarki et al. (1997)
Monoclonal antibody to chlamydial antigen	4–6 μg/dose (200 μl) orally twice, 2–3 weeks apart	Compared to s.c. particulate vaccine; similar protection post-ocular infection with *C. trachomatis*.	Whittum-Hudson et al. (1996)

Oral delivery refers to intragastric administration; *i.m.*, intramuscular; *i.p.*, intraperitoneal; *s.c.*, subcutaneous

3 Modifications of Microparticles for Mucosal Vaccine Delivery

There are currently several obstacles for the use of microparticles in mucosal vaccination. These include instability and degradation of the associated antigens in the mucosal lumen and the poor transport of particles across mucosal surfaces. Following mucosal uptake, PLG microparticles degrade slowly by non-enzymatic cleavage into the endogenous metabolites, lactic and glycolic acid. The slow dissolution provides a sustained release of incorporated antigen, which can be adjusted by selecting polymers with particular ratios of lactide and glycolide (Aguado and Lambert 1992; Lin et al. 2000; Watts et al. 1990). The main disadvantage of encapsulating antigen in PLG is that the acids released during hydrolysis generate a highly acidic microenvironment within the particle, which may denature the vaccine antigen (Park et al. 1995; Takahata et al. 1998). The most common method for manufacture of PLG/PLA microparticle vaccines is the emulsion/solvent evaporation process that utilizes conventional emulsifiers such as poly(vinyl alcohol) (PVA) to stabilize the emulsion. The manufacturing procedure involves the emulsification of antigens in organic solvents, followed by extraction or evaporation to form microparticles. This technique involves high-shear rates, elevated temperatures and the creation of large aqueous/organic solvent interfaces; all of which may degrade entrapped proteins or DNA (Ando et al. 1999; Gupta et al. 1998).

3.1 Attachment of Molecules to Particle Surfaces

One alternative to microencapsulation is to adsorb or covalently link antigen to the particle surface in order to preserve integrity (Coombes et al. 1999; Kazzaz et al. 2000). DNA, in particular, may be significantly damaged and lose its supercoiled structure following the microencapsulation process (Ando et al. 1999). To address this issue, cationic PLG microparticles have been developed for adsorption of negatively-charged DNA (Singh et al. 2000). Intranasal immunization of mice with HIV-1 gag-encoding DNA adsorbed onto cationic PLG microparticles induced potent local Th1 and systemic CTL responses and enhanced systemic antibodies when compared to i.n. immunization with naked plasmid DNA (Vajdy and O'Hagan 2001). Anionic PLG particles have also been developed for adsorption of positively-charged proteins (Kazzaz et al. 2000). Attachment of PLG to a PVA backbone results in three-dimensional branched polymeric structures which may be altered by substitution of PVA with negatively-charged sulfobutylated-PVA or positively-charged diethyl-aminoethyl-PVA derivatives. The negative charge on the surface of sulfobutylated-PVA particles increases antigen adsorption due to electrostatic interactions with positively charged proteins (Dailey et al. 2005). Intranasal or oral delivery of tetanus toxoid (TT) adsorbed to sulfobutylated PVA-graft-PLG particles generated higher serum IgG and IgA antibody titers in mice when compared to mucosal delivery of the same antigen in solution. However, the IgG titers induced after mucosal administration of particles with TT were lower than those elicited by parenteral immunization with the same formulations or with conventional Tetanol® vaccine (Jung et al. 2001).

3.2 Enteric Coating for Intestinal Delivery

Particles expressing vaccine antigen on their surfaces may be effective for i.n. delivery but not for oral administration as the antigen would be exposed to the harsh conditions of the gastrointestinal lumen. The coating of microparticles with enteric polymers has been shown to be an effective strategy for combating the problem of antigen degradation in the stomach following oral delivery. These enteric polymers, such as the methacrylic acid esters Eudragit® L100 and S100, have a pH-dependent solubility profile and only dissolve in the weakly acidic to alkaline medium of the intestine (Chourasia and Jain 2003). Their application on microparticles can protect surface-expressed or encapsulated antigen from degradation by stomach acid and can facilitate release in specific regions of the small intestine. Enhanced protection of encapsulated ovalbumin (OVA) against proteolysis in simulated gastric fluid was achieved by replacing the conventional PVA stabilizer with carboxymethylethylcellulose (CMEC) or Eudragit L100-55 enteric polymers. Furthermore, significantly greater antigen-specific salivary IgA responses were reported in mice orally immunized with OVA-loaded microparticles stabilized with CMEC compared to PVA (Delgado et al. 1999). More recently, Dea-Ayuela et al. (2006) reported enhanced serum IgG1 antibodies and protection against the nematode parasite *Trichinella spiralis* following three oral immunizations of mice with parasite proteins loaded in enterically-coated particles. Mice immunized with these starch/sugar particles coated with Eudragit® L100 showed a 50% decrease in worm/larvae burden following challenge when compared to non-immunized controls. However, the superiority of enterically-coated microparticles was not apparent in this study as other mice were not immunized with uncoated particles or with parasite antigens alone (Dea-Ayuela et al. 2006).

3.3 *Association of Particles with Bioadhesive Agents*

The microparticle surface may be modified by coating with bioadhesive polymers or surfactants (Fig. 1). Bioadhesive agents, including polyethylene glycol (PEG) and chitosan, may increase residence time on mucosal surfaces, and consequently, the uptake of particles following mucosal administration.

3.3.1 Polyethylene Glycol

PEG and its derivatives have been used widely for modifying particle surfaces or matrices in order to improve the stability and release profile of encapsulated molecules. The original idea was to provide a protective hydrophilic shell around encapsulated hydrophobic molecules, preventing their rapid clearance and degradation after intravenous delivery (Gref et al. 1994; Woodle and Lasic 1992). However, it is now known that coating particles with PEG is also beneficial for mucosal administration. The effect of PEG coating on the transport of particles across mucosal barriers has been investigated in numerous studies (Cu and Saltzman 2009; Tobio et al. 1998; Tobio et al. 2000; Wang et al. 2008).

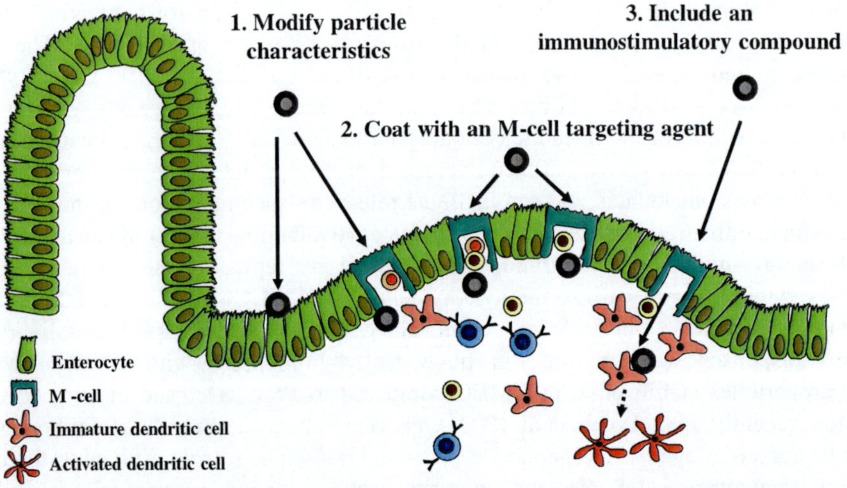

Fig. 1 *Strategies to enhance the efficacy of microparticles and nanoparticles for mucosal vaccine delivery.* 1. Particle characteristics, including size, surface charge and hydrophobicity, may be modified to increase their interaction with the mucosa and the intestinal epithelium. Particles may be enterically coated to protect the associated antigen from degradation under gastric conditions or they may be coated with bioadhesive polymers to enhance antigen bioavailability following mucosal administration. 2. Coating particles with specific targeting agents including lectins, microbial adhesins and antibodies may increase particle uptake by M cells. 3. Adjuvants, such as TLR agonists or other immunostimulatory compounds, may be included to promote DC activation and enhance innate and adaptive immunity to particulate antigen following uptake. It is likely that future mucosal vaccines based on microparticles will use a combination of these strategies to enhance their immunogenicity

Coating the surface of negatively-charged polystyrene nanoparticles with short-length PEG molecules increased their diffusion rate in cervico-vaginal mucus (Lai et al. 2007; Wang et al. 2008). Modification with PEG resulted in neutralization of the negative charge, thereby allowing these particles to diffuse readily in mucus gel when compared to their unmodified, negatively-charged counterparts (Wang et al. 2008). In rats given oral or i.n. immunizations with TT in PLA-PEG nanoparticles, it has been reported that the amount of TT recovered in blood, liver, draining lymph nodes and spleen was significantly higher than that in rats given non-PEGylated particles (Tobio et al. 1998; Tobio et al. 2000). It has also been reported that non-PEGylated particles aggregate strongly on contact with simulated digestive fluid (Tobio et al. 2000) or in aqueous solution containing lysozyme (Vila et al. 2004a). Vila et al. (2004b) also showed that i.n. delivery of TT-loaded PEGylated PLA microparticles in mice enhanced serum IgG and mucosal IgA responses when compared to soluble TT or TT encapsulated in non-PEGylated PLA particles. The authors have suggested that the enhanced immunogenicity of PEGylated particles may be due to decreased aggregation (Vila et al. 2004b).

Particles coated with PEG have also shown potential for mucosal delivery of DNA vaccines. Vila et al. (2002a) reported higher serum IgG antibody titers following i.n.

immunization of mice with a PLA-PEG encapsulated beta-galactosidase plasmid compared to those elicited by the plasmid alone. The PEG-coating of microparticles may also provide a basis for the attachment of ligands onto the particle surface. Garinot et al. (2007) attached integrin-binding, arginine-glycine-aspartate (RGD) peptides to PEGylated PLGA nanoparticles to successfully target human M cell-like epithelial cells in culture. Oral administration of these particles loaded with OVA induced an IgG antibody response in mice. However, RGD-labeling of PEGylated OVA-loaded particles did not produce significantly different OVA-specific IgG titers in serum when compared to the unlabeled particles (Garinot et al. 2007).

3.3.2 Chitosan

Chitosan has also been investigated for the surface modification of PLA/PLG microparticles because of its biocompatibility (Tharanathan and Kittur 2003), mucoadhesive properties (Singla and Chawla 2001) and ability to enhance the nasal absorption of drugs (Illum et al. 1994). In addition, chitosan has been reported to have immunostimulatory properties, including an ability to promote IL-1β and IL-18 cytokine secretion by immune cells (Li et al. 2008). A hydrophilic chitosan coating around nanoparticles was reported to enhance their resistance to aggregation (Vila et al. 2002b). The transport of TT across the nasal mucosa was enhanced by coating nanoparticles with chitosan, although this was less effective than PEG-coating (Vila et al. 2002b). Jaganathan and Vyas (2006) modified the surface of PLGA microspheres with chitosan to render them mucoadhesive and prolong their residence time in the nasal cavity. Intranasal immunization of mice with these surface-modified particles containing recombinant hepatitis B surface antigen (HBsAg) induced systemic and mucosal humoral immunity and cellular immune responses. After two i.n. immunizations, antigen-specific serum IgG antibodies were higher than those induced by chitosan-free HBsAg-particles, and they were comparable to the levels elicited by systemic immunization with an alum-adsorbed vaccine (Jaganathan and Vyas 2006).

3.3.3 Other Bioadhesive Strategies

In addition to chitosan and PEG, several other compounds have been evaluated recently for their ability to enhance the bioadhesive properties of microparticles for mucosal vaccine delivery. Salman et al. (2007) reported higher serum IgG1 and IgG2a titers and mucosal IgA antibodies following oral immunization of mice with thiamine-coated poly(anhydride) particles loaded with OVA, when compared to non-coated particles or to antigen in solution. Florindo et al. (2009) evaluated the immune responses induced after i.n. immunization of mice with PLA particles containing *Streptococcus equi* antigens which had been modified using a range of mucoadhesive polymers (glycol-chitosan and alginate) and absorption enhancers (spermine and oleic acid). Higher serum IgG titers were detected in mice immunized with the particle formulations compared to free antigen. The greatest IgA responses were observed in the lungs of mice immunized with antigens encapsulated in particles modified with spermine (Florindo et al. 2009). However, in this study a large vaccine volume (50 μl) was administered to anaesthetized mice, which may have resulted in some of the vaccine reaching the lungs.

4 Microparticle Vaccines Based on Alternative Polymers

A number of alternative polymers to PLG and PLA have been evaluated for the encapsulation or adsorption of antigens for mucosal delivery. Biodegradable calcium phosphate (CaP) nanoparticles, generated by combining calcium chloride, sodium phosphate and sodium citrate, have shown potential as parenteral vaccine delivery systems (He et al. 2000). A Phase I study in human volunteers demonstrated the safety of CaP nanoparticles following subcutaneous administration (Morcol et al. 2004). Calcium phosphate particles may additionally act as a mucosal adjuvant (He et al. 2002). Intranasal or intravaginal (i.vag.) immunization of mice with a CaP-based nanoparticle formulation containing a herpes simplex virus-2 (HSV-2) glycoprotein induced greater antigen-specific mucosal IgG and IgA and serum IgG when compared to the antigen alone. Furthermore, mice immunized i.vag. with HSV-2-containing CaP nanoparticles were protected against i.vag. HSV-2 challenge, as assessed by a reduction in clinical pathology when compared to mice immunized with the HSV-2 glycoprotein alone (He et al. 2002).

Intranasal immunization of mice with 1–100 μm polymer-grafted starch microparticles containing entrapped human serum albumin has also induced greater systemic humoral and local cellular immune responses when compared to administration of soluble antigen (Heritage et al. 1998). However, in contrast to CaP or PLG, these microparticles are less well characterized and their safety in humans has not been evaluated. Ideally, in studies evaluating novel microparticles for mucosal vaccine delivery, the immune responses or protective efficacy should be compared to those induced by vaccines based on well-characterized microparticles such as PLG/PLA.

Micro/nanoparticles composed of chitosan have also been used for mucosal vaccine delivery. Oral immunization of mice with DNA nanoparticles, synthesized by complexing chitosan with plasmid DNA encoding a peanut allergen, induced higher secretory IgA and serum IgG2a antibodies and greater protection against allergen-induced hypersensitivity compared to mice immunized with naked DNA alone (Roy et al. 1999). The efficacy of chitosan microparticles for i.n. vaccine delivery was evaluated by Iqbal et al. (2003), who reported the induction of CTL and protection against respiratory syncytial virus infection in mice nasally immunized with chitosan microparticles loaded with DNA encoding respiratory syncytial viral proteins. Sub-lingual administration of OVA-loaded chitosan particles to OVA-sensitized mice was reported to reduce airway hypersensitivity, eosinophil numbers in bronchoalveolar lavage and OVA-specific Th2-type responses in mediastinal lymph nodes (Saint-Lu et al. 2009). Interestingly, mucoadhesive particles formed from high molecular weight chitosan enhanced tolerance to a greater degree than particles consisting of low molecular weight polymers (Saint-Lu et al. 2009). Recently, the chitosan derivative *N*-trimethyl chitosan chloride (TMC), which has a better solubility profile than chitosan at physiological pH, was also shown to have potential as a mucosal vaccine delivery system. Oral immunization of mice with urease-loaded TMC nanoparticles generated greater serum IgG and intestinal IgA antibody responses when compared to urease antigen alone or urease co-administered with TMC solution (Chen et al. 2008). However, serum IgG titers induced by oral immunization with TMC/urease particles were weaker than those measured after systemic administration of the same vaccine (Chen et al. 2008). Many others have evaluated the efficacy of chitosan particles as mucosal vaccine delivery systems and this subject has been the focus of recent reviews (Bowman and Leong 2006; Kang et al. 2009).

5 Enhancing Particle Uptake Following Mucosal Delivery

The efficacy of microparticulate vaccines following oral or i.n. delivery in mice is partly due to their uptake into local lymphoid aggregates in the intestine or nasal cavity (Almeida and Alpar 1996; Beier and Gebert 1998). Detailed studies have shown that orally administered microparticles are preferentially taken up by specialized antigen-transporting epithelial cells called M cells, which overlie the Peyer's Patches (PP) lymphoid follicles in the small intestine (Jepson et al. 1993a; Jepson et al. 1993b). These M cells are characterized by a basolateral membrane that forms an intraepithelial pocket containing lymphocytes and phagocytic cells (Neutra and Kraehenbuhl 1992). Particulate vaccines taken up by M cells are subsequently transferred to underlying APC for presentation to T cells. Eldridge et al. (1990) demonstrated that microparticles of <10 μm are taken up by lymphoid tissue following oral delivery in mice. Larger particles (5–10 μm) were retained in the PP while smaller particles (<5 μm) left the PP and disseminated within cells (macrophages or DC) through the efferent lymphatics (Eldridge et al. 1990). Subsequently, other authors showed that the efficiency of particle absorption in the intestine increases with decreasing particle size (Damge et al. 1996; Desai et al. 1996; Jani et al. 1992; Sass et al. 1990). Using an in situ rat intestinal loop model, a significantly higher efficiency of uptake was reported for 100 nm PLG particles compared to 500 nm, 1 or 10 μm particles (Desai et al. 1996). Likewise, Jani et al. (1990) reported more efficient absorption of orally-administered polystyrene particles of less than 100 nm in diameter compared to larger particles in rats. However, increased particle uptake may not necessarily correlate with enhanced immune responses to encapsulated or associated antigens. Gutierro et al. (2002) reported that three oral immunizations of mice with bovine serum albumin in 1 μm PLG particles generated greater systemic IgG responses than smaller particles

(200 and 500 nm). In contrast, another study observed higher serum IgG and IgA antibody titers using 100 nm PVA-graft-PLG nanoparticles for the oral delivery of TT compared to particles of 500 nm or 1,500 nm diameter (Jung et al. 2001). Thus, other factors may play a role in the immunogenicity of microparticulate vaccines.

M cells similar to those in the intestine have also been reported in nasal-associated lymphoid tissue (NALT) and bronchus-associated lymphoid tissue (BALT) in a range of species (Fujimura 2000; Spit et al. 1989; Tango et al. 2000). Particulate vaccines delivered to the nasal mucosa are also preferentially taken up by M cells, and eventually reach the cervical lymph nodes where an immune response is induced (Brooking et al. 2001; Fujimura et al. 2006; Heritage et al. 1998). Although studies evaluating the effect of particle size specifically on M cell uptake in vivo following i.n. delivery have not been reported, the size of particles has been shown to influence the general internalization of nasally delivered microparticle-associated antigens and the magnitude of subsequent immune responses. Using an in vivo rat model, Brooking et al. (2001) found that the transport of nasally-applied polystyrene nanoparticles into the bloodstream was size-dependent, with the highest particle uptake observed for 20 nm particles compared to 500 and 1,000 nm beads. Similarly, Vila et al. (2004a) evaluated the effects of PLA-PEG particle size (200–10 μm) on the transport of encapsulated TT across the rat mucosa and found enhanced protein absorption following i.n. administration of smaller nanoparticles. Jung et al. (2001) found that serum IgG and IgA antibody responses to encapsulated TT were greater following i.n. immunization of mice with smaller PVA-graft-PLG nanoparticles (approximately 500 nm) compared to larger-sized particles (>1 μm). However, immunization with even smaller 100 nm particles did not further enhance the antibody titers (Jung et al. 2001). A significant factor in assessing the uptake of microparticle-based vaccines by mucosal tissue and cells is the difficulty in producing PLG/PLA microparticles of a narrow size range using conventional manufacturing techniques. Therefore, the use of polystyrene microparticles, which can be produced with a very narrow size distribution, may be advantageous for these studies.

5.1 Targeting Microparticles to M Cells

While it is well-established that M cells can take up particulates, such as PLG microparticles, it is now becoming clear that in many cases only low levels of particle uptake occurs via these cells in vivo. Improved confocal microscopy techniques and detection methods and enhanced models for assessing particle uptake by M cells have suggested that the levels of uptake are lower than previously thought (Brayden 2001). McClean et al. (1998) reported that only approximately 10% of the total number of PLG particles administered to intestinal loops of rabbits and rats actually bound to the gastrointestinal tract wall. This suggests that the majority of orally-delivered particles may become trapped in mucus, and that only a small fraction adsorb to epithelial cells, and an even smaller percentage will be translocated across M cells. This low-absorption efficiency may be the main reason why oral vaccines based on polymeric particles have not induced potent immunity. It is therefore possible that enhanced M cell targeting of particulate vaccines could enhance their efficacy. Particle uptake by lymphoid tissue may be enhanced by altering a range of parameters including particle size, surface charge and hydrophobicity (O'Hagan 1996) or by modifying the particle surface so as to allow specific interactions with mucosal cells (Fig. 1). This may be achieved by coating particles with molecules that selectively bind to M cell apical surfaces; including lectins, microbial adhesins and monoclonal antibodies.

5.1.1 Lectins for M Cell Targeting

Lectins are proteins or glycoproteins that recognize and bind reversibly to specific carbohydrates, some of which are expressed on the surface of M cells. Both *Ulex europaeus* agglutinin I (UEA-I), a lectin from the gorse plant *Ulex europaeus*, and *Aleuria aurantia* lectin (AAL) from the edible orange peel fungus have specificity for fucose residues expressed on apical membranes of murine M cells (Giannasca et al. 1994), and thus, have the potential to target microparticles to these cells in vivo. Covalent attachment of UEA-1 to 0.5 μm polystyrene microspheres resulted in specific targeting to M cells in PP of mice and rapid endocytosis of the particles after oral gavage or injection into ligated gut loops of mice (Foster et al. 1998). Similarly, targeting to murine M cells using a gut loop model or to human M-like cells in vitro has been reported after conjugation of UEA-1 to the surface of polymerized liposomes (Clark et al. 2001) or AAL coating of PLG particles (Roth-Walter et al. 2005), respectively.

A number of studies have assessed the ability of UEA-I to enhance immune responses to both soluble antigens and particle-associated antigens following mucosal administration in mice. Foster and Hirst (2005) reported enhanced levels of serum IgG and IgM antibodies after oral immunization of mice with latex particles coated with OVA and UEA-I compared to particles coated with OVA alone. Higher antigen-specific serum IgG and mucosal IgA antibody titers were also reported following oral immunization of mice with PLGA nanoparticles loaded with HBsAg and anchored with UEA-I compared to non-targeted particles (Gupta et al. 2007). Interestingly, in this study, mice orally immunized with particulate lectinized vaccine on three consecutive days and boosted 3 weeks later with the same formulation generated titers of antigen-specific serum IgG which were comparable to those in mice immunized twice by the intramuscular (i.m.) route with antigen and alum (Gupta et al. 2007).

The plant lectin, concavalin A (Con A), has also been investigated as an M cell targeting agent. Coating PLGA microparticles with this lectin enhanced particle uptake following oral administration in rats (Russell-Jones 2001). The induction of antiviral mucosal IgA responses has also been reported following i.vag. or i.n.

immunization of mice with Con A-conjugated polystyrene methacrylate particles coated with inactivated HIV-1 (Akagi et al. 2003; Kawamura et al. 2002). Moreover, i.n. immunization of macaques with similar carriers bearing inactivated chimeric simian/human immunodeficiency virus (SHIV) generated antigen-specific IgA and IgG antibodies in the genital tract and some protection after intravenous challenge with SHIV (Miyake et al. 2004). However, the non-biodegradability of these particles as well as the toxicity of Con A would prevent the clinical application of this delivery system.

The main limitations for the clinical use of lectins as targeting agents are concerns over toxicity and doubts regarding expression of their ligands on human M cells. It may be possible to avert toxicity issues by selecting lectins from edible fruits or plants, such as tomato lectin or AAL. However, edible lectins in mucosal vaccines could induce allergic responses due to their inherent immunogenicity. Alternatively, the component of the lectin directly responsible for M cell binding may be isolated. In a competitive binding assay, stable low molecular weight fragments of the UEA-1 lectin were identified that mimic the binding of UEA-I and may have potential to target drugs and vaccines to M cells (Hamashin et al. 2003). Lambkin et al. (2003) showed that polystyrene particles coated with one of these UEA-I mimetics adhered to murine M cells in vivo. Recently, Misumi et al. (2009) demonstrated by immunofluorescence that a peptide mimetic of UEA-I, called tetragalloyl lysine dendrimer (TGDK), was transported efficiently into rhesus macaque M cells in PP following intestinal inoculation. Furthermore, three oral immunizations of non-human primates with enteric-coated capsules containing a rhesus CCR5 cyclic peptide conjugated to TGDK induced antigen-specific IgA in feces, which inhibited SIV infection of a simian lymphocytic cell line in vitro. The TGDK dendrimer also binds to human M cell-like intestinal epithelial cells in an in vitro M cell culture model (Misumi et al. 2009).

5.1.2 M cell Targeting with Antibodies

Another strategy which may be used to enhance M cell absorption of particles is to coat them with antibodies that selectively recognize specific M cell surface antigens. The uptake of polystyrene particles (1 μm) by rabbit M cells was enhanced by coating with an antibody directed against an antigen expressed on M cells. In contrast, coating the particles with an isotype-matched monoclonal antibody of irrelevant specificity had no effect on particle uptake (Pappo et al. 1991).

A novel, particulate oral cholera vaccine has been developed by Nochi et al. (2007) using protein organelles (1–2 μm) of rice seeds expressing the B subunit of cholera toxin (MucoRice-CTB). MucoRice-CTB is stable at room temperature for over 18 months, obviating the requirement for cold-storage of the vaccine, and it is also resistant to the harsh environment of the gastrointestinal lumen. Oral immunization of mice with MucoRice-CTB induced antigen-specific serum IgG and mucosal IgA responses and protected against an oral challenge with cholera toxin as assessed by a decrease in intestinal fluid levels (Nochi et al. 2007; Yuki et al. 2009). MucoRice-CTB was taken up by M cells after oral administration to mice (Nochi et al. 2007) and Kiyono et al. are now exploiting this by further developing a vaccine variant expressing a monoclonal antibody that specifically targets murine M cells (Cranage and Manoussaka 2009).

5.1.3 M cell Targeting using Microbial Adhesins

Enteric pathogens such as *Listeria monocytogenes* and *Yersinia pseudotuberculosis* naturally target M cells during invasion. The bacteria express adhesins at their surface which allow binding to and uptake by M cells (Kerr 1999). These adhesins are naturally resistant to proteolytic degradation and several studies have investigated these natural M cell pathways for the targeting of particulate delivery systems. Coating inert, carboxylated microparticles with the protein invasin from *Y. pseudotuberculosis* was reported to augment particle binding and uptake by canine epithelial kidney cells in vitro (Haltner et al. 1997). In addition, enhanced absorption of orally administered, latex nanoparticles across rat epithelium was shown after coating with the cell-binding fragment of the Yersinia invasin protein (Hussain and Florence 1998). Further studies are required to determine the safest and most effective M cell targeting agents to use in order to reliably enhance protective immunity to microparticle-associated antigens, particularly in larger animal models and in humans.

5.2 Targeting to Antigen-Presenting Cells

While numerous studies have demonstrated the importance of M cells in particle uptake following mucosal delivery, other cells such as enterocytes, macrophages and DC are also involved. Ligands suitable for targeting microparticles to enterocytes include tomato lectin (Florence et al. 1995; Naisbett and Woodley 1994) and microbial adhesins. The uptake of microparticles by phagocytic antigen-presenting cells (APC) has been reported on several occasions and it is likely that these cells are crucial for the induction of immunity to particle-associated antigens. Dendritic cells are critical in the activation of na T cells, and they have been shown to take up biodegradable PLGA particles directly both in vitro (Elamanchili et al. 2004) and in vivo following systemic delivery to mice (Lunsford et al. 2000; Newman et al. 2002). Latex particles were also shown to be taken up by immature DC after intravenous administration to rats (Matsuno et al. 1996). Furthermore, $CD11c^{+}$ DC in PP were reported to phagocytose latex beads (0.28 μm) after oral administration to mice (Shreedhar et al. 2003). An inverse relationship between particle size and the levels of uptake by DC has been reported (Reece et al. 2001). Foged et al. (2005) showed that human DC could internalize polystyrene particles between 0.04 and 15 μm in diameter, although larger beads (1–15 μm) were phagocytosed by a smaller percentage of cells. Another study demonstrated enhanced IL-1β production, which was dependent on particle uptake, by bone marrow-derived DC incubated with smaller polystyrene particles (430 nm and 1 μm) compared to larger-sized particles (Sharp et al. 2009). Macrophages can also readily internalize PLG microparticles (Luzardo-Alvarez et al. 2005) and, as with DC, maximal uptake has been reported for smaller particles (<2 μm) (Tabata and Ikada 1988). In addition to particle size, the surface charge is also important for uptake. Cationic, polyamine-coated microparticles have been reported to be more efficiently internalized by APC than anionic, hydrophilic microparticles (Thiele et al. 2003). Targeting particles to APC may therefore be achieved by modifying their characteristics and also by coating the surface with specific biological moieties that can interact with these cells. In particular, a number of groups have reported enhanced immunogenicity of particulate vaccines that target DC following systemic delivery using monoclonal antibodies directed to DC surface receptors such as DEC205 (Kwon et al. 2005; van Broekhoven et al. 2004). It remains to be seen if targeting microparticulate vaccines to APC may also be beneficial for mucosal delivery.

6 Inclusion of Immunmostimulatory Agents in Microparticle Vaccines

Recent studies have shown that, contrary to what was previously thought, microparticles do not simply function as antigen delivery systems. They may also activate innate immune responses (Sharp et al. 2009). Both PLG and inert, polystyrene microparticles synergize with adjuvants such as lipopolysaccharide (LPS) to promote the secretion of the pro-inflammatory cytokine IL-1β by murine DC in vitro. This occurs through activation of a protein complex called the NLRP3 inflammasome (Sharp et al. 2009). Although microparticles can therefore have direct effects on the immune system, adjuvants may additionally be included with particulate delivery systems to further activate innate responses, and thus, enhance the magnitude of the adaptive immune response (Fig. 1). In particular, adjuvants derived from microbial compounds may stimulate APC directly, resulting in the secretion of inflammatory cytokines and the upregulation of co-stimulatory molecules on the cell surface. Addition of these adjuvants may also induce the migration of APC to the T cell area of the draining lymph node (O'Hagan and De Gregorio 2009). Microbial adjuvants or pathogen-associated molecular patterns (PAMP) engage receptors known as pathogen recognition receptors (PRR) expressed on cells such as DC and macrophages (Janeway and Medzhitov 2002). Toll-like receptors (TLR) are the best characterized group of PRR, and many microbial compounds which have demonstrated potential as vaccine adjuvants are TLR agonists (van Duin et al. 2006).

The beneficial effect of formulating TLR agonists in microparticles for systemic vaccine delivery has been demonstrated on numerous occasions. A potent immunostimulatory effect was reported by formulating anionic PLG microparticles, containing meningococcal or HIV antigens, with monophosphoryl lipid A (MPL) or synthetic forms (RC-529) of LPS. In particular, mice immunized i.p. with HIV gp120 protein adsorbed onto PLG microparticles in combination with microparticle-entrapped MPL or RC-529 generated higher IgG antibody titers than those immunized with particulate vaccines alone or with soluble forms of the adjuvants (Kazzaz et al. 2006). Strong CTL responses were generated by i.m. immunization of mice with anionic PLG microparticles containing adsorbed HIV-1 antigens in combination with CpG on the surface of cationic particles (Kazzaz et al. 2006). Expression of TLR has been reported on nasal (Dong et al. 2005) and lung epithelial cells (Muir et al. 2004) and also on gut epithelial cells (Cario et al. 2000; Chabot et al. 2006), M cells (Shimosato et al. 2005) and DC (Monteleone et al. 2008). Furthermore, TLR agonists have shown potential as adjuvants for the mucosal delivery of soluble antigens (Gallichan et al. 2001; McCluskie et al. 2000). However, to date, there is little evidence that co-entrapping TLR agonists in microparticles is beneficial for mucosal vaccine administration. Co-encapsulation of CpG with TT in alginate microparticles did not potentiate serum IgG or anti-toxin titers following i.n. administration in rabbits. However, the antigen-specific IgA in nasal lavage was higher in rabbits immunized with microparticles formulated with CpG compared to particles with TT alone (Tafaghodi et al. 2006). A recent study by Pun et al. (2009) did show some enhancement of antigen-specific IgG and IgA antibodies in sera (3–4 fold increases) and IgA in mucosal secretions following a single i.n. immunization of mice with CpG co-encapsulated in microparticles with HIV peptides compared to microparticles with peptides alone (Pun et al. 2009). It is likely that a second i.n. immunization would have increased antibody responses to an even greater extent.

In addition to TLR agonists, ligands for other receptors which are expressed on mucosal tissues and cells may have potential as mucosal adjuvants. One such ligand is mannose, which has high affinity for mannose-binding lectins expressed by lymphoid and non-lymphoid cells of various organs including the intestine (Wagner et al. 2003). Recently, it was shown that oral immunization of mice with 300–400 nm OVA-loaded poly(anhydride) particles coated with mannose or the TLR5 agonist flagellin elicited a stronger and more balanced IgG1 and IgG2a response than non-coated OVA-loaded particles (Salman et al. 2009). Furthermore, higher levels of OVA-specific intestinal IgA were detected in mice immunized with coated particles. Interestingly, in this study a single oral dose of OVA-loaded particles was sufficient for induction of an immune response (Salman et al. 2009).

In another study, lymphotactin, which has chemotactic activity for lymphocytes, was encapsulated in chitosan particles and co-administered intranasally to mice with chitosan microparticles loaded with DNA encoding a coxsackievirus B3 (CVB3) protein. In comparison to particulate DNA vaccine alone, immunization with lymphotactin in chitosan particles significantly enhanced serum IgG and mucosal IgA antibody titers and promoted CVB3-specific CTL activity and Th1 type immunity as well as enhanced resistance to viral myocarditis after challenge (Yue et al. 2009).

7 Concluding Remarks

Recent clinical studies have demonstrated the feasibility and enhanced immunogenicity of systemic vaccines based on a combination of particulate adjuvants, such as alum, with TLR agonists or other immunostimulatory reagents. A recently licensed vaccine against human papillomavirus (Cervarix) and an improved hepatitis B vaccine (Fendrix^{TM}) contain alum and MPL as key components (Boland et al. 2004; Monie et al. 2008). Moreover, a candidate malaria vaccine, which was reported to provide protection against malaria in a Phase II clinical trial, is based on a combination of liposomes with both MPL and QS21 saponin (Bejon et al. 2008). It is likely that new generation subunit vaccines for mucosal delivery will also require combinations of particulates such as micro/nanoparticles with immunostimulatory compounds. Furthermore, targeting agents will probably be required to direct microparticle vaccines to mucosal inductive sites and to enhance their uptake. In recent years, modifications in the design of polymeric microparticle vaccines have enhanced immunogenicity in rodents and small animals. There is now a need to increase our understanding of the role of mucosal M cells, DC and other APC in particle uptake and in promoting mucosal innate responses in order to develop more efficacious microparticle-based vaccines for mucosal delivery to humans. This information will be vital to inform targeted approaches for particulate mucosal vaccines. The challenge remains to identify the best combination of adjuvants and/or targeting agents with particulates to promote optimal immune activation without the induction of adverse reactions.

Acknowledgments Edel McNeela is funded by Enterprise Ireland and Sigmoid Pharma through the Innovation Partnerships Programme (IP20090046). Ed Lavelle's work on danger signals, mucosal immunity and vaccines is also funded by Science Foundation Ireland (08/RFP/BMT1363, 07/RFP/BICF537, 07/SRC/B1144), and the Meningitis Research Foundation (0610.0).

References

Aguado MT, Lambert PH (1992) Controlled-release vaccines–biodegradable polylactide/polyglycolide (PL/PG) microspheres as antigen vehicles. Immunobiology 184:113–125

Akagi T, Kawamura M, Ueno M et al (2003) Mucosal immunization with inactivated HIV-1-capturing nanospheres induces a significant HIV-1-specific vaginal antibody response in mice. J Med Virol 69:163–172

Allaoui-Attarki K, Pecquet S, Fattal E et al (1997) Protective immunity against *Salmonella typhimurium* elicited in mice by oral vaccination with phosphorylcholine encapsulated in poly(DL-lactide-co-glycolide) microspheres. Infect Immun 65:853–857

Almeida AJ, Alpar HO (1996) Nasal delivery of vaccines. J Drug Target 3:455–467

Ando S, Putnam D, Pack DW et al (1999) PLGA microspheres containing plasmid DNA: preservation of supercoiled DNA via cryopreparation and carbohydrate stabilization. J Pharm Sci 88:126–130

Beier R, Gebert A (1998) Kinetics of particle uptake in the domes of Peyer's patches. Am J Physiol 275:G130–G137

Bejon P, Lusingu J, Olotu A et al (2008) Efficacy of RTS, S/AS01E vaccine against malaria in children 5 to 17 months of age. N Engl J Med 359:2521–2532

Boland G, Beran J, Lievens M et al (2004) Safety and immunogenicity profile of an experimental hepatitis B vaccine adjuvanted with AS04. Vaccine 23:316–320

Bowman K, Leong KW (2006) Chitosan nanoparticles for oral drug and gene delivery. Int J Nanomed 1:117–128

Brandtzaeg P, Johansen F-E (2008) The mucosal B-cell system. In: Vajdy M (ed) Immunity against mucosal pathogens. Springer-Verlag, New York, pp 33–76

Brayden DJ (2001) Oral vaccination in man using antigens in particles: current status. Eur J Pharm Sci 14:183–189

Brooking J, Davis SS, Illum L (2001) Transport of nanoparticles across the rat nasal mucosa. J Drug Target 9:267–279

Cahill ES, O'Hagan DT, Illum L et al (1995) Immune responses and protection against *Bordetella pertussis* infection after intranasal immunization of mice with filamentous haemagglutinin in solution or incorporated in biodegradable microparticles. Vaccine 13:455–462

Carcaboso AM, Hernandez RM, Igartua M et al (2003) Immune response after oral administration of the encapsulated malaria synthetic peptide SPf66. Int J Pharm 260:273–282

Carcaboso AM, Hernandez RM, Igartua M et al (2004) Potent, long lasting systemic antibody levels and mixed Th1/Th2 immune response after nasal immunization with malaria antigen loaded PLGA microparticles. Vaccine 22:1423–1432

Cario E, Rosenberg IM, Brandwein SL et al (2000) Lipopolysaccharide activates distinct signaling pathways in intestinal epithelial cell lines expressing Toll-like receptors. J Immunol 164:966–972

Carpenter ZK, Williamson ED, Eyles JE (2005) Mucosal delivery of microparticle encapsulated ESAT-6 induces robust cell-mediated responses in the lung milieu. J Control Release 104:67–77

Chabot S, Wagner JS, Farrant S et al (2006) TLRs regulate the gatekeeping functions of the intestinal follicle-associated epithelium. J Immunol 176:4275–4283

Challacombe SJ, Rahman D, Jeffery H et al (1992) Enhanced secretory IgA and systemic IgG antibody responses after oral immunization with biodegradable microparticles containing antigen. Immunology 76:164–168

Chen F, Zhang ZR, Yuan F et al (2008) In vitro and in vivo study of N-trimethyl chitosan nanoparticles for oral protein delivery. Int J Pharm 349:226–233

Chourasia MK, Jain SK (2003) Pharmaceutical approaches to colon targeted drug delivery systems. J Pharm Pharm Sci 6:33–66

Clark MA, Blair H, Liang L et al (2001) Targeting polymerised liposome vaccine carriers to intestinal M cells. Vaccine 20:208–217

Cleland JL (1999) Single-administration vaccines: controlled-release technology to mimic repeated immunizations. Trends Biotechnol 17:25–29

Conway MA, Madrigal-Estebas L, McClean S et al (2001) Protection against *Bordetella pertussis* infection following parenteral or oral immunization with antigens entrapped in biodegradable particles: effect of formulation and route of immunization on induction of Th1 and Th2 cells. Vaccine 19:1940–1950

Coombes AG, Lavelle EC, Davis SS (1999) Biodegradable lamellar particles of poly(lactide) induce sustained immune responses to a single dose of adsorbed protein. Vaccine 17: 2410–2422

Cranage MP, Manoussaka M (2009) Modern mucosal vaccines, adjuvants and microbicides. Expert Rev Anti Infect Ther 7:21–23

Cu Y, Saltzman WM (2009) Controlled surface modification with poly(ethylene)glycol enhances diffusion of PLGA nanoparticles in human cervical mucus. Mol Pharm 6:173–181

Czerkinsky C, Holmgren J (2011) Mucosal delivery routes for optimal immunization: targeting immunity to the right tissues. Curr Top Microbiol Immunol (in press)

Dailey LA, Wittmar M, Kissel T (2005) The role of branched polyesters and their modifications in the development of modern drug delivery vehicles. J Control Release 101:137–149

Damge C, Aprahamian M, Marchais H et al (1996) Intestinal absorption of PLAGA microspheres in the rat. J Anat 189(Pt 3):491–501

Dea-Ayuela MA, Rama-Iniguez S, Torrado-Santiago S et al (2006) Microcapsules formulated in the enteric coating copolymer Eudragit L100 as delivery systems for oral vaccination against infections by gastrointestinal nematode parasites. J Drug Target 14:567–575

Delgado A, Lavelle EC, Hartshorne M et al (1999) PLG microparticles stabilised using enteric coating polymers as oral vaccine delivery systems. Vaccine 17:2927–2938

Desai MP, Labhasetwar V, Amidon GL et al (1996) Gastrointestinal uptake of biodegradable microparticles: effect of particle size. Pharm Res 13:1838–1845

Dong Z, Yang Z, Wang C (2005) Expression of TLR2 and TLR4 messenger RNA in the epithelial cells of the nasal airway. Am J Rhinol 19:236–239

Douce G, Giannelli V, Pizza M et al (1999) Genetically detoxified mutants of heat-labile toxin from *Escherichia coli* are able to act as oral adjuvants. Infect Immun 67:4400–4406

Elamanchili P, Diwan M, Cao M et al (2004) Characterization of poly(D, L-lactic-co-glycolic acid) based nanoparticulate system for enhanced delivery of antigens to dendritic cells. Vaccine 22:2406–2412

Eldridge JH, Meulbroek JA, Staas JK et al (1989) Vaccine-containing biodegradable microspheres specifically enter the gut-associated lymphoid tissue following oral administration and induce a disseminated mucosal immune response. Adv Exp Med Biol 251: 191–202

Eldridge JH, Hammond CJ, Meulbroek JA, Staas JK et al (1990) Controlled vaccine release in the gut-associated lymphoid tissues. I. Orally administered biodegradable microspheres target the Peyer's patches. J Controlled Release 11:205–214

Fattal E, Pecquet S, Couvreur P et al (2002) Biodegradable microparticles for the mucosal delivery of antibacterial and dietary antigens. Int J Pharm 242:15–24

Florence AT, Hillery AM, Hussain N et al (1995) Factors affecting the oral uptake and translocation of polystyrene nanoparticles: histological and analytical evidence. J Drug Target 3:65–70

Florindo HF, Pandit S, Goncalves LM et al (2009) New approach on the development of a mucosal vaccine against strangles: systemic and mucosal immune responses in a mouse model. Vaccine 27:1230–1241

Foged C, Brodin B, Frokjaer S et al (2005) Particle size and surface charge affect particle uptake by human dendritic cells in an in vitro model. Int J Pharm 298:315–322

Foster N, Hirst BH (2005) Exploiting receptor biology for oral vaccination with biodegradable particulates. Adv Drug Deliv Rev 57:431–450

Foster N, Clark MA, Jepson MA et al (1998) Ulex europaeus 1 lectin targets microspheres to mouse Peyer's patch M-cells in vivo. Vaccine 16:536–541

Fujimura Y (2000) Evidence of M cells as portals of entry for antigens in the nasopharyngeal lymphoid tissue of humans. Virchows Arch 436:560–566

Fujimura Y, Akisada T, Harada T et al (2006) Uptake of microparticles into the epithelium of human nasopharyngeal lymphoid tissue. Med Mol Morphol 39:181–186

Gallichan WS, Woolstencroft RN, Guarasci T et al (2001) Intranasal immunization with CpG oligodeoxynucleotides as an adjuvant dramatically increases IgA and protection against herpes simplex virus-2 in the genital tract. J Immunol 166:3451–3457

Garinot M, Fievez V, Pourcelle V et al (2007) PEGylated PLGA-based nanoparticles targeting M cells for oral vaccination. J Control Release 120:195–204

Giannasca PJ, Giannasca KT, Falk P et al (1994) Regional differences in glycoconjugates of intestinal M cells in mice: potential targets for mucosal vaccines. Am J Physiol 267: G1108–G1121

Giudice EL, Campbell JD (2006) Needle-free vaccine delivery. Adv Drug Deliv Rev 58:68–89

Gref R, Minamitake Y, Peracchia MT et al (1994) Biodegradable long-circulating polymeric nanospheres. Science 263:1600–1603

Gupta RK, Singh M, O'Hagan DT (1998) Poly(lactide-co-glycolide) microparticles for the development of single-dose controlled-release vaccines. Adv Drug Deliv Rev 32:225–246

Gupta PN, Khatri K, Goyal AK et al (2007) M-cell targeted biodegradable PLGA nanoparticles for oral immunization against hepatitis B. J Drug Target 15:701–713

Gutierro I, Hernandez RM, Igartua M et al (2002) Size dependent immune response after subcutaneous, oral and intranasal administration of BSA loaded nanospheres. Vaccine 21: 67–77

Haltner E, Easson JH, Lehr CM (1997) Lectins and bacterial invasion factors for controlling endo- and transcytosis of bioadhesive drug carrier systems. Eur J Pharm Biopharm 44:3–13

Hamashin C, Spindler L, Russell S et al (2003) Identification of novel small-molecule Ulex europaeus I mimetics for targeted drug delivery. Bioorg Med Chem 11:4991–4997

He Q, Mitchell AR, Johnson SL et al (2000) Calcium phosphate nanoparticle adjuvant. Clin Diagn Lab Immunol 7:899–903

He Q, Mitchell A, Morcol T et al (2002) Calcium phosphate nanoparticles induce mucosal immunity and protection against herpes simplex virus type 2. Clin Diagn Lab Immunol 9:1021 1024

Heritage PL, Brook MA, Underdown BJ et al (1998) Intranasal immunization with polymer-grafted microparticles activates the nasal-associated lymphoid tissue and draining lymph nodes. Immunology 93:249–256

Herrmann JE, Chen SC, Jones DH et al (1999) Immune responses and protection obtained by oral immunization with rotavirus VP4 and VP7 DNA vaccines encapsulated in microparticles. Virology 259:148–153

Hussain N, Florence AT (1998) Utilizing bacterial mechanisms of epithelial cell entry: invasin-induced oral uptake of latex nanoparticles. Pharm Res 15:153–156

Illum L, Farraj NF, Davis SS (1994) Chitosan as a novel nasal delivery system for peptide drugs. Pharm Res 11:1186–1189

Iqbal M, Lin W, Jabbal-Gill I et al (2003) Nasal delivery of chitosan-DNA plasmid expressing epitopes of respiratory syncytial virus (RSV) induces protective CTL responses in BALB/c mice. Vaccine 21:1478–1485

Jaganathan KS, Vyas SP (2006) Strong systemic and mucosal immune responses to surface-modified PLGA microspheres containing recombinant hepatitis B antigen administered intranasally. Vaccine 24:4201–4211

Janeway CA Jr, Medzhitov R (2002) Innate immune recognition. Annu Rev Immunol 20:197–216

Jani P, Halbert GW, Langridge J, Florence AT (1990) Nanoparticle uptake by the rat gastrointestinal mucosa: quantitation and particle size dependency. J Pharm Pharmacol 42:821–826

Jani PU, Florence AT, McCarthy DE (1992) Further histological evidence of the gastrointestinal absorption of polystyrene nanospheres in the rat. Int J Pharm 84:245–252

Jepson MA, Simmons NL, O'Hagan DT et al (1993a) Comparison of poly(DL-lactide-co-glycolide) and polystyrene microsphere targeting to intestinal M cells. J Drug Target 1:245–249

Jepson MA, Simmons NL, Savidge TC et al (1993b) Selective binding and transcytosis of latex microspheres by rabbit intestinal M cells. Cell Tissue Res 271:399–405

Jones DH, McBride BW, Thornton C et al (1996) Orally administered microencapsulated *Bordetella pertussis fimbriae* protect mice from B. pertussis respiratory infection. Infect Immun 64:489–494

Jung T, Kamm W, Breitenbach A et al (2001) Tetanus toxoid loaded nanoparticles from sulfobutylated poly(vinyl alcohol)-graft-poly(lactide-co-glycolide): evaluation of antibody response after oral and nasal application in mice. Pharm Res 18:352–360

Kaneko H, Bednarek I, Wierzbicki A et al (2000) Oral DNA vaccination promotes mucosal and systemic immune responses to HIV envelope glycoprotein. Virology 267:8–16

Kang ML, Cho CS, Yoo HS (2009) Application of chitosan microspheres for nasal delivery of vaccines. Biotechnol Adv 27:857–865

Katz DE, DeLorimier AJ, Wolf MK et al (2003) Oral immunization of adult volunteers with microencapsulated enterotoxigenic Escherichia coli (ETEC) CS6 antigen. Vaccine 21: 341–346

Kawamura M, Naito T, Ueno M et al (2002) Induction of mucosal IgA following intravaginal administration of inactivated HIV-1-capturing nanospheres in mice. J Med Virol 66:291–298

Kazzaz J, Neidleman J, Singh M, Ott G, O'Hagan DT (2000) Novel anionic microparticles are a potent adjuvant for the induction of cytotoxic T lymphocytes against recombinant p55 gag from HIV-1. J Control Release 67:347–356

Kazzaz J, Singh M, Ugozzoli M et al (2006) Encapsulation of the immune potentiators MPL and RC529 in PLG microparticles enhances their potency. J Control Release 110:566–573

Kende M, Yan C, Hewetson J et al (2002) Oral immunization of mice with ricin toxoid vaccine encapsulated in polymeric microspheres against aerosol challenge. Vaccine 20:1681–1691

Kerr JR (1999) Cell adhesion molecules in the pathogenesis of and host defence against microbial infection. Mol Pathol 52:220–230

Kwon YJ, James E, Shastri N et al (2005) In vivo targeting of dendritic cells for activation of cellular immunity using vaccine carriers based on pH-responsive microparticles. Proc Natl Acad Sci USA 102:18264–18268

Lai SK, O'Hanlon DE, Harrold S et al (2007) Rapid transport of large polymeric nanoparticles in fresh undiluted human mucus. Proc Natl Acad Sci USA 104:1482–1487

Lambert JS, Keefer M, Mulligan MJ et al (2001) A Phase I safety and immunogenicity trial of UBI microparticulate monovalent HIV-1 MN oral peptide immunogen with parenteral boost in HIV-1 seronegative human subjects. Vaccine 19:3033–3042

Lambkin I, Pinilla C, Hamashin C et al (2003) Toward targeted oral vaccine delivery systems: selection of lectin mimetics from combinatorial libraries. Pharm Res 20:1258–1266

Lavelle EC (2001) Targeted delivery of drugs to the gastrointestinal tract. Crit Rev Ther Drug Carrier Syst 18:341–386

Lavelle EC (2005) Generation of improved mucosal vaccines by induction of innate immunity. Cell Mol Life Sci 62:2750–2770

Li H, Willingham SB, Ting JP et al (2008) Cutting edge: inflammasome activation by alum and alum's adjuvant effect are mediated by NLRP3. J Immunol 181:17–21

Lin SY, Chen KS, Teng HH et al (2000) In vitro degradation and dissolution behaviours of microspheres prepared by three low molecular weight polyesters. J Microencapsul 17: 577–586

Lunsford L, McKeever U, Eckstein V et al (2000) Tissue distribution and persistence in mice of plasmid DNA encapsulated in a PLGA-based microsphere delivery vehicle. J Drug Target 8:39–50

Luzardo-Alvarez A, Blarer N, Peter K et al (2005) Biodegradable microspheres alone do not stimulate murine macrophages in vitro, but prolong antigen presentation by macrophages in vitro and stimulate a solid immune response in mice. J Control Release 109:62–76

Macpherson AJ, McCoy KD, Johansen FE et al (2008) The immune geography of IgA induction and function. Mucosal Immunol 1:11–22

Maloy KJ, Donachie AM, O'Hagan DT et al (1994) Induction of mucosal and systemic immune responses by immunization with ovalbumin entrapped in poly(lactide-co-glycolide) microparticles. Immunology 81:661–667

Matsuno K, Ezaki T, Kudo S et al (1996) A life stage of particle-laden rat dendritic cells in vivo: their terminal division, active phagocytosis, and translocation from the liver to the draining lymph. J Exp Med 183:1865–1878

McClean S, Prosser E, Meehan E et al (1998) Binding and uptake of biodegradable poly-DL-lactide micro- and nanoparticles in intestinal epithelia. Eur J Pharm Sci 6:153–163

McCluskie MJ, Weeratna RD, Krieg AM et al (2000) CpG DNA is an effective oral adjuvant to protein antigens in mice. Vaccine 19:950–957

Mestecky J, Russell MW (2009) Specific antibody activity, glycan heterogeneity and polyreactivity contribute to the protective activity of S-IgA at mucosal surfaces. Immunol Lett 124:57–62

Minne A, Louahed J, Mehauden S et al (2007) The delivery site of a monovalent influenza vaccine within the respiratory tract impacts on the immune response. Immunology 122:316–325

Minor P (2009) Vaccine-derived poliovirus (VDPV): impact on poliomyelitis eradication. Vaccine 27:2649–2652

Misumi S, Masuyama M, Takamune N et al (2009) Targeted delivery of immunogen to primate m cells with tetragalloyl lysine dendrimer. J Immunol 182:6061–6070

Miyake A, Akagi T, Enose Y et al (2004) Induction of HIV-specific antibody response and protection against vaginal SHIV transmission by intranasal immunization with inactivated SHIV-capturing nanospheres in macaques. J Med Virol 73:368–377

Moldoveanu Z, Novak M, Huang WQ et al (1993) Oral immunization with influenza virus in biodegradable microspheres. J Infect Dis 167:84–90

Monie A, Hung CF, Roden R et al (2008) Cervarix: a vaccine for the prevention of HPV 16, 18-associated cervical cancer. Biologics 2:97–105

Monteleone I, Platt AM, Jaensson E et al (2008) IL-10-dependent partial refractoriness to Toll-like receptor stimulation modulates gut mucosal dendritic cell function. Eur J Immunol 38:1533–1547

Moore A, McGuirk P, Adams S et al (1995) Immunization with a soluble recombinant HIV protein entrapped in biodegradable microparticles induces HIV-specific CD8+ cytotoxic T lymphocytes and CD4+ Th1 cells. Vaccine 13:1741–1749

Morcol T, Nagappan P, Nerenbaum L et al (2004) Calcium phosphate-PEG-insulin-casein (CAPIC) particles as oral delivery systems for insulin. Int J Pharm 277:91–97

Muir A, Soong G, Sokol S et al (2004) Toll-like receptors in normal and cystic fibrosis airway epithelial cells. Am J Respir Cell Mol Biol 30:777–783

Naisbett B, Woodley J (1994) The potential use of tomato lectin for oral drug delivery. 1. Lectin binding to rat small intestine in vitro. Int J Pharm 107:223–230

Neutra MR, Kraehenbuhl JP (1992) Transepithelial transport and mucosal defence I: the role of M cells. Trends Cell Biol 2:134–138

Newman KD, Elamanchili P, Kwon GS et al (2002) Uptake of poly(D, L-lactic-co-glycolic acid) microspheres by antigen-presenting cells in vivo. J Biomed Mater Res 60:480–486

Nochi T, Takagi H, Yuki Y et al (2007) Rice-based mucosal vaccine as a global strategy for cold-chain- and needle-free vaccination. Proc Natl Acad Sci USA 104:10986–10991

O'Hagan DT (1996) The intestinal uptake of particles and the implications for drug and antigen delivery. J Anat 189(Pt 3):477–482

O'Hagan DT (1998) Recent advances in vaccine adjuvants for systemic and mucosal administration. J Pharm Pharmacol 50:1–10

O'Hagan DT, De Gregorio E (2009) The path to a successful vaccine adjuvant—'the long and winding road'. Drug Discov Today 14:541–551

O'Hagan DT, Singh M, Ulmer JB (2006) Microparticle-based technologies for vaccines. Methods 40:10–19

Pappo J, Ermak TH, Steger HJ (1991) Monoclonal antibody-directed targeting of fluorescent polystyrene microspheres to Peyer's patch M cells. Immunology 73:277–280

Park TG, Lu W, Crotts G (1995) Importance of in vitro experimental conditions on protein release kinetics, stability and polymer degradation in protein encapsulated poly (D, L-lactic acid-co-glycolic acid) microspheres. J Controlled Release 33:211–222

Pun PB, Bhat AA, Mohan T et al (2009) Intranasal administration of peptide antigens of HIV with mucosal adjuvant CpG ODN coentrapped in microparticles enhances the mucosal and systemic immune responses. Int Immunopharmacol 9:468–477

Reece JC, Vardaxis NJ, Marshall JA et al (2001) Uptake of HIV and latex particles by fresh and cultured dendritic cells and monocytes. Immunol Cell Biol 79:255–263

Roth-Walter F, Bohle B, Scholl I et al (2005) Targeting antigens to murine and human M-cells with Aleuria aurantia lectin-functionalized microparticles. Immunol Lett 100:182–188

Roy K, Mao HQ, Huang SK et al (1999) Oral gene delivery with chitosan—DNA nanoparticles generates immunologic protection in a murine model of peanut allergy. Nat Med 5:387–391

Russell-Jones GJ (2001) The potential use of receptor-mediated endocytosis for oral drug delivery. Adv Drug Deliv Rev 46:59–73

Rydell N, Stertman L, Stalenheim G et al (2006) Use of an oral diphtheria vaccine in human. Vaccine 24:5928–5930

Saint-Lu N, Tourdot S, Razafindratsita A et al (2009) Targeting the allergen to oral dendritic cells with mucoadhesive chitosan particles enhances tolerance induction. Allergy 64:1003–1013

Salerno-Goncalves R, Pasetti MF, Sztein MB (2002) Characterization of CD8(+) effector T cell responses in volunteers immunized with Salmonella enterica serovar Typhi strain Ty21a typhoid vaccine. J Immunol 169:2196–2203

Salman HH, Gamazo C, Agueros M, Irache JM (2007) Bioadhesive capacity and immunoadjuvant properties of thiamine-coated nanoparticles. Vaccine 25:8123–8132

Salman HH, Irache JM, Gamazo C (2009) Immunoadjuvant capacity of flagellin and mannosamine-coated poly(anhydride) nanoparticles in oral vaccination. Vaccine 27: 4784–4790

Sass W, Dreyer HP, Seifert J (1990) Rapid insorption of small particles in the gut. Am J Gastroenterol 85:255–260

Seong SY, Cho NH, Kwon IC et al (1999) Protective immunity of microsphere-based mucosal vaccines against lethal intranasal challenge with *Streptococcus pneumoniae*. Infect Immun 67:3587–3592

Sharp FA, Ruane D, Claass B et al (2009) Uptake of particulate vaccine adjuvants by dendritic cells activates the NALP3 inflammasome. Proc Natl Acad Sci USA 106:870–875

Shimosato T, Tohno M, Kitazawa H et al (2005) Toll-like receptor 9 is expressed on follicle-associated epithelia containing M cells in swine Peyer's patches. Immunol Lett 98:83–89

Shreedhar VK, Kelsall BL, Neutra MR (2003) Cholera toxin induces migration of dendritic cells from the subepithelial dome region to T- and B-cell areas of Peyer's patches. Infect Immun 71:504–509

Singh M, Briones M, Ott G et al (2000) Cationic microparticles: A potent delivery system for DNA vaccines. Proc Natl Acad Sci USA 97:811–816

Singla AK, Chawla M (2001) Chitosan: some pharmaceutical and biological aspects—an update. J Pharm Pharmacol 53:1047–1067

Spit BJ, Hendriksen EG, Bruijntjes JP et al (1989) Nasal lymphoid tissue in the rat. Cell Tissue Res 255:193–198

Tabata Y, Ikada Y (1988) Effect of the size and surface charge of polymer microspheres on their phagocytosis by macrophage. Biomaterials 9:356–362

Tabata Y, Inoue Y, Ikada Y (1996) Size effect on systemic and mucosal immune responses induced by oral administration of biodegradable microspheres. Vaccine 14:1677–1685

Tacket CO, Reid RH, Boedeker EC et al (1994) Enteral immunization and challenge of volunteers given enterotoxigenic. E.coli CFA/II encapsulated in biodegradable microspheres. Vaccine 12:1270–1274

Tafaghodi M, Sajadi Tabassi SA, Jaafari MR (2006) Induction of systemic and mucosal immune responses by intranasal administration of alginate microspheres encapsulated with tetanus toxoid and CpG-ODN. Int J Pharm 319:37–43

Takahata H, Lavelle EC, Coombes AG et al (1998) The distribution of protein associated with poly(DL-lactide co-glycolide) microparticles and its degradation in simulated body fluids. J Control Release 50:237–246

Tango M, Suzuki E, Gejyo F et al (2000) The presence of specialized epithelial cells on the bronchus-associated lymphoid tissue (BALT) in the mouse. Arch Histol Cytol 63:81–89

Tharanathan RN, Kittur FS (2003) Chitin—the undisputed biomolecule of great potential. Crit Rev Food Sci Nutr 43:61–87

Thiele L, Merkle HP, Walter E (2003) Phagocytosis and phagosomal fate of surface-modified microparticles in dendritic cells and macrophages. Pharm Res 20:221–228

Thompson AH, McRoberts JG, Crowe SR et al (1999) Optimal induction of upper respiratory tract immunity to reovirus 1/L by combined upper and lower respiratory tract inoculation. Vaccine 17:1404–1415

Tobio M, Gref R, Sanchez A et al (1998) Stealth PLA-PEG nanoparticles as protein carriers for nasal administration. Pharm Res 15:270–275

Tobio M, Sanchez A, Vila A et al (2000) The role of PEG on the stability in digestive fluids and in vivo fate of PEG-PLA nanoparticles following oral administration. Colloids Surf B Biointerfaces 18:315–323

Ugozzoli M, O'Hagan DT, Ott GS (1998) Intranasal immunization of mice with herpes simplex virus type 2 recombinant gD2: the effect of adjuvants on mucosal and serum antibody responses. Immunology 93:563–571

Vajdy M, O'Hagan DT (2001) Microparticles for intranasal immunization. Adv Drug Deliv Rev 51:127–141

van Broekhoven CL, Parish CR, Demangel C et al (2004) Targeting dendritic cells with antigen-containing liposomes: a highly effective procedure for induction of antitumor immunity and for tumor immunotherapy. Cancer Res 64:4357–4365

van Duin D, Medzhitov R, Shaw AC (2006) Triggering TLR signaling in vaccination. Trends Immunol 27:49–55

Vila A, Sanchez A, Perez C, Alonso MJ (2002a) PLA-PEG nanospheres: new carriers for transmucosal delivery of proteins and plasmid DNA. Polym Adv Technol 13:851–858

Vila A, Sanchez A, Tobio M et al (2002b) Design of biodegradable particles for protein delivery. J Control Release 78:15–24

Vila A, Gill H, McCallion O et al (2004a) Transport of PLA-PEG particles across the nasal mucosa: effect of particle size and PEG coating density. J Control Release 98:231–244

Vila A, Sanchez A, Evora C et al (2004b) PEG-PLA nanoparticles as carriers for nasal vaccine delivery. J Aerosol Med 17:174–185

Vyas SP, Gupta PN (2007) Implication of nanoparticles/microparticles in mucosal vaccine delivery. Expert Rev Vaccines 6:401–418

Wagner S, Lynch NJ, Walter W et al (2003) Differential expression of the murine mannose-binding lectins A and C in lymphoid and nonlymphoid organs and tissues. J Immunol 170:1462–1465

Wang YY, Lai SK, Suk JS et al (2008) Addressing the PEG mucoadhesivity paradox to engineer nanoparticles that "slip" through the human mucus barrier. Angew Chem Int Ed Engl 47:9726–9729

Watts PJ, Davies MC, Melia CD (1990) Microencapsulation using emulsification/solvent evaporation: an overview of techniques and applications. Crit Rev Ther Drug Carrier Syst 7:235–259

Whittum-Hudson JA, An LL, Saltzman WM et al (1996) Oral immunization with an anti-idiotypic antibody to the exoglycolipid antigen protects against experimental Chlamydia trachomatis infection. Nat Med 2:1116–1121

Woodle MC, Lasic DD (1992) Sterically stabilized liposomes. Biochim Biophys Acta 1113: 171–199

Yeh MK, Liu YT, Chen JL et al (2002) Oral immunogenicity of the inactivated *Vibrio cholerae* whole-cell vaccine encapsulated in biodegradable microparticles. J Control Release 82: 237–247

Yue Y, Xu W, Hu L et al (2009) Enhanced resistance to coxsackievirus B3-induced myocarditis by intranasal co-immunization of lymphotactin gene encapsulated in chitosan particle. Virology 386:438–447

Yuki Y, Tokuhara D, Nochi T et al (2009) Oral MucoRice expressing double-mutant cholera toxin A and B subunits induces toxin-specific neutralising immunity. Vaccine 27:5982–5988

Plant-Derived Antigens as Mucosal Vaccines

H. S. Mason and M. M. Herbst-Kralovetz

Abstract During the last two decades, researchers have developed robust systems for recombinant subunit vaccine production in plants. Stably and transiently transformed plants have particular advantages that enable immunization of humans and animals via mucosal delivery. The initial goal to immunize orally by ingestion of plant-derived antigens has proven difficult to attain, although many studies have demonstrated antibody production in both humans and animals, and in a few cases, protection against pathogen challenge. Substantial hurdles for this strategy are low-antigen content in crudely processed plant material and limited antigen stability in the gut. An alternative is intranasal delivery of purified plant-derived antigens expressed with robust viral vectors, especially virus-like particles. The use of pattern recognition receptor agonists as adjuvants for mucosal delivery of plant-derived antigens can substantially enhance serum and mucosal antibody responses. In this chapter, we briefly review the methods for recombinant protein expression in plants, and describe progress with human and animal vaccines that use mucosal delivery routes. We do not attempt to compile a comprehensive list, but focus on studies that progressed to clinical trials or those that showed strong indications of efficacy in animals. Finally, we discuss some regulatory concerns regarding plant-based vaccines.

H. S. Mason (✉) · M. M. Herbst-Kralovetz
Center for Infectious Diseases and Vaccinology, Biodesign Institute,
Arizona State University, Tempe, AZ 85287, USA
e-mail: hugh.mason@asu.edu

H. S. Mason
School of Life Sciences, Arizona State University, Tempe, AZ 85287, USA

M. M. Herbst-Kralovetz
Department of Basic Medical Sciences,
University of Arizona College of Medicine-Phoenix,
Phoenix, AZ 85004, USA

Current Topics in Microbiology and Immunology (2012) 354: 101–120
DOI: 10.1007/82_2011_158

Published Online: 3 August 2011

Keywords Plant viral vector · Oral immunization · Nasal immunization · Toll-like receptor agonist · Norovirus

Contents

1 Introduction

Advances in plant biotechnology in the last two decades have facilitated production of recombinant proteins in plants, including subunit vaccine antigens. Several good review articles (Rybicki 2009; Streatfield 2006; Thanavala et al. 2006; Yusibov and Rabindran 2008) have summarized much of this work and have focused attention on the utility of plants for subunit vaccine expression. During the twenty years since the seminal work that demonstrated the potential of plant-derived vaccines (Curtiss and Cardineau 1990; Mason et al. 1992), a large body of literature has demonstrated expression of antigens in many plants, including edible plants like corn, potato, and tomato, as well as tobacco and its relatives. And yet, commercial development of plant-derived vaccine products has been very slow, for a variety of reasons, as discussed previously (Rybicki 2009). One of the biggest obstacles is the reluctance of the pharmaceutical industry to invest in a new technology when the existing seems adequate. However, a steady accumulation of promising data has shown that plant-based expression has great potential, especially if a few hurdles can be overcome.

The original and oft-touted goal for plant-derived vaccines was to provide cheap and conveniently delivered oral recombinant subunit vaccines to underdeveloped countries where poor economic conditions limit the application of modern medical science. The hypothesis was that ingestion of edible plant material, either raw or minimally processed, could induce protective immune responses via activation of immune effectors in gut-associated lymphoid tissue (GALT) (Streatfield 2006; Thanavala et al. 2006). Oral delivery of bacterial antigens has generated protective immunity against enteric pathogens. However, there is scarce evidence that protection against respiratory or urogenital tract infectious disease can be achieved using the oral vaccine delivery route.

Digestive acids and proteases that degrade proteins for nutrient absorption are a substantial problem for oral vaccine development. Antigens must be relatively resistant to gut proteases, and typically very large antigen doses be administered. Encapsulation might better protect immunogens and their delivery into GALT (Streatfield 2006). However, little work in this area has been done with plant-derived antigens.

Another problem for edible vaccines is that accumulation of antigens in transgenic plant tissues is usually rather low ($\leq$1% of total soluble protein, TSP), creating a requirement for processing of plant material to concentrate the antigen. Moreover, the inherent plant-to-plant variability in antigen content requires processing of plant material to produce a well-characterized batch of antigen that can be administered in controlled dosages. Thus, plant-derived oral vaccine immunogens will require substantial purification and concentration, and probable delivery in capsules that protect them from proteolytic degradation in the small intestine.

Recently, plant-based recombinant protein production has been revolutionized by transient expression of antigens in plants using viral vectors (Gleba et al. 2007; Yusibov et al. 2006). The plant host is usually the tobacco relative *Nicotiana benthamiana* (Goodin et al. 2008), which is remarkably permissive to many plant viruses. Expression levels obtained with viral vectors in *N. benthamiana* leaves are variable depending on the protein, but are generally ten-fold greater than in stable transformants of the nuclear genome, and frequently in the range of 1–2 mg/kg of leaf mass. Thus, the prospect of plant-based expression and purification of vaccine antigens, especially virus-like particles (VLP) (Huang et al. 2009), for mucosal delivery is substantially brighter than that obtained using stably integrated transgenes. Moreover, the high yields of recombinant antigens that can be obtained using viral vectors may facilitate intranasal delivery, which requires smaller volumes and hence, more concentrated vaccine solutions than the oral delivery route.

An ideal mucosal vaccine would induce both antibody- and cell-mediated protection, not only at the relevant mucosal site, but also throughout the body. The most convenient means to achieve mucosal immunity in global health programs is oral delivery. Oral vaccination eliminates the possibility of transmission of other infectious diseases by contaminated needles, as well as elimination of pain associated with injections and the need for trained personnel to deliver the vaccines (Holmgren and Czerkinsky 2005; Lavelle 2005). However, nasal vaccines are not hampered by the physical and chemical barriers of the gut. Nasal vaccination has demonstrated particular potential with regard to induction of broadly disseminated immunity (Neutra and Kozlowski 2006; Staats et al. 1997). In humans, monkeys, and mice, nasal immunization induced antigen-specific mucosal IgA responses in salivary glands, upper and lower respiratory tracts, small and large intestines, and most notably male and female reproductive tracts (Harandi et al. 2003; Imaoka et al. 1998; Kozlowski et al. 2002; Rudin et al. 1999; Staats et al. 1997). In addition, the nasal route of immunization can induce cytotoxic T lymphocytes (CTL) in distant mucosal tissues including the female reproductive tract (Gallichan and Rosenthal 1998). In both humans and mice, nasal immunization has produced greater systemic antibody responses than other mucosal immunization routes (Kozlowski et al. 1997, 2002; Staats et al. 1997). Kunkel and Butcher (2002) provided evidence from naïve human vaccine recipients that mucosal immunization can prime the immune system for both mucosal and systemic responses by inducing the expression of both mucosal and systemic homing receptors in responding lymphocytes. Thus, delivery of subunit antigens or VLP via the nasal route has excellent prospects as a vaccine strategy. For further reading on VLP vaccines, readers are directed to "Recent Advances in Microparticle and Nanoparticle Delivery Vehicles for Mucosal Vaccination" of this volume.

2 Plant Expression Systems

The strategies used for recombinant protein expression in plants are conceptually similar to those used for mammalian, yeast, or other eukaryotic hosts (Rybicki 2009; Thanavala et al. 2006; Yusibov and Rabindran 2008). They include stably integrated transgenes in the nuclear or chloroplast genomes, and transient expression using vectors that are either non-replicating or that utilize plant virus replication elements to amplify the mRNA for the target gene. Nuclear genes behave in a Mendelian fashion, and utilize the typical eukaryotic pathways of protein translation, processing, and subcellular localization. Organ- and development stage-specific promoters can be utilized, such that foreign proteins can be directed to accumulate in seeds (Nochi et al. 2007; Streatfield et al. 2003; Wu et al. 2007). Expression of antigens in seeds has a particular advantage in regard to protein stability due to drying of the storage tissue during seed development. Thus, seeds can be stored at ambient temperatures for months to years with little loss of protein activity.

Although site-specific recombination of plant nuclear genomes has been studied intensively (Hanin and Paszkowski 2003), it is currently not routine and usually rather inefficient. In most cases, the recombinant construct is delivered as DNA using *Agrobacterium tumefaciens*, a plant pathogen that has the ability to transfer genes into the plant cell nucleus (Gelvin 2003). The foreign DNA may be integrated stably into the host nuclear chromosomal DNA by non-homologous recombination at random sites, although some work suggests that transcriptionally active sites may be preferentially targeted. The transferred DNA may also reside in the nucleus without integration for several days, and can thus act as a template for transcription to effect transient expression. Unless the foreign DNA is constructed as a viral replicon, it will remain in low-copy numbers, but can be used to evaluate expression of foreign antigens (Huang and Mason 2004).

Agrobacterium-mediated DNA transfer can also be used to deliver viral replicons. DNA viruses such as geminiviruses have been used to develop gene amplification systems (Huang et al. 2009). Genomes of RNA viruses such as tobacco mosaic virus (TMV) can be constructed as cDNA fused to a plant promoter, which is transcribed in the nucleus to produce viral RNA that then moves to the cytoplasm to establish replication (Gleba et al. 2007). A method called "Magnifection" was developed to allow whole-plant inoculation of *N. benthamiana* by vacuum infiltration with *Agrobacterium* lines containing recombinant TMV replicons that lack the coat protein, resulting in foreign gene expression in all leaves (Gleba et al. 2005). Recombinant viral genomes can also be delivered directly as RNA after in vitro transcription from a plasmid by simply abrading the leaf surface and applying a solution of RNA (Gleba et al. 2007; Yusibov et al. 2006). In this case, the replicon needs to contain viral elements that mediate long-distance transport in the plant vasculature so that expression is not restricted only to the site of inoculation.

Chloroplast transformation is routine in only a few laboratories, but can yield very high-expression levels of some antigens, due to the high gene copy numbers from many chloroplasts per cell and genome molecules per chloroplast (Arlen et al. 2008; Singh et al. 2009). The DNA construct is delivered by micro projectile bombardment (gene gun), and site-specific recombination allows targeted gene insertion. One great advantage of chloroplast transgenes is that they are not usually subject to gene silencing mediated by RNA interference, which is a common problem with nuclear transgenes. Another advantage is that the chloroplast genome is exclusively maternally inherited, making gene containment much easier because pollen grains are devoid of plastids. However, the chloroplast genetic system is a prokaryotic one; thus, some protein processing events, notably glycosylation, will not occur.

3 Plant-Derived Human Vaccines

3.1 Norovirus

Noroviruses are non-enveloped positive-sense RNA members of Caliciviridae, and are enteric pathogens that cause gastroenteritis. The capsid protein of Norwalk virus (NVCP) can be expressed in insect cells (Jiang et al. 1992) or plants (Mason et al. 1996), and self-assembles into VLP (rNV) that are orally immunogenic. A clinical study evaluated the antibody responses after ingestion of 2 or 3 doses of 150 g raw potato tubers expressing rNV (Tacket et al. 2000). Although 19 of 20 subjects who ingested the rNV expressing potato developed measurable increases in circulating antibody-secreting cells, the overall response was rather weak. The variable rNV content of the tubers (215–750 μg per dose) and relatively poor VLP assembly in the potato (effective rNV dose of ≤325 μg per dose) were likely limiting factors. However, a detrimental effect of the potato vehicle, perhaps due to poor release of VLP in the gut lumen, cannot be discounted. A clinical trial using orally delivered purified insect cell-derived rNV (i-rNV) produced stronger antibody responses at 250 μg per dose than were obtained with potato (Tacket et al. 2003), suggesting that purified rNV is a more potent oral immunogen.

Later, rNV was expressed at higher levels in transgenic tomato fruit using a plant codon-optimized NVCP gene (Zhang et al. 2006). Oral immunogenicity in mice was excellent: 4 doses of 0.4 g freeze–dried tomato fruit containing 64 μg NVCP (40 μg rNV) induced anti-rNV serum IgG and fecal IgA in ≥80% of mice, and 0.8 g doses generated systemic and mucosal antibodies in all mice. It was also shown that air-dried tomato fruit was at least as active in mice as freeze–dried tomato, indicating that sophisticated drying technology is not required for rNV in tomato. Interestingly, rNV delivered in freeze–dried potato tuber was less orally immunogenic in mice, due to oxidation by phenolic compounds and polyphenol oxidase in potato (Zhang et al. 2006). Tomato is much better in this respect, having low-phenolic content, as well as a high level of ascorbic acid that can act as antioxidant. Thus, dried rNV tomato fruit would be worthy of study in humans.

In recent years, our group has been experimenting with viral vectors for transient expression of rNV in plants because of the potential for high-level expression and the rapidity of protein production (Gleba et al. 2005; Marillonnet et al. 2004). We used the Magnifection system to express NVCP in the tobacco relative *N. benthamiana* at levels of 800 mg/kg leaf tissue (Santi et al. 2008). Further, we developed a VLP purification process that did not require ultracentrifugation but instead utilized pH 5.3 precipitation of the major leaf proteins, followed by filtration through a 100 kDa membrane to remove unassembled NVCP subunits. In the absence of adjuvant, the tobacco-derived rNV (t-rNV) was orally immunogenic in mice at a 100 μg dose, generating systemic and mucosal anti-rNV antibodies (Santi et al. 2008). Inclusion of cholera toxin adjuvant with t-rNV substantially increased anti-rNV responses.

In Velasquez et al. 2010 studies with mice, we have found that nasal co-delivery of t-rNV and a Toll-like receptor (TLR) agonist can produce robust systemic and mucosal antigen-specific antibody responses. We undertook these experiments to evaluate the potential of these VLP to induce distal mucosal IgA responses with or without adjuvant. In unpublished studies we examined the TLR9 agonist, CpG-containing oligodeoxynucleotides (CpG-ODN) as adjuvant because it is known to trigger an immunostimulatory cascade that culminates in the maturation, differentiation, and proliferation of multiple cell types, including B cells, and CpG-ODN had been used previously in mice by the nasal route (Abe et al. 2006; Balmelli et al. 1998; McCluskie et al. 2000). We nasally immunized conscious female BALB/c mice with 25 μg purified t-rNV alone or t-rNV with 10 μg type B CpG-ODN. Nasal immunization of conscious mice with VLP has been shown to target antigen to the nasopharyngeal-associated lymphoid tissue (NALT) but not deeper respiratory tract tissues (BALT); whereas nasal immunization of sedated mice is more analogous to intratracheal administration

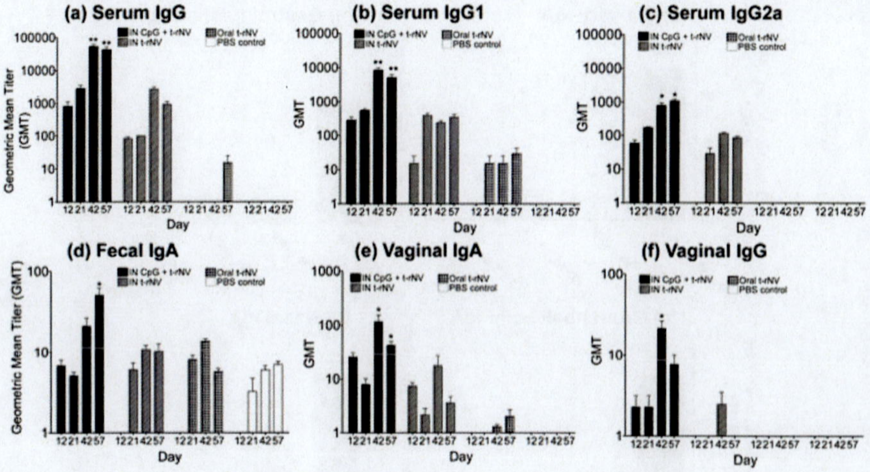

Fig. 1 TLR agonist significantly increases rNV-specific antibody production in mice immunized with tobacco-derived Norwalk virus-like particles (t-rNV). Conscious female BALB/c mice were immunized intranasally (IN) on days 0 and 21 with 25 μg t-rNV with or without 10 μg CpG ODN (10 μg), or orally (ORAL) on days, 0, 21, and 42 with 100 μg t-rNV or PBS vehicle alone. Serum (**a–c**), feces (**d**), and vaginal lavages (**e–f**) were collected at days 0, 12, 21, 42, and 56 and analyzed by ELISA for rNV-specific IgG or IgA. Data are geometric mean titers (GMT). Significantly higher levels of rNV-specific antibody production were observed throughout the time course in mice immunized IN with t-rNV and CpG ODN compared to t-rNV alone or vehicle alone-immunized mice. Prism software from GraphPad was used to conduct one-way ANOVA with Bonferroni post test ($p < 0.05$ was considered significant)

(Balmelli et al. 1998). We also immunized mice orally with 100 μg t-rNV alone. The rNV-specific IgG1 and IgG2a antibodies induced in serum were analyzed to determine if immunization had produced a Th1, Th2, or mixed Th1/Th2 immune response. Overall, rNV-specific serum IgG levels were higher in nasally versus orally immunized mice, with greatest levels achieved by nasal co-delivery of CpG-ODN with rNV (Fig. 1a–c). Within the nasal groups, both anti-rNV IgG1 and IgG2a in serum were significantly increased in the CpG-ODN immunization group relative to controls. This suggests that CpG-ODN drives a mixed Th1/Th2 response with respect to the production of anti-rNV antibodies.

In these immunized animals, IgG levels had increased by 12 days following a single immunization and continued to rise following booster immunizations at days 21 (intranasal and oral) and 42 (oral only). Antibody levels began to plateau by day 57 (Fig. 1a–c). The orally delivered t-rNV at 100 μg was not very immunogenic; however, nasal immunization with 25 μg t-rNV produced robust immune responses. Fecal IgA was produced only in the CpG-ODN immunization groups (Fig. 1d). In addition, the levels of rNV-specific IgA and IgG in vaginal lavages were significantly elevated ($p < 0.001$) in nasal groups given rNV with CpG-ODN (Fig. 1e and f). To further characterize distal induction of antigen-specific IgA, we

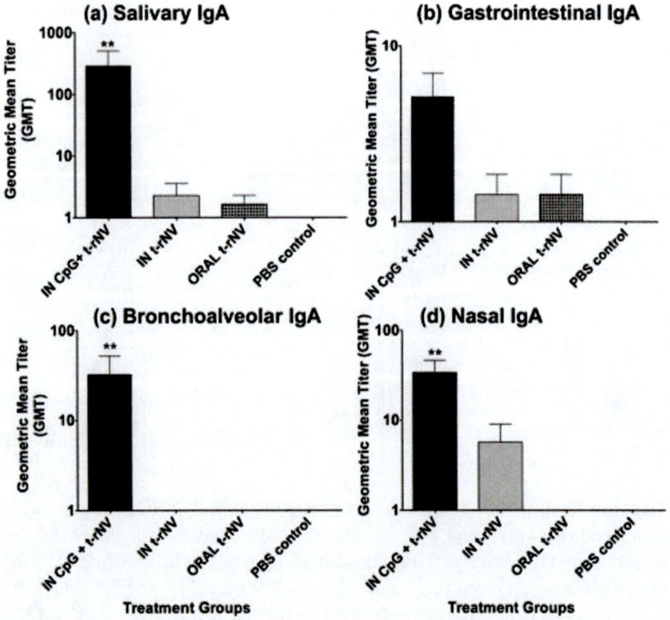

Fig. 2 Induction of antigen-specific IgA at distal mucosal sites following intranasal, but not oral administration of tobacco-derived Norwalk virus-like particles (t-rNV). Female BALB/c mice were immunized as described in the Fig. 1. Salivary samples (**a**), gastrointestinal lavages (**b**), bronchoalvelolar lavages (**c**), and nasal lavages (**d**) were collected from mice on day 56 and analyzed for rNV-specific IgA production by ELISA (presented as GMT). Distal mucosal sites contained significantly higher ($p < 0.001$) levels of antigen-specific IgA in CpG ODN + t-rNV IN vaccinated groups relative to t-rNV alone delivered via IN or ORAL routes

evaluated IgA production at additional mucosal sites, including salivary samples, gastrointestinal lavages, nasal washes, and bronchoalveolar lavages. At each of these distal mucosal sites, IgA production was significantly increased relative to controls in the rNV/CpG-ODN-immunized mice (Fig. 2a–d). These results demonstrate that t-rNV co-delivered with TLR agonist by the nasal route can induce robust antigen-specific IgA production at distal mucosal sites that would be important for mucosal protection against not only enteric organisms, but also respiratory and sexually–transmitted pathogens. Overall, the data demonstrate that immunization with t-rNV by the nasal route is more effective than the oral route for inducing robust rNV-specific systemic IgG and mucosal IgA antibody responses in upper and lower respiratory (nasal and bronchoalveolar), gastrointestinal (salivary, intestine and fecal), and female reproductive (vaginal) tracts. We are now planning a Phase I clinical trial to evaluate systemic and mucosal antibody responses to t-rNV after nasal delivery with a selected adjuvant.

3.2 Hepatitis B Virus

Chronic infection with hepatitis B virus (HBV) can result in liver cancer, accounting for up to one million deaths per year among approximately 350 million chronic carriers worldwide. HBV is transmitted mainly by blood or through sexual contact, but vertical transmission occurs frequently when HBV–infected mothers give birth. In this regard, a mucosal HBV vaccine may be an improvement over the current intramuscular hepatitis B surface antigen (HBsAg) vaccine made in recombinant yeast (McAleer et al. 1984). Moreover, an orally delivered plant-derived vaccine could improve patient compliance for multiple doses due to the convenience, and it would obviate the need for needles. However, we must take care to avoid interference with current efforts to expand HBV vaccination in the developing world, and move forward with a plant-derived vaccine only if distinct advantages are demonstrated.

The perception among plant vaccinologists that a plant-derived HBV vaccine is important is apparent from the large body of work demonstrating expression of HBsAg in a variety of plants including potato, lettuce, tomato, tomatillo, corn, and banana (Streatfield 2005). The first publication on plant-based vaccine antigen expression was with HBsAg in transgenic tobacco (Mason et al. 1992). After optimization of HBsAg expression in transgenic potato tubers (Richter et al. 2000), its oral immunogenicity in mice (albeit dependent upon inclusion of CT; Kong et al. 2001), encouraged a human trial. Due to FDA concerns that immunologically naïve subjects might experience antigenic tolerance after ingestion of HBsAg, the clinical study used HBsAg seropositive volunteers who had been previously vaccinated with the yeast recombinant HBsAg (Thanavala et al. 2005). Titers of anti-HBsAg in serum were increased in 9/17 and 10/16 volunteers who consumed 2 or 3 doses of transgenic potatoes, respectively, with each dose containing roughly 850 μg HBsAg. This finding suggests that oral boosting with plant-derived HBsAg could be incorporated as a viable component of immunization programs. Oral delivery of HBsAg can activate systemic memory cells generated by intramuscular immunization, However, the possibility of priming immunization by HBsAg potato ingestion cannot be excluded. An earlier study had shown that presumably naïve human subjects who ingested transgenic lettuce expressing low levels of HBsAg underwent seroconversion (Kapusta et al. 1999). It is interesting to note that neither of these clinical trials employed an adjuvant, which suggests that oral delivery can be substantially optimized in further work.

The fear of oral tolerance is one that must be taken seriously; however, very little work has addressed this issue with plant-derived vaccines. One recent paper examined regulatory T cells (Tregs) in humanized mice orally immunized with transgenic HBsAg tobacco (Kostrzak et al. 2009). T regulatory cells mediate immunological unresponsiveness to self-antigens and are implicated in oral tolerance (Sakaguchi et al. 2008). The humanized mice were immunized by gavage with different amounts of powdered tobacco leaves, and Foxp3 + CD3 +CD4 + Tregs were measured in spleen and peripheral lymph nodes (Kostrzak et al. 2009).

Serum IgG and fecal IgA were inversely correlated with antigen dose, while the frequency of Tregs positively correlated with tobacco dose, leading the authors to conclude that oral tolerance occurred at higher doses. While the data are not strongly conclusive due to the relatively poor antibody response rate among groups, they do suggest that, in the absence of adjuvant, oral plant vaccines may induce tolerance, and that higher-vaccine dosages are not necessarily better. Nonetheless, much more work is needed with different antigens, plant vehicles, and dosages in order to make firm conclusions regarding the potential of plant-derived antigens to induce oral tolerance.

3.3 Rabies Virus

Rabies is a zoonotic disease that is invariably fatal after development of clinical symptoms (Nagarajan et al. 2008). Because most human deaths from rabies occur in developing countries, new technologies like plant-derived recombinant antibodies and vaccines could make a significant impact. Yusibov and colleagues (Yusibov et al. 2002) have shown that oral delivery of rabies virus epitopes expressed in spinach is immunogenic in humans. A chimeric peptide containing determinants from rabies virus glycoprotein (G protein) and nucleoprotein (N protein) was fused to the N-terminus of the alfalfa mosaic virus coat protein, and expressed with viral vectors in tobacco and spinach. Virus particles were expressed at 0.4 mg per g leaf tissue, of which 70% was recovered in purified form. In mice, 3 intraperitoneal doses of recombinant virus particles (with 35 μg of rabies peptide) generated neutralizing antibodies and protected against lethal rabies virus challenge.

Thus, a human study was performed using 10 volunteers who had previously received the conventional rabies vaccine (as with the HBV potato vaccine, there were concerns about potential oral tolerance). Five subjects were fed 20 g raw recombinant spinach leaves (0.6 mg of recombinant virus with 84 μg chimeric rabies peptide per dose) a total of 3 times at biweekly intervals, while another five subjects ingested control vector-only spinach. Three of the antigen-treated volunteers, but none of the individuals in the control group, showed significant boosting of anti-rabies virus antibody in serum. Based on these results, naïve subjects were tested. Nine volunteers consumed 3 doses of raw rabies-recombinant spinach leaves (150 g per dose) and 5 were fed control spinach. All subjects then received a single dose of commercial rabies vaccine 7 days after the last oral dose. Six of the subjects who ate the rabies antigen-containing spinach showed significant increases in serum IgG or IgA specific for rabies virus (Yusibov et al. 2002). These results are similar to those obtained with HBsAg-expressing potatoes (Thanavala et al. 2005), and although a greater response rate would be desirable, the studies demonstrate the potential for successful oral delivery of plant-derived vaccines in humans.

Little further work on rabies vaccines has been reported, but in one study (Loza-Rubio et al. 2008) the rabies virus G protein was expressed in transgenic maize seeds at 1% TSP. Mice were fed a single dose of transgenic seeds containing 50 μg of G protein, and challenged 90 days later with a lethal dose of rabies virus (100 LD_{50}). The vaccine induced virus-neutralizing antibodies and impressively protected all mice against challenge. These results suggest that maize seeds may be an ideal vehicle for expression and delivery of rabies G protein.

3.4 Measles Virus

Measles virus (MV) causes substantial morbidity and mortality worldwide, but developing countries carry the heaviest burden due to the instability of the attenuated virus vaccine and the requirement for inoculation needles (Webster et al. 2005). Moreover, evidence indicates that vaccinated individuals generate less robust and long-lasting antibody titers than individuals who recovered from a natural MV infection (Muller et al. 2003). Thus, boosting with a convenient mucosally delivered MV vaccine would be a great boon to health, especially in resource-poor countries. Two groups of researchers have approached this problem using plant-derived vaccines. Webster and colleagues expressed a soluble form of the MV hemagglutinin (MV-H) surface protein in stable transgenic tobacco and lettuce (Webster et al. 2006, 2005). The MV-H was stable in freeze–dried lettuce leaf stored at room temperature for 6 months, and showed only 30–40% loss after 13 months (Webster et al. 2006). Moreover, the dried MV-H was orally immunogenic in mice after resuspension and delivery by gavage with a crude saponin adjuvant. Since no reference standard was available, the amount of MV-H antigen in the lettuce could not be accurately determined. Best results were obtained when mice were systemically primed with a MV-H DNA vaccine, then orally boosted five times with lettuce expressing MV-H. The mean titers of MV-specific serum IgG were boosted tenfold by the oral doses, while control lettuce had no effect. The virus-neutralizing titers were roughly 3.5-fold higher in MV-H lettuce boosted mice than in control lettuce mice. These data indicate the potential for oral boosting with plant-derived MV-H for humans that have been intramuscularly vaccinated but experience waning of anti-MV antibody titer.

Another group has used a MV polyepitope strategy, expressing four copies of the loop–forming hemagglutinin protective B cell epitope fused to four repeats of the human promiscuous T cell epitope of tetanus toxoid in transgenic carrots (Bouche et al. 2005). Although the vaccine was delivered by the intraperitoneal route and not mucosally, the antigen was immunogenic and generated serum antibodies that neutralized ten different MV strains. This approach might be developed for oral or nasal delivery, with appropriate mucosal adjuvants, in order to produce a vaccine that is more convenient for populations in developing countries. No plant-derived MV vaccines have been tested in humans yet, but the data above show very promising indications that oral boosting could provide substantial benefits.

3.5 Enteric Bacterial Infections

The first plant-derived vaccine immunogen to be tested in humans was the B subunit protein of the enterotoxigenic *Escherichia coli* heat–labile toxin (LT) expressed in transgenic potatoes (Mason et al. 1998; Tacket et al. 1998). The non-toxic LTB protein mediates binding of the LT holotoxin to epithelial cells, triggering intracellular delivery of the toxic A subunit. The rationale for a mucosal vaccine rationale presumes that oral delivery of LTB will induce local secretion of anti-LTB antibodies in the gut, which will prevent the binding of the holotoxin to enterocytes. Data from mouse studies supports this hypothesis, and mice that ingested LTB-containing potato tubers were partially protected against LT challenge, as indicated by reduced fluid secretion in the small intestine (Mason et al. 1998). The clinical trial showed that ingestion of LTB in potatoes stimulated anti-LT serum IgG in 9 of 11 subjects, serum IgA in six subjects, and fecal IgA in 5 of 10 subjects; and further showed that the antibodies could neutralize LT (Tacket et al. 1998). Another clinical trial using transgenic maize germ (embryo of seeds) expressing LTB yielded similar results (Tacket et al. 2004). The fact that LTB is one of the most orally immunogenic proteins known does not diminish the impact of these findings, which provide clear evidence that the ingestion of crude plant material, in the absence of adjuvant, could potentially stimulate protective antibody responses to enteric pathogens in humans.

Recently, transgenic rice seeds expressing the structurally and functionally similar B subunit of cholera toxin were developed (Nochi et al. 2007). Cholera toxin B subunit (CTB) was expressed in rice seeds using the *GluB*-1 seed storage protein promoter at up to 30 μg per seed (2.1% TSP). It was localized in protein storage bodies, which allowed high stability (immunogenicity after 1.5 years at room temperature), and resistance to pepsin treatment. Thus, rice and corn appear to be good vehicles for delivery of antigens in the gut.

A plant-derived vaccine against enterohemorrhagic *E. coli* (O157:H7) has also been created by expressing part of the bacterial adhesin intimin in cultured transgenic tobacco cells (Judge et al. 2004). The C-terminal domain of intimin (Int261) mediates binding to the translocated intimin receptor, as well as host–specific surface molecules, for bacterial colonization in the gut. Oral immunization of mice by ingestion of Int261 expressing tobacco cells after intraperitoneal priming with plant-derived Int261 stimulated specific fecal IgA in 7 of 10 mice, and reduced bacterial shedding after challenge with O157:H7 (Judge et al. 2004). However, low expression of Int261 in the transgenic tobacco cells limited the amount of antigen that could be produced. Using viral vectors and transient expression, our research team has substantially enhanced Int261 expression in leaves of *N. benthamiana* (E. Topal & H. Mason, manuscript in preparation).

Further testing in more appropriate hosts, such as cattle, will be needed to assess the efficacy of this and other intimin expressing plant-based vaccines for preventing infection by *E. coli* 0157:H7.

4 Plant-Derived Animal Vaccines

Plant-derived vaccines for animals are likely to be realized sooner than those for humans, due to more relaxed regulations (Rybicki 2009). In fact, the only licensed plant-derived vaccine is for prevention of Newcastle disease virus (NDV) in chickens, comprising recombinant hemagglutinin–neuraminidase protein expressed in cultured transgenic tobacco cells and prepared as an injectable vaccine for chickens (Dow AgroSciences, www.dowagro.com/animalhealth/resources/faq.htm#faq11). As discussed below, several other plant-derived mucosally delivered vaccines against animal diseases have shown potential.

4.1 Foot-and-Mouth Disease Virus

Foot-and-mouth disease virus (FMDV) is a very important veterinary pathogen because it is highly infectious in animals and has economically devastating effects on meat and milk production. The FMDV VP1 capsid protein contains virus-neutralizing determinants (Wigdorovitz et al. 1999). Several studies have shown expression of VP1 in various plant hosts (Yusibov and Rabindran 2008). Transgenic VP1 alfalfa leaves were immunogenic in mice by intraperitoneal or oral delivery (Wigdorovitz et al. 1999). For oral delivery, mice were fed 0.3 g of fresh leaves three times per week for 2 weeks. Ten days later serum was obtained. All mice in two separate experiments developed serum antibodies against FMDV particles, at titers ranging up to 320. Moreover, 14 of 17 mice were protected against intraperitoneal challenge with FMDV, as measured by the absence of viremia 36 h later, while none of the control mice were protected.

A different strategy fused a VP1 epitope (amino acids 135–160) to β-glucuronidase (GUS), a stable enzyme that is readily measured using a fluorometric assay (Dus Santos et al. 2002). Expression in transgenic alfalfa plants ranged from 0.05 to 0.1% of TSP, and crude extracts injected by the intraperitoneal route elicited completely protective immune responses in mice. Another fusion protein study used VP1 amino acids 128–164 replacing the N-terminal 35 residues of bamboo mosaic virus coat protein, and the recombinant virus used to infect leaves of *Chenopdium quinoa* (a spinach relative) (Yang et al. 2007). Infected leaves produced chimeric virions expressing VP1 epitopes in its coat protein. Although the yield of recombinant protein was not quantified, the data suggest accumulation to $\sim$5–10% TSP (Yang et al. 2007). Intramuscular immunization of pigs with 5 mg of VP1 virions resulted in the induction of anti-FMDV neutralizing antibodies, VP1-specific IFN-γ-producing cells, and complete protection against

FMDV challenge. The high antigen dose used in these studies indicates robust expression of this viral coat protein fusion.

In view of the promising results obtained through oral delivery of plant-derived VP1 (Wigdorovitz et al. 1999), it is perhaps surprising that these later fusion protein strategies that yielded improved expression were not tested by the oral route. Further investigation is needed in order to evaluate oral delivery with adjuvants, and in animal species that have more economic relevance.

4.2 Transmissible Gastroenteritis Virus

Transmissible gastroenteritis virus (TGEV) is a coronavirus that significantly affects swine production (Hammond and Nemchinov 2009). The disease is highly infectious, and the severe diarrhea and vomiting produce high mortality in young piglets. The envelope spike (S) protein is a target for neutralizing antibody, and thus has been expressed in plant systems for oral delivery (Howard 2004; Lamphear et al. 2004). Transgenic corn seed expressing TGEV-S protein fed to piglets stimulated antibody production and partially protected animals from viral challenge (Howard 2004). The truncated soluble S protein product was targeted to the cell wall instead of protein bodies, which allowed accumulation of antigen at 13 mg/kg seed, and a dose of 20–30 mg S protein in a single feeding. Further studies examined the potential to immunize gilts (young sows) and stimulate anti-S antibody secretion in the milk for protection of suckling piglets (Lamphear et al. 2004). Oral dosing by ingestion of TGEV-S corn by gilts on days −35 and −14 before farrowing (day 0), after having received the modified live TGEV vaccine orally at days −115 and −102, stimulated significantly higher TGEV-neutralizing activity in serum, colostrum (day 0), and milk (day 3) compared to a placebo group. Antibody isotypes were not determined, but the authors suggest that the milk antibodies later than day two are mostly IgA (Lamphear et al. 2004). Protective efficacy was not examined, but the neutralizing titers in milk suggest that suckling piglets would have been protected. However, the milk titers dropped precipitously at day 7–14, suggesting that continued boosting would be necessary to maintain protection.

An interesting chimeric antibody against TGEV was expressed in plants and tested for its ability to protect piglets after oral delivery (Monger et al. 2006). These investigators fused an anti-TGEV single-chain antibody (scFv) to the CH4 domain of IgE to mediate dimerization. The protein was expressed in cowpea leaves using a cowpea mosaic virus vector, achieving accumulation of ~2%TSP. This plant-derived antibody (dubbed "ε-small immune protein" or εSIP) showed similar TGEV-neutralizing activity as the parent antibody 6A.C3 or the εSIP expressed in mammalian cells. Moreover, oral gavage in piglets reduced viral titers in lung and gut of piglets challenged with TGEV, though less effectively than antibody 6A.C3. These studies illustrate the potential for plant-derived antibodies to provide mucosal protection against enteric viral disease, and deserve further attention for application in veterinary and human medicine.

4.3 Infectious Bursal Disease Virus

Infectious bursal disease virus (IBDV) is highly contagious and deadly in young chickens. It thus has a major economic impact on the poultry industry. IBDV is a member of the *Birnaviridae* with two double–stranded RNA genome segments (Wu et al. 2007). The VP2 viral capsid protein is the immunodominant antigen that generates antiviral neutralizing antibodies. The currently used vaccines are either attenuated or killed viruses, but suffer problems regarding the potential for the live virus vaccine to recombine and generate variants, or poor efficacy in the case of the whole-killed vaccine.

One of the more compelling plant-derived vaccine successes to date is recombinant VP2 delivered orally. The VP2 was expressed in leaves of *Arabidopsis thaliana* at levels up to 4.8% TSP (Wu et al. 2004a), which is among the highest obtained for a recombinant subunit vaccine in stably transformed plants. Leaves of transgenic plants were dried, powdered, and resuspended in water for oral delivery (Wu et al. 2004b). One-week old birds received five oral doses at 3 days intervals (~5 μg VP2 per dose), or the live intermediate vaccine Bursine-2, or priming with Bursine-2 followed by boosting with oral VP2. Although the Bursine-2 primed birds developed serum anti-VP2 antibodies earlier, the titers were similar in all three groups after 5 weeks. Furthermore, all groups exhibited similar protection (80–90%) after challenge with virulent IBDV (Wu et al. 2004b).

Later, VP2 was expressed in stable transgenic rice seeds at up to 4.5% TSP, or 40 μg per seed (Wu et al. 2007). Two week old chickens were fed 4 weekly doses of 1, 3, or 5 g rice seed, or they received the B87 live attenuated nasal virus vaccine. Anti-VP2 serum antibodies increased during the 2 weeks following immunization, with the 5 g oral group attaining levels similar to those in the B87 nasal vaccine group. Among the different VP2-rice oral groups, antibody levels were positively correlated with the dosage. Interestingly, the 5 g oral VP2 group was better protected against virulent IBDV challenge than the B87 vaccine group (5/6 vs. 2/6, respectively). Although the bursal lesion score used to calculate efficacy could be considered somewhat subjective, efficacy was correlated with oral antigen dose (Wu et al. 2007). We have estimated that the 5 g rice seed contained roughly a 10 mg dose VP2 protein, which is rather high. In this regard, seeds have a distinct advantage over leaves, by enabling a high dose as well as excellent protein stability on long-term storage.

4.4 Actinobacillus Pleuropneumoniae

Actinobacillus pleuropneumoniae is an agent of porcine pleuropneumonia, which is an important swine disease. Although the pathogenic mechanism is not fully understood, Apx toxins are associated with bacterial virulence (Shin et al. 2005). The Apx I, II, and III toxins mediate virulence by inserting into host cell membranes and creating pores; thus they may be good targets for immune intervention in this disease. One group has demonstrated the protective potential of ApxIA and ApxIIA proteins as vaccine antigens after oral delivery in mice (Lee et al. 2006; Shin et al. 2005, 2007). Their first study used the yeast *Saccharomyces cerevisiae* for expression of ApxIIA and oral delivery in mice, showing ApxIIA-specific IgA production in lung and intestine, as well as partial ($\leq$50%) and dose-dependent protection against challenge with *A. pleuropneumoniae*.

In a second study, stable transgenic tobacco was used to express ApxIIA at relatively low levels ($\leq$0.1% TSP) (Lee et al. 2006). Mice were gavaged with 4 weekly doses of dried tobacco leaf (1 mg or 5 mg dry mass, which we estimate contained 30 or 150 ng ApxIIA) suspended in PBS, which evoked modest serum IgG specific for ApxIIA in the higher dose group. Challenge of the mice by intraperitoneal injection of *A. pleuropneumoniae* killed all mice in the control non-transgenic tobacco group within 72 h, while 50% of the higher–dose ApxIIA tobacco group survived. By comparison, 90% of mice immunized subcutaneously with recombinant *E. coli*-expressed ApxIIA survived (Lee et al. 2006). Although the ultimate fate of the mice beyond 72 h was not reported, it appears that oral delivery of ApxIIA tobacco afforded some protection. A later oral immunization study using both ApxIA and ApxIIA expressed in yeast showed enhanced protective efficacy over either toxin delivered alone, suggesting that multiple toxins should be included in a swine vaccine (Shin et al. 2007). Certainly, the levels of antigen expression in plants must be increased in order to facilitate more robust protection by oral delivery. Moreover, testing in swine must be performed in order to examine the potential for protection by oral delivery of the Apx antigens.

5 Conclusion

Plant-based expression of vaccine antigen and oral delivery of crude or minimally processed plant tissues is most promising for antigens expressed in seeds, such as rice or corn. The seed vehicle provides a stable environment for accumulated proteins, thus the need for refrigeration could be obviated or minimized. Nonetheless, only a few antigens have been expressed in seeds at sufficient levels to afford protection in animals upon ingestion. Due to the variable nature of protein structure and biochemical characteristics, it is difficult to predict which proteins will accumulate well and be correctly folded to display protective epitopes. The generation and screening for optimal expression in stable transgenic plant lines is a time- and labor-intensive process, but in some cases may yield excellent results.

Regulatory agencies have a substantial concern regarding the use of plants, especially plants used as food for humans, for the production of pharmaceutical proteins and vaccines. This issue was discussed in a recent review (Rybicki 2009). Although the World Health Organization, United States Department of Agriculture, and the Food and Drug Administration agree that applicable regulatory and good manufacturing practice requirements are in place for plant-derived vaccines, enthusiasm is dimmed by fears that noncompliance could compromise food security. Thus, investment of funds for commercial development of vaccines in food crops is likely to suffer.

Meanwhile, much recent work has focused on the use of non-food plants (tobacco and relatives) for production of vaccine antigens using robust transient expression via plant virus replicons (Gleba et al. 2007; Huang et al. 2009; Santi et al. 2006). These systems provide expression levels high enough to facilitate purification of antigens in good yield and concentrated enough to use for intranasal delivery, or to incorporate into oral delivery formulations. Ongoing work to develop mucosal adjuvants will synergize with these efficient plant expression systems to provide more alternatives for vaccination and, ultimately, vaccines tailored for particular pathogens and their hosts. Agonists for pattern recognition receptors (e.g. Toll-like receptors) show great promise as mucosal adjuvants, and deserve further research and development.

References

Abe N, Kodama S, Hirano T et al (2006) Nasal vaccination with CpG oligodeoxynucleotide induces protective immunity against non-typeable Haemophilus influenzae in the nasopharynx. Laryngoscope 116:407–412

Arlen PA, Singleton M, Adamovicz JJ et al (2008) Effective plague vaccination via oral delivery of plant cells expressing F1-V antigens in chloroplasts. Infect Immun 76:3640–3650

Balmelli C, Roden R, Potts A et al (1998) Nasal immunization of mice with human papillomavirus type 16 virus-like particles elicits neutralizing antibodies in mucosal secretions. J Virol 72:8220–8229

Bouche FB, Steinmetz A, Yanagi Y et al (2005) Induction of broadly neutralizing antibodies against measles virus mutants using a polyepitope vaccine strategy. Vaccine 23:2074–2077

Curtiss RI, Cardineau GA (1990) Oral immunisation by transgenic plants. World Intellectual Property Organization. Washington University

Dus Santos MJ, Wigdorovitz A, Trono K et al (2002) A novel methodology to develop a foot and mouth disease virus (FMDV) peptide-based vaccine in transgenic plants. Vaccine 20:1141–1147

Gallichan WS, Rosenthal KL (1998) Long-term immunity and protection against herpes simplex virus type 2 in the murine female genital tract after mucosal but not systemic immunization. J Infect Dis 177:1155–1161

Gelvin SB (2003) Agrobacterium-mediated plant transformation: the biology behind the "gene-jockeying" tool. Microbiol Mol Biol Rev 67:16–37

Gleba Y, Klimyuk V, Marillonnet S (2005) Magnifection–a new platform for expressing recombinant vaccines in plants. Vaccine 23:2042–2048

Gleba Y, Klimyuk V, Marillonnet S (2007) Viral vectors for the expression of proteins in plants. Curr Opin Biotechnol 18:134–141

Goodin MM, Zaitlin D, Naidu RA et al (2008) Nicotiana benthamiana: its history and future as a model for plant-pathogen interactions. Mol Plant Microbe Interact 21:1015–1026

Hammond RW, Nemchinov LG (2009) Plant production of veterinary vaccines and therapeutics. Curr Top Microbiol Immunol 332:79–102

Hanin M, Paszkowski J (2003) Plant genome modification by homologous recombination. Curr Opin Plant Biol 6:157–162

Harandi AM, Eriksson K, Holmgren J (2003) A protective role of locally administered immunostimulatory CpG oligodeoxynucleotide in a mouse model of genital herpes infection. J Virol 77:953–962

Holmgren J, Czerkinsky C (2005) Mucosal immunity and vaccines. Nat Med 11:S45–S53

Howard JA (2004) Commercialization of plant-based vaccines from research and development to manufacturing. Anim Health Res Rev 5:243–245

Huang Z, Mason HS (2004) Conformational analysis of hepatitis B surface antigen fusions in an Agrobacterium-mediated transient expression system. Plant Biotechnol J 2:241–249

Huang Z, Chen Q, Hjelm B et al (2009) A DNA replicon system for rapid high-level production of virus-like particles in plants. Biotechnol Bioeng 103:706–714

Imaoka K, Miller CJ, Kubota M et al (1998) Nasal immunization of nonhuman primates with simian immunodeficiency virus p55gag and cholera toxin adjuvant induces Th1/Th2 help for virus-specific immune responses in reproductive tissues. J Immunol 161:5952–5958

Jiang X, Wang M, Graham DY et al (1992) Expression, self-assembly, and antigenicity of the Norwalk virus capsid protein. J Virol 66:6527–6532

Judge NA, Mason HS, O'Brien AD (2004) Plant cell-based intimin vaccine given orally to mice primed with intimin reduces time of *Escherichia coli* O157:H7 shedding in feces. Infect Immun 72:168–175

Kapusta J, Modelska A, Figlerowicz M et al (1999) A plant-derived edible vaccine against hepatitis B virus. Faseb J 13:1796–1799

Kong Q, Richter L, Yang YF et al (2001) Oral immunization with hepatitis B surface antigen expressed in transgenic plants. Proc Natl Acad Sci U S A 98:11539–11544

Kostrzak A, Cervantes-Gonzalez M, Guetard D et al (2009) Oral administration of low doses of plant-based HBsAg induced antigen-specific IgAs and IgGs in mice, without increasing levels of regulatory T cells. Vaccine 27:4798–4807

Kozlowski PA, Cu-Uvin S, Neutra MR et al (1997) Comparison of the oral, rectal, and vaginal immunization routes for induction of antibodies in rectal and genital tract secretions of women. Infect Immun 65:1387–1394

Kozlowski PA, Williams SB, Lynch RM et al (2002) Differential induction of mucosal and systemic antibody responses in women after nasal, rectal, or vaginal immunization: influence of the menstrual cycle. J Immunol 169:566–574

Kunkel E, Butcher E (2002) Homeostatic chemokines and the targeting of regional immunity. Adv Exp Med Biol 512:65–72

Lamphear BJ, Jilka JM, Kesl L et al (2004) A corn-based delivery system for animal vaccines: an oral transmissible gastroenteritis virus vaccine boosts lactogenic immunity in swine. Vaccine 22:2420–2424

Lavelle EC (2005) Generation of improved mucosal vaccines by induction of innate immunity. Cell Mol Life Sci 62:2750–2770

Lee K-Y, Kim D-H, Kang T-J et al (2006) Induction of protective immune responses against the challenge of *Actinobacillus pleuropneumoniae* by the oral administration of transgenic tobacco plant expressing ApxIIA toxin from the bacteria. FEMS Immunol Med Microbiol 48:381–389

Loza-Rubio E, Rojas E, Gomez L et al (2008) Development of an edible rabies vaccine in maize using the Vnukovo strain. Dev Biol (Basel) 131:477–482

Marillonnet S, Giritch A, Gils M et al (2004) In planta engineering of viral RNA replicons: Efficient assembly by recombination of DNA modules delivered by Agrobacterium. Proc Natl Acad Sci U S A 101:6852–6857

Mason HS, Lam DM-K, Arntzen CJ (1992) Expression of hepatitis B surface antigen in transgenic plants. Proc Natl Acad Sci U S A 89:11745–11749

Mason HS, Ball JM, Shi J-J et al (1996) Expression of Norwalk virus capsid protein in transgenic tobacco and potato and its oral immunogenicity in mice. Proc Natl Acad Sci U S A 93:5335–5340

Mason HS, Haq TA, Clements JD et al (1998) Edible vaccine protects mice against *Escherichia coli* heat-labile enterotoxin (LT): potatoes expressing a synthetic LT-B gene. Vaccine 16:1336–1343

McAleer WJ, Buynak EB, Maigetter RZ et al (1984) Human hepatitis B vaccine from recombinant yeast. Nature 307:178–180

McCluskie MJ, Weeratna RD, Davis HL (2000) Intranasal immunization of mice with CpG DNA induces strong systemic and mucosal responses that are influenced by other mucosal adjuvants and antigen distribution. Mol Med 6:867–887

Monger W, Alamillo JM, Sola I et al (2006) An antibody derivative expressed from viral vectors passively immunizes pigs against transmissible gastroenteritis virus infection when supplied orally in crude plant extracts. Plant Biotechnol J 4:623–631

Muller CP, Marquet-Blouin E, Fack F et al (2003) Immunogenic measles antigens expressed in plants: role as an edible vaccine for adults. Vaccine 21:816–819

Nagarajan T, Rupprecht CE, Dessain SK et al (2008) Human monoclonal antibody and vaccine approaches to prevent human rabies. Curr Top Microbiol Immunol 317:67–101

Neutra MR, Kozlowski PA (2006) Mucosal vaccines: the promise and the challenge. Nat Rev Immunol 6:148–158

Nochi T, Takagi H, Yuki Y et al (2007) Rice-based mucosal vaccine as a global strategy for cold-chain- and needle-free vaccination. Proc Natl Acad Sci U S A 104:10986–10991

Richter LJ, Thanavala Y, Arntzen CJ et al (2000) Production of hepatitis B surface antigen in transgenic plants for oral immunization. Nat Biotechnol 18:1167–1171

Rudin A, Riise GC, Holmgren J (1999) Antibody responses in the lower respiratory tract and male urogenital tract in humans after nasal and oral vaccination with cholera toxin B subunit. Infect Immun 67:2884–2890

Rybicki EP (2009) Plant-produced vaccines: promise and reality. Drug Discov Today 14:16–24

Sakaguchi S, Yamaguchi T, Nomura T et al (2008) Regulatory T cells and immune tolerance. Cell 133:775–787

Santi L, Huang Z, Mason H (2006) Virus-like particles production in green plants. Methods 40:66–76

Santi L, Batchelor L, Huang Z et al (2008) An efficient plant viral expression system generating orally immunogenic Norwalk virus-like particles. Vaccine 26:1846–1854

Shin SJ, Bae JL, Cho YW et al (2005) Induction of antigen-specific immune responses by oral vaccination with Saccharomyces cerevisiae expressing Actinobacillus pleuropneumoniae ApxIIA. FEMS Immunol Med Microbiol 43:155–164

Shin SJ, Shin SW, Kang ML et al (2007) Enhancement of protective immune responses by oral vaccination with Saccharomyces cerevisiae expressing recombinant Actinobacillus pleuropneumoniae ApxIA or ApxIIA in mice. J Vet Sci 8:383–392

Singh ND, Ding Y, Daniell H (2009) Chloroplast-derived vaccine antigens and biopharmaceuticals: protocols for expression, purification, or oral delivery and functional evaluation. Methods Mol Biol 483:163–192

Staats HF, Montgomery SP, Palker TJ (1997) Intranasal immunization is superior to vaginal, gastric, or rectal immunization for the induction of systemic and mucosal anti-HIV antibody responses. AIDS Res Hum Retroviruses 13:945–952

Streatfield SJ (2005) Oral hepatitis B vaccine candidates produced and delivered in plant material. Immunol Cell Biol 83:257–262

Streatfield SJ (2006) Mucosal immunization using recombinant plant-based oral vaccines. Methods 38:150–157

Streatfield SJ, Lane JR, Brooks CA et al (2003) Corn as a production system for human and animal vaccines. Vaccine 21:812–815

Tacket CO, Mason HS, Losonsky G et al (1998) Immunogenicity in humans of a recombinant bacterial antigen delivered in a transgenic potato. Nat Med 4:607–609

Tacket CO, Mason HS, Losonsky G et al (2000) Human immune responses to a novel norwalk virus vaccine delivered in transgenic potatoes. J Infect Dis 182:302–305

Tacket CO, Sztein MB, Losonsky GA et al (2003) Humoral, mucosal, and cellular immune responses to oral Norwalk virus-like particles in volunteers. Clin Immunol 108:241–247

Tacket CO, Pasetti MF, Edelman R et al (2004) Immunogenicity of recombinant LT-B delivered orally to humans in transgenic corn. Vaccine 22:4385–4389

Thanavala Y, Mahoney M, Pal S et al (2005) Immunogenicity in humans of an edible vaccine for hepatitis B. Proc Natl Acad Sci U S A 102:3378–3382

Thanavala Y, Huang Z, Mason HS (2006) Plant-derived vaccines: a look back at the highlights and a view to the challenges on the road ahead. Expert Rev Vaccines 5:249–260

Velasquez LS, Hjelm BE, Arntzen CJ, Herbst-Kralovetz MM (2010) An intranasally delivered Toll-like receptor 7 agonist elicits robust systemic and mucosal responses to Norwalk virus-like particles. Clin Vaccine Immunol 17(12):1850–1858

Webster DE, Thomas MC, Huang Z, Wesselingh SL (2005) The development of a plant-based vaccine for measles. Vaccine 23:1859–1865

Webster DE, Smith SD, Pickering RJ et al (2006) Measles virus hemagglutinin protein expressed in transgenic lettuce induces neutralising antibodies in mice following mucosal vaccination. Vaccine 24:3538–3544

Wigdorovitz A, Carrillo C, Dus Santos MJ et al (1999) Induction of a protective antibody response to foot and mouth disease virus in mice following oral or parenteral immunization with alfalfa transgenic plants expressing the viral structural protein VP1. Virology 255:347–353

Wu H, Singh NK, Locy RD et al (2004a) Expression of immunogenic VP2 protein of infectious bursal disease virus in Arabidopsis thaliana. Biotechnol Lett 26:787–792

Wu H, Singh NK, Locy RD et al (2004b) Immunization of chickens with VP2 protein of infectious bursal disease virus expressed in Arabidopsis thaliana. Avian Dis 48:663–668

Wu J, Yu L, Li L et al (2007) Oral immunization with transgenic rice seeds expressing VP2 protein of infectious bursal disease virus induces protective immune responses in chickens. Plant Biotechnol J 5:570–578

Yang CD, Liao JT, Lai CY et al (2007) Induction of protective immunity in swine by recombinant bamboo mosaic virus expressing foot-and-mouth disease virus epitopes. BMC Biotechnol 7:62

Yusibov V, Rabindran S (2008) Recent progress in the development of plant derived vaccines. Expert Rev Vaccines 7:1173–1183

Yusibov V, Hooper DC, Spitsin SV et al (2002) Expression in plants and immunogenicity of plant virus-based experimental rabies vaccine. Vaccine 20:3155–3164

Yusibov V, Rabindran S, Commandeur U et al (2006) The Potential of Plant Virus Vectors for Vaccine Production. Drugs R D 7:203

Zhang X, Buehner NA, Hutson AM et al (2006) Tomato is a highly effective vehicle for expression and oral immunization with Norwalk virus capsid protein. Plant Biotechnol J 4:419–432

Dry Powder Vaccines for Mucosal Administration: Critical Factors in Manufacture and Delivery

Sheena H. Wang, Afton L. Thompson, Anthony J. Hickey and Herman F. Staats

Abstract Dry powder vaccine formulations have proved effective for induction of systemic and mucosal immune responses. Here we review the use of dry vaccines for immunization in the respiratory tract. We discuss techniques for powder formulation, manufacture, characterization and delivery in addition to methods used for evaluation of stability and safety. We review the immunogenicity and protective efficacy of dry powder vaccines as compared to liquid vaccines delivered by mucosal or parenteral routes. Included is information on mucosal adjuvants and mucoadhesives that can be used to enhance nasal or pulmonary dry vaccines. Mucosal immunization with dry powder vaccines offers the potential to provide a needle-free and cold chain-independent vaccination strategy for the induction of protective immunity against either systemic or mucosal pathogens.

Contents

S. H. Wang · A. J. Hickey
Division of Molecular Pharmaceutics, School of Pharmacy,
University of North Carolina, Chapel Hill, NC 27599, USA

A. L. Thompson · H. F. Staats (✉)
Department of Pathology, Duke University Medical Center, Durham, NC 27710, USA
e-mail: Herman.staats@duke.edu

Current Topics in Microbiology and Immunology (2012) 354: 121–156

DOI: 10.1007/82_2011_167

Published Online: 6 August 2011

1 Introduction

1.1 The Need for Needle-Free and Cold Chain-Independent Vaccines

Most vaccines are administered in humans using the intramuscular (IM) or subcutaneous (SC) routes, which has proved effective over the years. However, the ability to immunize without needles would be desirable for several reasons. First, in developing countries, needles are frequently re-used without adequate sterilization, which contributes to the spread of blood-borne pathogens such as hepatitis B, hepatitis C and human immunodeficiency virus (HIV) (Giudice and Campbell 2006; Hutin and Chen 1999; Levine 2003). The World Health Organization (WHO) recently reported that "...each year unsafe injections [in developing countries] cause an estimated 1.3 million early deaths, a loss of 26 million years of life, and an annual burden of US $535 million in direct medical costs" (Hutin and Chen 1999). In some countries, fear of injection may cause people to avoid vaccination (Giudice and Campbell 2006; Logullo et al. 2008). Thus, the development of needle-free vaccines could dramatically reduce the transmission of disease.

Many infectious diseases are acquired in the respiratory tract (Brankston et al. 2007; Seto et al. 2003; Tellier 2006; Van Hoeven et al. 2009). Anthrax spores and other pathogens used as biological weapons are also likely to initiate infection after first contacting upper or lower respiratory tract surfaces. To generate protective immune responses at these sites, local delivery of vaccine via the nasal or pulmonary route is likely to be optimal to parenteral immunization. Immunization

Table 1 Diseases that could potentially be prevented by nasal or pulmonary vaccine delivery

Bacterial respiratory infections	Viral respiratory infections	Sexually-transmitted or blood-borne	Other
B. anthracis	Influenza	HIV/AIDS	Malaria
Streptococcus pneumoniae	Severe acute respiratory syndrome	Herpes	Tetanus
Haemophilus influenzae		Papillomavirus	Plague
Moraxella catarrhalis		Hepatitis	Alzheimer's
Neisseria meningitides		Chlamydia	West Nile virus
Bordetella pertussis			
Pseudomonas aeruginosa			Dengue
Mycobacterium tuberculosis			
Diphtheria			

in the nasal cavity or lung has been a topic of research for many years with promising results regarding the induction of antigen-specific mucosal immune responses and protective immunity (Alpar et al. 2001; Baumann 2008; Hornick and Eigelsbach 1966; Kasel et al. 1968; Lu and Hickey 2007; Mann et al. 2009; Oliveira et al. 2007; Sullivan et al. 2006; Waldman et al. 1969; Wigley et al. 1969). Importantly, immunization in the respiratory tract can produce strong immune responses in the systemic compartment and in the distal reproductive tract mucosa (Porgador et al. 1997; Staats et al. 1994, 1996, 1997, 2001; Staats and McGhee 1996; Staats and Ennis 1999). Therefore, nasal or pulmonary immunization could be employed for practical mass vaccination against systemic diseases or sexually transmitted infections (Table 1) without safety concerns related to the use and disposal of needles (Clements et al. 2004; Hutin and Chen 1999; Lu and Hickey 2007). Recently, Flumist™, a live-attenuated influenza vaccine that is delivered nasally (Ambrose et al. 2011), was approved by the Food and Drug Administration (FDA), demonstrating that safe and efficacious nasal vaccines can be developed for use in humans.

Most vaccines require constant refrigeration ("cold chain") (Baker et al. 2002; Bhuyan 2000; Kendal et al. 1997) since high temperatures can aggregate or denature protein components (Wang 1999). Lack of refrigeration is often responsible for reduced vaccine immunogenicity, and it results in significant vaccine wastage (Baker et al. 2002; Gold et al. 1998; Setia et al. 2002). Vaccines that maintain potency in the absence of refrigeration would decrease wastage and increase the number of vaccinated people in developing countries. It is unlikely that vaccination of an entire population against bioterrorist agents would be cost-effective (Zohrabian et al. 2006). Therefore, vaccines for select agents are likely to be stockpiled and administered first to health care providers and others at greatest risk at the time of a suspected exposure. For efficacy under these conditions, a vaccine must maintain stability when stored for long periods, and it must quickly induce protective immunity.

The most common method used to stabilize vaccine components is to prepare them in a dry powder form, which reduces mobility of the macromolecules and eliminates degradation pathways such as hydrolysis (Wang 2000). In addition, dry powder formulations are superior to liquid formulations in sterility, cost effectiveness and lack of cold chain requirement. Dry powder vaccination in the respiratory tract is not a novel concept. In 1925, Sewall reviewed nasal immunization and mentioned nasal delivery of powders containing killed cultures of bacilli of typhoid, cholera or dysentery for the induction of resistance to bacilli (Sewall 1925). Evidence for the utility of dry powder formulations is found in their application for vaccine delivery by the nasal, pulmonary, epidermal (Chen et al. 2002; Dean and Chen 2004) and oral (Lazzell et al. 1984) routes. The interest in generating local mucosal immunity and the stability of powders has renewed interest in dry powder vaccine delivery in the respiratory tract. Here we discuss the formulation, manufacturing, characterization, stability and delivery strategies of dry powder vaccines in addition to their immunogenicity when delivered by a mucosal or parenteral route.

1.2 Mucosal Adjuvants and Bioadhesives

Mucosal delivery of protein immunogens in the absence of adjuvant generally induces tolerance or low-to-undetectable antigen-specific immune responses (Czerkinsky et al. 1999; Xiao and Link 1997). Hence, many mucosal vaccines will require an adjuvant (Freytag and Clements 2005). The most widely used experimental mucosal adjuvant is cholera toxin (CT) (Elson 1996). However, CT and other enterotoxin-based adjuvants (Chen et al. 2002; Freytag and Clements 2005) cannot be safely administered in the human nasal cavity due to their propensity to cause Bell's palsy (Couch 2004; Lewis et al. 2009; Mutsch et al. 2004). In an attempt to develop non-toxic adjuvants for mucosal vaccines, our laboratory has determined that the cytokines interleukin (IL)-1α, IL-1β, IL-12, IL-18 or granulocyte–macrophage colony stimulating factor (GM-CSF) or small-molecule mast cell activators can be used as effective as CT for adjuvant mucosal vaccines (Bradney et al. 2002; Egan et al. 2004; McGowen et al. 2009; McLachlan et al. 2008; Staats et al. 2001; Staats and Ennis 1999).

Cells of the innate immune system recognize pathogen-derived molecules using Toll-like receptors (TLR). The ligands for TLR2, TLR3, TLR4, TLR5 and TLR9 include microbial lipopeptides, double-stranded RNA, lipopolysaccharide, flagellin and cytosine-to-guanine oligodeoxynucleotides (CpG ODN), respectively (Lien and Ingalls 2002; Modlin 2002). Signaling pathways triggered by TLR binding induce the maturation of immature dendritic cells (DC), with consequent increases in surface expression of MHC and costimulatory molecules (CD80, CD86) and synthesis of proinflammatory cytokines IL-1, IL-6 and Tumor Necrosis Factor-α by these cells (Barton and Medzhitov 2002). Since mature DC are the most potent antigen-presenting cells (APC) for activation of na T cells (Jenkins et al. 2001;

Reid et al. 2000), it is not surprising that TLR ligands exhibit adjuvant activity when co-administered with antigens.

The TLR ligands that have been tested in human vaccine studies include CpG ODN and monophosphoryl lipid A (MPL), ligands for TLR9 and TLR4, respectively (Daubenberger 2007; Jiang and Koganty 2003; Persing et al. 2002; Seya et al. 2006). Monphosphoryl lipid A was recently approved for IM administration in the European Union (Sesardic and Dobbelaer 2004) and Australia (Casella and Mitchell 2008). In animals, MPL has proved successful as a mucosal adjuvant, and its adjuvant activity has been linked to activation of APC (Freytag and Clements 2005). Unlike alum, MPL is a T helper cell type 1 (Th1)-inducing adjuvant, although the degree of this response is dependent on the antigen co-administered and the route of delivery (Casella and Mitchell 2008). The CpG adjuvant is also a potent Th1-inducer (Tengvall et al. 2005; Weeratna et al. 2001). Although CpG has not yet been licensed for use in humans, it has been used for more than a decade in animal studies (Klinman et al. 2004; Peng et al. 2001; Teloni et al. 1994; Xu et al. 2008) and more recently, in several clinical trials (Cooper et al. 2005, 2004a, b; Halperin et al. 2003). Although CpG has primarily been used as an intradermal or IM adjuvant, it has demonstrated activity as a mucosal adjuvant in animals (Boyaka et al. 2003; McCluskie and Davis 1999; Uddowla et al. 2007). Both CpG and MPL have been utilized as adjuvants in nasally administered dry powder vaccines (see anthrax vaccine section below).

The immunogenicity of mucosal vaccines can be further increased through formulation with products that enhance vaccine internalization. For example, antigen-specific immune responses have been augmented by supplementing vaccines with carboxymethylcellulose (Hamajima et al. 1998), chitosan (Mills et al. 2003), poloxamer/polyethylene oxide (Park et al. 2003), poloxamers and polycarbophil (Oh et al. 2003), sucrose acetate isobutyrate (Nally et al. 2000) or esterified hyaluronic acid microspheres (Singh et al. 2001). These substances typically act as bioadhesives and function to adhere the vaccine to the mucosal surface of the host. We have determined that the addition of hydroxypropylmethylcellulose to a liquid nasal vaccine can augment the immunogenicity of HIV-1 peptide immunogens (Nordone et al. 2006).

Chitosan stands out as an additive for dry powder vaccine formulations. Chitosan is a positively charged deacetylation product of chitin that was originally described in 1859 (van der Lubben et al. 2001). It has been reviewed in depth elsewhere (Kurita 2006; van der Lubben et al. 2001). Chitosan is a strong mucoadhesive (van der Lubben et al. 2001) as its positive charge, carried on an amino group, facilitates interaction with negatively charged portions of mucosal epithelial cell surfaces. This results in a loosening of tight junctions, which allows large molecules or particles to cross the mucosal barrier. As such, chitosan is a valuable absorption enhancer, and it has been shown to increase the absorption of several drugs (van der Lubben et al. 2001). There is also evidence that chitosan can act as an adjuvant, increasing cytokine production and macrophage activation (Kurita 2006; van der Lubben et al. 2001). However, this activity seems to be dependent on the degree of acetylation, with less acetylated chitosan increasing cellular and humoral immune responses, as well as cytokine production. The chitosan formulation also plays a role. Phagocytosable chitosan induces macrophage activation and cytokine production, while fully soluble chitosan does not (van der Lubben et al. 2001). Chitosan is extremely useful for dry powder vaccines as it can act as a mucoadhesive, absorption enhancer and adjuvant, all of which enhance the immune response.

2 Dry Powder Vaccine Manufacturing

Dry powder preparations are suitable for protein subunit vaccines, whole virus vaccines and DNA vaccines. There are several potential methods available to prepare powder formulations, and their suitability for biopharmaceutical preparation and respiratory delivery are discussed below.

2.1 Spray Drying and Freeze Drying

Historically, several methods have been used to prepare dry powder vaccine formulations: spray drying, freeze drying (FD) (lyophilization) and spray-freeze drying (SFD). Spray drying (SD) involves atomization of the liquid feed into small droplets and then drying by feeding it through hot gas. One advantage of SD is that process parameters can be controlled to engineer particles with different physical properties. The particle size prepared by this method is often in the range of 1–10 microns (μm), which is suitable for pulmonary delivery (Maa et al. 1999; Shoyele and Cawthorne 2006; Weers et al. 2007). Spray drying may be more suitable for conventional small-molecule pharmaceutics than vaccines because the high temperature required for drying may induce heat stress, which can cause crystallization of the excipient or denaturation/aggregation of bioactive molecules, resulting in loss of adjuvant activity and/or antigen immunogenicity.

FD has been the most convenient and popular drying method for biopharmaceuticals (Wang 2000). In this method, an aqueous solution containing biomaterial is first frozen, followed by removal of water by sublimation under reduced pressure. Several process parameters including freezing rate and drying steps need to be controlled to ensure product integrity (Cameron 1997; Wang 2000). Different sugars/polyols (see Table 2) are often added in bulk as stabilizers to prevent potential damage during freezing, drying and storage. Disaccharides, such as trehalose, have been used with whole inactivated influenza virus during the FD preparation of a nasal dry powder influenza vaccine (Huang et al. 2004) as well as an anthrax vaccine (Jiang et al. 2006). The mechanism of stabilization provided by the bulking agent can be two fold. Upon lyophilization, bioactive macromolecules are incorporated inside a glass state of the sugar matrix. This reduces the molecular mobility of each molecule (Duddu et al. 1997; Hagen et al. 1995) and provides a physical barrier between molecules (Molina et al. 2004; Wang 2000), thereby

Table 2 Excipients and the stabilizing effect for solid state biopharmaceuticals preparation and storage

Common excipients/bulking agents		Possible advantages	Possible disadvantages
Polyols	Mannitol	Water replacement property during drying	Low T_g, high concentration of mannitol display increased crystallization tendency, same is true at elevated temperature and moisture level
	Sorbitol		Low T_g
Non-reducing sugars	Trehalose	High T_g, around 120°C, disaccharide with a good water replacement property, non-reducing sugar	Formation of fused and sticky agglomerates
	Sucrose	Good water replacement property for drying	Fairly hygroscopic
	Inulin	High T_g, low crystallization rate, low number of reducing groups	Bulkiness, steric hindrance, lacks a good water replacement property
	Dextran		
Reducing sugars	Fructose		Reducing sugars, potential for Maillard reaction and causes protein glycation, moisture-induced crystallization
	Glucose (dextrose)		
	Lactose	Safety: FDA-approved excipients for inhalation	
	Maltodextrin		
	Maltose		
Polymers	poly(D-lactide-co-glycolide) (PLG)	High-matrix T_g	Requires the use of organic solvents
	PLGA		
Amino acids	Glycine	Hydrophobic properties that benefit the powder flow property	
	Isoleucine		
Surfactant	Tween80	Prevent protein aggregation	
	Brij 30		
Salts	PBS	Provide a buffering effect during freezing or drying	
	HBS		

preventing aggregation and denaturation during the process. Furthermore, the hydroxyl groups on the sugar molecules can replace H-bonding interaction provided by water molecules, which helps maintain the tertiary structure of the macromolecules as water is removed (Carpenter and Crowe 1989). However, freezing stress introduced during this process should be considered. The large ice/liquid interface created during FD can cause protein adsorption that result in conformational changes and loss of immunogenicity. Moreover, as the solute concentration increases during freezing, there is an acceleration of the reaction kinetics, which can increase hydrolytic degradation. Changes in ionic strength can further destabilize the vaccine (Pikal 1999; Pikal et al. 1991; Wang 2000).

Buffer selection for the lyophilization process is also important. Freezing-induced pH changes can be dependent on buffer type and concentration, freezing rate and the presence of sugar and other excipients (Amorij et al. 2007; Croyle et al. 1998; Eriksson et al. 2003; Gomez et al. 2001; Orii and Morita 1977; Van Den Berg and Rose 1959). The pH will normally drop to a more acidic value during lyophilization, and the shift can be as large as 3 pH units. This means that the selection of buffer for lyophilization is crucial for maintaining the integrity of pH-sensitive bioactive macromolecules. Amorij et al. (2007) reported a conformational change of influenza virus hemagglutinin (HA) protein during freezing in phosphate-buffered saline (PBS) due to a change to an acidic pH (which makes HA more prone to hydrolysis by trypsin), whereas the pH shift in HEPES-buffered saline was smaller and the resulting freeze-dried powder was more stable.

FD does not have the flexibility required for particle engineering. After lyophilization, further milling and mixing is necessary to break up the lyophilized 'cake' and reduce the particle size for enhancing the dispersion properties of the powder for nasal application (Klas et al. 2008). This process introduces mechanical forces, which could potentially cause a loss of activity.

2.2 *Spray-Freeze Drying*

SFD is a relatively new process for the production of dry powder biopharmaceuticals that combines conventional SD and FD. In the SFD process, atomizing nitrogen gas with a fixed back pressure is used to force the aqueous solution containing the active ingredients through a spray nozzle that produces small droplets of liquid that are collected in a container with liquid nitrogen. The large surface area of the liquid droplets and their direct contact with the freezing medium leads to rapid vitrification, which prevents possible phase separation. Once the liquid nitrogen has evaporated, the frozen droplets are dried under a vacuum. The large surface area of the frozen particles allows rapid drying, which is more energy efficient than FD. SFD frequently produces porous spherical particles that are larger than those produced by SD (Maa et al. 1999). Spray-freeze-dried particles rarely require further particle size reduction and can either be used directly or after blending with other vaccine components. When SFD is carried out under optimized conditions, by adjusting and selecting process parameters including nitrogen flow rate, liquid feed rate and atomization pressure, particles with desired sizes and in narrow ranges are produced and may be used directly for nasal application. For example, SFD powders for nasal influenza vaccination have been prepared with a target size of approximately 25 μm for the rat nasal cavity (Garmise et al. 2007).

2.3 Vacuum Drying and Supercritical Drying

Other techniques, such as vacuum drying and supercritical drying, provide alternative methods that are to some extent complimentary to the above methods for dry powder preparation. According to the water phase diagram, the boiling point of water is lowered at high pressure. Vacuum drying takes advantage of this physical phenomenon and dries biopharmaceuticals at room temperature, which eliminates the freeze stress and atomization stress associated with FD and SFD. However, this process may require extended times, and it may increase the risk of sugar glass transition to a rubbery state.

Supercritical drying or supercritical fluid (SCF) drying is a relatively new method (Jovanovic et al. 2004; Kompella and Koushik 2001) that involves the use of fluid that is in supercritical (SC) state with both pressure and temperature above the critical pressure (P_c) and critical temperature (T_c). Supercritical CO_2 (SC-CO_2) has the most desirable properties for pharmaceutical application (Amorij et al. 2008). The drying process can be operated according to two principles. The vaccine solution can be sprayed into SC-CO_2 and dried via an anti-solvent effect. Alternatively, SC-CO_2 can be dissolved in the vaccine solution and then together sprayed to atmospheric conditions. Rapid expansion of CO_2 breaks the solution into small droplets, which can be efficiently dried by a flow of nitrogen. This process can be operated at moderate temperature above the T_c (31.5°C) of CO_2 and it can shorten the duration of drying when compared to FD and SFD (Jovanovic et al. 2004).

3 Nasal Residence Time and Mucoadhesives

Mucociliary clearance of the nasal cavity is an important defense mechanism against inhaled pathogens. Cilia, which line the nasal epithelium, are covered by a thin layer of mucus, and beat rapidly in a coordinated fashion, propelling particles trapped in the mucus layer to the posterior nasopharynx. In humans, the average clearance rate is about 8 mm per minute, with a normal clearance half-life of approximately 15–20 min (Soane et al. 1999). Mucociliary clearance presents one of the major challenges in nasal drug/vaccine delivery. The nasal residence time may be increased by the addition of mucoadhesives, and this is considered a key strategy to improve the performance of products delivered by the nasal route. When a dry powder formulation is delivered to the nasal cavity, local dehydration of the mucus may occur, thereby reducing the ciliary beat frequency and

Table 3 Mucoadhesives and mucoadhesion mechanisms adapted from Smart (2005)

First generation mucoadhesives		*Possible mucoadhesion mechanisms*
Natural polymers	Chitosan	Positive charge interacts with negative charge on sialic acid in mucin
	Sodium alginate	Hydrogen bonding
	Cellulose and its derivatives	Hydrogen bonding
Synthetic polymers	polyacrylic acid and its derivatives	Hydrogen bonding, physical entanglement, dehydration
Second generation mucoadhesives		
Modification to first generation materials	Addition of thiol functional group	Disulfide bond formation within the polymer or between the polymer and mucin
	Copolymer with ethyl hexyl acrylate	Increase hydrophobicity, reduce polymer hydration to allow polymer-mucus interaction
	Grafting PEG	Promote interpenetration
Novel materials	Poloxomer: Pluronics	Thermal induced phase transition
	Amino acid: Dihydroxyphenylalanine	Found in mussel adhesive protein
	Glyceryl monooleate	Forms liquid crystalline phase with water
	Glycoproteins: Lectins	Weak (secondary) interaction with specific sugar residue

increasing the local residence time. To prolong nasal residence time, mucoadhesive compounds such as natural and synthetic polymers may be included in the formulation. Recently, mucoadhesive compounds and their possible mechanisms of action have been reviewed (Smart 2005) (see Table 3).

First generation mucoadhesives have been studied extensively since 1970. However, they may be associated with significant formulation challenges such as high viscosity, pH sensitivity, or low concentration in aqueous solutions (Illum et al. 2001). Second generation mucoadhesive materials were developed to address the issues associated with their physicochemical properties. These molecules interact with mucus in a number of ways. Chitosan has been widely used in liquid formulations or prepared as microparticulate delivery systems to enhance nasal bioavailability. The salt form of chitosan is positively charged in solution, which has a strong electrostatic interaction with the negatively charged sialic acid in mucin (Illum et al. 2001). Powder formulations of trehalose and chitosan have also been prepared by (Huang et al. 2004) for a nasal influenza vaccine, which elicited significantly greater serum HA inhibition titers than vaccine formulated with trehalose alone, and anti-HA titers comparable to those induced by IM injection (Huang et al. 2004). Starch and Carbopol (polyacrylic acid) mixtures have been shown to enhance the bioavailability of nasally administered insulin in rabbits (Callens et al. 2003; Callens and Remon 2000; Pringels et al. 2006), and this mixture has been used to develop an influenza vaccine for nasal delivery (Coucke et al. 2009). A more rapid development of anti-HA IgG antibodies has been demonstrated with a higher proportion of Carbopol in the mixture (Coucke et al. 2009).

There are three important characteristics in the mucoadhesion scenario: the mucoadhesive compound, the nasal mucosa and the antigen. The residence time of the antigen is enhanced through interaction with the mucoadhesive compound. It may be speculated that the antigen release profile from the delivery system will play a role in the immune response elicited. However, the relationship between the antigen release rate and antigen absorption window is poorly understood. In some studies, there was no correlation between the in vitro antigen release profile and the in vivo immune response; similar immune responses were detected when comparing delivery systems that had a rapid and extended in vitro antigen release (Amidi et al. 2006; Spiers et al. 2000).

4 Characterization of Antigen/Adjuvant Stability in Dry Powder Preparations

Dry powder vaccine development encompasses a series of processes in which the biologically active component is incorporated into pharmaceutical ingredients to become the final vaccine product. The structural and functional activity of the antigen is a prerequisite for a successful dosage form. It is important to monitor the structural and functional integrity of the antigen and adjuvant during manufacturing and storage. In this section, we focus on proteinaceous antigens, though the methods may also apply to other macromolecular entities utilized as vaccine antigens.

4.1 Structural Integrity

It is known that the structural properties of proteins are closely correlated to their biological activity and stability. Freezing, drying, pH shifts and interaction with excipients can all cause structural changes to vaccine components (Chang et al. 1996a, b; Gomez et al. 2001; Kueltzo et al. 2008; Li et al. 1996), which might lead to aggregation and degradation. While more advanced biophysical methods are now available to study protein structure or interactions (Shriver 2009; Uversky and Permyakov 2007), basic spectroscopic techniques such as circular dichroism (CD) and Fourier Transform infrared (FTIR) spectroscopy are most often utilized due to ease and simplicity of performance. These techniques provide a global view of the protein secondary structure and may be sufficient for discriminating structural changes caused by the manufacturing process and storage. Circular dichroism spectroscopy is a form of light absorption spectroscopy that measures the difference in the absorbance of right- and left-circularly polarized light due to asymmetric components in the protein structure, such as the peptide bond and the amino acid side chains. Protein secondary structure, in terms of protein backbone conformation, is most sensitive in the far-UV region (190–250 nm), where the peptide bonds have dominant contributions. The CD spectrum is obtained for 0.2–0.5 mg/ml samples of protein in solution, while maintaining the total UV absorbance of the cell, buffer and protein at less than one. Amorij et al. (2007) employed CD to investigate the conformational changes of HA during freezing and FD. The CD spectra of HA had a negative absorption in the far-UV region, and the intensity of the absorption was lower for HA exposed to freezing, whereas freeze drying induced a more substantial loss of negative absorption that can be attributed to the conformational change of an α-helix to a more β-sheet structure (Amorij et al. 2007; Luykx et al. 2004). In the same report, CD was utilized to demonstrate that the structure of HA can be stabilized by the addition of sugars, such as trehalose and inulin, to the freeze-drying mixture (Amorij et al. 2007). Circular dichroism can also be used to monitor the physical stability of protein immunogens at different pH and temperatures, and it can aid in the screening of stabilizers and excipients (Jiang et al. 2006). Circular dichroism does not give absolute structural information, but different secondary structure contents can be estimated with the selection of reference proteins using computational analysis (Sreerama and Woody 2000, 2004a, b).

Fourier Transform infrared spectroscopy can be done with samples in either the liquid or solid state. Like CD spectra, similar information can be derived from FTIR spectroscopy. The FTIR technique is based on the sample absorption of electromagnetic energy at the infrared region where molecules vibrate and rotate at discrete energy levels. The basic structural repeat of a protein is the peptide (amide) bond. Different vibration modes of amide bonds give rise to characteristic absorption bands in different regions of the infrared spectrum. The most intensive absorption is the amide I band (1,600–1,700 cm^{-1}), which originates mainly from the carbonyl stretching of the amide group. The carbonyl group is prone to hydrogen bonding and thus is directly related to the protein backbone conformation. Different secondary structure content can be obtained through analysis of the amide I region. Schüle et al. (2007) used FTIR to study the secondary structure of IgG before and after spray drying. No major change was observed for the reconstituted IgG powder, which was consistent with CD results (Schule et al. 2007). Analysis of the IR absorbance of the spray-dried solid IgG using attenuated total reflectance (ATR) FTIR indicated an increase in the β-sheet elements, which has been recognized as a favored conformation in a dehydrated state (Prestrelski et al. 1993). The structural change appeared to be reversible upon rehydration. The ATR-FTIR technique employs novel sample preparation method, which allows liquid or solid sample to be loaded directly onto the surface of an optical dense crystal, where the IR beam can be directed through the crystal at a certain angle to create reflectance on the surface, which generates an evanescent wave on the surface. The evanescent wave penetrates into the sample in close contact to the surface and, as a result, is attenuated and altered due to sample absorption in the IR region. This technique requires only a small sample (as little as one drop) and permits fast analysis without potassium bromide processing. Multiple reflections of the IR beam dramatically increase the optical path and sensitivity on a small quantity of sample. Facilitated by developments in data processing, FTIR and CD have become robust methods for protein structure analysis. These methods are complementary and can be used together to ensure accuracy in the analysis.

4.2 Aggregation Detection

Aggregation may occur at various stages throughout vaccine formulation, storage and transportation. It has been a major concern and challenge in liquid vaccine formulations and should be closely monitored for dry powder vaccines. Although CD and FTIR are the most sensitive techniques for detection of protein secondary structural changes, they may not always be sensitive to the different aggregation states of a protein (Hawe et al. 2009; Schule et al. 2007). This may be explained by the presence of small quantities of aggregates or by unfolding that occurs in some areas and may affect tertiary structure but not secondary structure (Fink 1995; Mahler et al. 2005). Depending on the nature of the aggregates, different analytical techniques are available to detect, characterize and quantify them (Mahler et al. 2009). The simplest method is based on the concept of Rayleigh scattering, which requires UV measurements of the turbidity or opalescence of a protein solution at optical densities (OD) around 340–360 nm and at 550 nm (Mahler et al. 2005). By measuring the OD at 360 nm, Jiang et al. compared the aggregation levels of recombinant anthrax protective antigen (PA) in different trehalose concentrations and identified stabilizing excipients (Jiang et al. 2006).

Sodium dodecyl (lauryl) sulfate–polyacrylamide gel electrophoresis chromatography (SDS–PAGE) is another method that separates protein based on its size and can resolve protein content on a microgram scale. It is the most useful for detection of covalently linked aggregates or SDS non-dissociable aggregates. Jiang et al. demonstrated the retention of rPA integrity during the SFD process using reducing and non-reducing conditions (Jiang et al. 2006). For SDS–PAGE, protein samples must be heated at high temperatures, which might introduce artifacts due to dissolution of existing aggregates or formation of new aggregates, as in the case of membrane proteins (Thomas and McNamee 1990). Alternatively, Native-PAGE involves preparing samples under mild conditions without heating or addition of the SDS denaturizing agent. Proteins may be separated using their inherent charge or by addition of the negatively charged protein-binding Coomassie Brilliant Blue G-250 dye (Schagger and von Jagow 1991). The migration of a protein will not only depend on its size but also on its shape and hydrodynamic radius, so the band location with respect to the molecular weight marker might not reflect its true size except for globular proteins.

Size exclusion chromatography (SEC) or gel filtration is essential for protein purification. This method can be coupled with high-performance liquid chromatography (HP-SEC) for increased selectivity and efficiency in separation. Buffer type, pH and the ionic strength of the mobile phase need to be carefully selected to limit the introduction of artifacts. The detection method can be UV, light scattering, fluorescence or mass spectrum with increased sensitivity and accuracy. Hawe et al. (2009) quantified aggregate formation using HP-SEC, and their results demonstrated that the heat stress during SD induced more aggregation compared to freeze thawing. Using a combination of techniques, further analysis showed the different nature of the aggregates. Freeze thawing tended to produce a greater proportion of aggregates in the μm size range, whereas heating produced more structurally perturbed aggregates, which were evidenced by CD and ATR-FTIR. Furthermore, the shape and morphology of the aggregation can be closely examined by microscopic methods such as TEM and AFM (McAllister et al. 2005), providing understanding of the causes and pathways of aggregation with the aim of better controlling protein aggregation and ensuring successful products.

4.3 *Functional Stability*

Instrumental analyses (as described above) of the antigen after powder formulation can provide quick and general information on the stability. However, it is important to confirm that the antigen or adjuvant maintains its functional activity (potency). The functional stability of the bioactive component of the antigen and adjuvant can be tested with various biological assays in vitro using reconstituted powder, e.g., macrophage toxicity assay for rPA activity (Boyaka et al. 2003; Cui and Sloat 2006; Staats et al. 2007), hemagglutination titer for HA (Schild et al. 1975; Wood et al. 1977). It is very important to monitor the effects of the bulking agent (sugar), mucoadhesives and excipients on the in vitro activity of the antigen. A well-designed in vitro biological assay gives definitive information on the potency of the antigen or adjuvant after being prepared and stored as a dry powder. However, biological assays may be more time consuming and highly variable. A practical approach would be to establish a quantitative correlation between the structural activity characterization and in vitro biological performance so that the former can be used to monitor stability.

5 Pharmaceutical Characterization of Dry Powder Vaccines

It is very important to characterize and control the pharmaceutical properties of powder formulations to achieve a successful and reproducible delivery of dry vaccine components. Particle size, bulk density and device-associated parameters such as spray pattern and plume geometry are the most important variables that affect powder deposition. These factors and those important for powder stability are discussed below.

5.1 *Particle Size*

Particle size distribution is one of the most important parameters that dictates the performance of dry powder inhalation (Telko and Hickey 2005) and nasal products. However, the requirements for nasal sprays are less stringent and not well established (US Department of Health and Human Services, Food and Drug

Administration, and Center for Drug Evaluation and Research 2002). In general, particles designed for nasal delivery should be large enough to impact in the nasal cavity with minimal deposition in the pulmonary airway. It is believed that particles greater than 10 μm localize in the upper respiratory tract, those less than 5 μm are inhaled, and those less than 0.5 μm are exhaled (Ugwoke et al. 2001). There are few descriptions of the particle size properties of dry powder nasal vaccines used in animals. A D_{50} (volume median diameter) of 37 μm was reported for influenza vaccination in rats (Huang et al. 2004), a FD mixture of Amioca® starch/Carbopol® 947P with a D_{50} of approximately 60 μm was used for influenza vaccination in rabbits (Coucke et al. 2009) and D_{50} of roughly 50 and 70 μm were reported, respectively, for FD and SFD anthrax powder vaccines delivered to rabbits (Mikszta et al. 2005). Mostly notably, (Garmise et al. 2007) prepared dry powder particles under optimized conditions of SFD, which produced particles with a target volume median diameter of 26.9 μm for influenza vaccination in rats.

Deposition in the human nasal cavity has been characterized with nasal spray devices using nasal airway replicas (Cheng et al. 2001), silicone human nose models (Pringels et al. 2006) or a computational fluid dynamics (CFD) model of human nasal passages (Kimbell et al. 2007). General findings in these studies are that large particles (50–60 μm) tend to deposit mainly in the anterior region of the nose with a small proportion reaching the turbinate or nasopharynx, while smaller particles, such as 20 μm, better penetrate beyond the nasal valve.

The anatomy of the nose and the site of action should be considered before selecting a size range for nasal or pulmonary dry powder vaccines. The nasal cavity can anatomically be segregated into five different regions: nasal vestibule, atrium, respiratory area, olfactory region and the nasopharynx (Arora et al. 2002). The respiratory region, including the inferior turbinate, middle turbinate and superior turbinate, is the most permeable region due to its large surface area and rich vasculature. This has been the target site for nasal drug delivery. However, the site of action for nasally delivered vaccines in humans is believed to be toward the back of the nasal cavity and includes the Waldeyer's ring (Brandtzaeg 2003; Davis 2001). Two types of deposition were described for nasal uptake of insulin powder (Pringels et al. 2006), and these may also be the pathways utilized in antigen delivery. Direct deposition in the nasopharynx region can be limited given that the powder has to pass the narrow nasal valve and the highly humid and structured turbinate region. It is more likely that antigen is brought to the nasopharynx by mucociliary clearance. The site and pattern of powder deposition in the nasal cavity can lead to different biologic or pharmacologic outcomes as evidenced by studies with nasal insulin dry powders where the bioavailability of insulin increased with anterior deposition of the formulation (Pringels et al. 2006). Similarly, it is reasonable to predict that the location of particle deposition with dry powder vaccines might have a significant influence on the overall immune response elicited. However, this hypothesis is yet to be tested. It is important to understand the diversity in the anatomy and physiology of different animal species when designing the study and interpreting the results (Harkema et al. 2006; Ugwoke et al. 2001). Extrapolation to human situations can become complicated.

5.2 Bulk Density

Bulk density (the density of powder without tapping) is another variable that may affect dispersion and therefore, deposition of the powder. Pringels et al. (2006) reported that the plume pattern from a powder device is influenced by bulk density. However, no effect on the bioavailability of insulin was observed. Garmise et al. (2006) reported the bulk density of SFD trehalose powder to be 0.26 mg/mm^3, and a similar bulk density (0.12–0.18 mg/mm^3 depending on the solid fraction) was reported by Pringels et al. (2006) for a FD mixture of Amioca® starch/Carbopol® 947P. Bulk density and other powder properties such as tap density (the density after tapping), static angle of repose and specific surface area are indicative of surface properties of the powder that can influence flow properties (Garmise et al. 2007) and dispersion behavior. These should be closely monitored to ensure the performance of the final product.

5.3 Particle Sizing Techniques

Laser diffraction (LD) is a widely used particle sizing technique in aerosol development, and it is rapidly becoming a standard method in the pharmaceutical industry for inhalation and nasal formulations (Mitchell et al. 2006). Laser diffraction can measure a wide size range (0.5–1000 μm) and provides information on the volume equivalent diameter. However, deviation might occur with the presence of non-spherical particles in the dry powder products, since the assumption of spherical particles in the algorithm is invalid. In addition, the diameter measured by LD is not directly related to the particle volume or surface. Thus, the size measured may not represent primary particle size but rather the size of aggregates. Complementary techniques, such as scanning electron microscopy (SEM) are often used in conjunction with LD, which are useful for determining primary particle size, shape and morphology.

While the particle size of nasal dry powders is often determined by LD, the most appropriate measure of aerosol particle size is the aerodynamic diameter (D_{ae}), which combines particle density and shape factored into a measure of the particle dynamic behavior, and which can lead to important information on particle deposition. Since dry powders produced by SFD and FD are often porous particles with a low density, they often have a smaller D_{ae} compared to particles in the same volume produced by other methods. It is known that even for particles with D_{ae} up to 20 μm, as much as 10% of the particle mass is able to escape the nasal cavity and deposit in the lungs, an undesirable outcome for nasal products (Bates et al. 1966). It is important to characterize the aerodynamic size of the dry powder formulation to ensure that the minimum quantity of respirable particles appears in the product. Conventional Andersen cascade impaction (CI) is an ideal technique for sizing pulmonary aerosols. However, this method does not cover the entire size range that has the potential to enter the lungs. A modified CI with a reduced flow rate was developed by Garmise and Hickey (2008), which extended the upper limit of the size range to 16.5 μm and is more suitable for the characterization of nasal products.

5.4 Delivery Device and Related Parameters

Nasal dry powders can be delivered via passive and active systems. Passive systems require patients to sniff (inhale through the nose) to deliver the powder. In contrast, for an active system, dry powder delivery is driven by a flow of pressured air, which passes through the container and carries the powder into the nasal cavity. Most devices used in animals are active devices. In a nasal vaccination study for anthrax, a Valois Monopowder device (Valois Pharmaceutical Division, Le Vaudreuil, France) was employed to deliver 10 mg of powder to the rabbit nasal cavity (Klas et al. 2008). In a separate study, a syringe containing 1 ml compressed air was used to deliver 10 mg of influenza vaccine powder through polyethylene tubes (Medisize, Hillegom, The Netherlands) into each nostril of rabbits (Coucke et al. 2009). The Monopowder device has also been used in a clinical study of diphtheria vaccine (McNeela et al. 2004). A similar device has been developed by BD Technologies that includes a housing unit for a powder-filled capsule at the end of the syringe instead of polyethylene tube. Upon depressing the syringe plunger, the compressed air will rupture the capsule film and deliver the powder through the diffuser (Huang et al. 2004). The diffuser can be modified to fit the narrow nasal passages of different animal models, such as rabbits (Mikszta et al. 2005) and rats (Huang et al. 2004).

As mentioned, the deposition of the dry powder is very important in nasal vaccine delivery, which is not only affected by the inherent properties of the powder, but also affected by the device used. Device-associated parameters such as spray pattern and plume geometry (i.e., plume width, plume length, spray cone angle, and spray velocity) are often characterized for nasal spray products, as required by the FDA. Spray pattern looks at the shape and the cross section of the plume at a specified distance from the spray nozzle. Experimental data on nasal sprays with nasal casts showed that larger spray angle of 60–70° resulted in an increased deposition in the anterior region, whereas reducing the spray angle to 30 or 35° leads to a more posterior deposition (Cheng et al. 2001; Newman et al. 1987; Pringels et al. 2006). Similar findings were implicated in a powder study by Pringles et al., where the spray pattern of the powder delivered through the polyethylene tube was examined (Pringels et al. 2006). In a separate study using a computational fluid dynamic model of the human nasal cavity, (Kimbell et al. 2007) simulated 48 different spray conditions with 8 different spray variables based on 18 different commercially available nasal spray devices. The authors predicted the best nasal valve penetration condition as a particle size of 20 μm and spray velocity of 1 m/sec with the spray nozzle 1 cm from the nose and a gentle inspiratory airflow at a larger spray angle of 79° (Kimbell et al. 2007). This is, however, somewhat contradictory to the experimental findings described above.

Nasal dry powder formulation development is still a relatively new area and little has been done in terms of characterization of deposition from nasal dry powder devices, which should be emphasized in future studies. A few experimental studies looked at patient variables such as inhaler orientation (Newman et al. 1987), head position (Bateman et al. 2002) and inspiratory flow (Newman et al. 1994), which appeared to have no significant effect on spray distribution or patterns.

5.5 Storage Stability of Dry Powder Formulation

Dry powder formulations of protein/peptide vaccines can provide greater stability than liquid formulations. However, chemical and physical degradation can still occur in the solid state leading to loss of immunogenicity or powder delivery failure. Chemical degradation pathways observed for proteins/peptides in the solid state are very similar to possible degradation pathways for liquid formulations, which involve covalent modifications such as deamidation, oxidation, disulfide exchange and hydrolysis. In addition, protein/peptides are often susceptible to physical degradation due to non-covalent interactions such as hydrophobic interactions that lead to protein denaturization and aggregation (Yoshioka et al. 1993; Yoshioka and Stella 2002). Chemical and physical degradation may both occur during dry powder manufacturing and storage. Various factors that affect the stability of dry powder formulation during the manufacturing process have been mentioned in the earlier sections. It is also of great importance to examine factors that could influence the storage stability of the dry powder formulation.

The matrix glass transition temperature (T_g) is a critical parameter for solid-state protein/peptide stability, and refers to the transition temperature between the glassy (solid-like) states and the rubbery (liquid-like) states. In general, for excipients of the same kind, a higher matrix T_g often affords greater stability. Increasing T_g for the excipients sucrose, trehalose, raffinose and stachyose has been correlated with an increase in the storage stability of lyophilized recombinant human interleukin-2 (Prestrelski et al. 1995). As it is true for any solid-state pharmaceutical, the protein formulation needs to be stored at a temperature well below T_g in order to ensure long-term storage stability. More specifically, a T_g of at least 20°C higher than the ambient storage temperature has been recommended for solid protein pharmaceuticals (Franks 1994). The preferential use of trehalose rather than other sugars and polyols in dry powder protein formulations (Garmise et al. 2006; Jiang et al. 2006) is in part due to the amorphous trehalose having a high T_g of around 120°C (Maa et al. 1999). An extensive list has been generated by Wang regarding the glass transition and collapse temperatures of commonly used buffers, excipients and proteins reported in the literature (Wang 2000). Many factors, such as the concentration of the excipient (sugar/polyols or polymers), moisture content and the presence of buffer salts and other excipients can greatly influence the overall matrix T_g. During formulation development, T_g is one of the most important physicochemical properties of the product, which can be determined by differential scanning calorimetry (DSC). It is often evaluated as part of the screening process for different excipient combinations (Garmise et al. 2006; Schule et al. 2008).

The effect of moisture on the stability of solid-state protein or peptide has been studied extensively since the late 1980s (Hageman 1988). Moisture-induced aggregation has been a well-known phenomena for lyophilized pharmaceutical proteins, especially recombinant human albumin (Costantino et al. 1995) and lyophilized insulin (Costantino et al. 1994). Three possible roles have been proposed for water during the aggregation process: it might act as reactant, reaction media or plasticizer (Shalaev and Zografi 1996). Sugars/polyols are known as cryoprotectants, which have wonderful stabilizing effects during freezing and drying, and also for long-term storage of lyophilized proteins. It has been proposed that sugars/polyols stabilize proteins by forming an amorphous glassy matrix and providing hydrogen bonding to the protein, thereby limiting molecular mobility (Prestrelski et al. 1993), by providing physical separation and dilution of the protein, which prevents protein intermolecular interactions and aggregation (Fox 1995), and through the substitution of the water-protein interaction with a water-excipient interaction (Costantino et al. 1995). However, the hygroscopic nature of the sugars/polyols in combination with the large surface area of the particles prepared by SFD or FD renders the powder formulation very susceptible to moisture uptake during storage. Increased moisture content can significantly decrease the T_g of the matrix and increase the free volume of the protein, thereby accelerating the degradation rate and possible product collapse (Hancock and Zografi 1994; Oksanen and Zografi 1990; Strickley and Anderson 1997). Solid-state water content is known to cause increased covalent aggregation for lyophilized bovine serum albumin (Jordan et al. 1994), recombinant human IL-1 receptor agonist (Chang et al. 1996a, b) and recombinant HA (Costantino et al. 1995). Residual moisture after manufacture and the moisture content throughout storage should be closely monitored. The most common methods used for this purpose are mass loss on drying or Karl Fischer titration.

Many amorphous sugar/polyol excipients also have a tendency to crystallize during storage, especially under elevated temperature and moisture. Spray-dried amorphous sucrose, trehalose and lactose can crystallize at 25°C under relative humidity $\geq$52% (Naini et al. 1998). Crystallization of the excipient can cause phase separation and destabilize the protein during storage. For example, the storage stability of an anti-IgE monoclonal antibody was drastically decreased at 5 or 30°C due to mannitol crystallization (Costantino et al. 1998). The crystallization tendency of amorphous excipient can be affected by multiple factors, such as the amount used, interaction with a second excipient or the SD process. For a detailed review, see (Wang 2000). Crystallization can be inhibited by many polymer excipients, such as maltodextrins, PVP, dextran and carboxymethyl cellulose (Wang 2000).

Many factors contribute to the storage stability of powder formulations. The aggregation state of the protein/peptide is often indicative of antigen stability, which can be easily measured by SEC-high-pressure liquid chromatography, providing a robust method to assess the storage stability quantitatively. Loss of powder stability can also be reflected in the change of particle size distribution and powder flow properties, which could cause deterioration of powder performance by changing the deposition and powder delivery efficiency.

6 Immunogenicity and Efficacy of Mucosal Dry Powder Vaccines

Dry powder vaccines have been demonstrated to induce protective immunity against several pathogens in animals. Recent studies of nasal or pulmonary powder vaccine formulations are discussed here with an emphasis on comparison of dry and liquid vaccines for the induction of immune responses and protective immunity.

6.1 Anthrax Vaccines

Nasal immunization studies with dry powder anthrax vaccines have provided convincing data that the nasal powder vaccination strategy can be used for the induction of protective immunity to anthrax (Huang et al. 2007; Jiang et al. 2006; Klas et al. 2008; Mikszta et al. 2005; Wimer-Mackin et al. 2006; Mikszta et al. 2005) demonstrated that nasal immunization of rabbits on days 0, 21 and 42 with powder formulations of anthrax PA (50 μg) containing CpG and chitosan protected all rabbits against a lethal B. anthracis spore challenge. In this same study, nasal immunization with a liquid vaccine formulation (lacking chitosan) protected only 67% of rabbits against spore challenge (Mikszta et al. 2005). Interestingly, the rabbits immunized by the nasal route with dry powder vaccine had lower anthrax toxin neutralizing antibodies in serum than rabbits immunized by the IM route, suggesting that the nasal route may have induced a local immune response that contributed to protection. However, minimal antigen-specific IgA was detected in nasal secretions of these animals (Huang et al. 2007). In a subsequent study, nasal immunization of rabbits with a dry powder anthrax vaccine containing 10 μg PA with CpG and chitosan on days 0 and 28 induced complete protection against anthrax aerosol spore challenge on day 80 (Huang et al. 2007). In contrast, only 86% of rabbits immunized IM with PA plus alum and 63% of rabbits immunized nasally with liquid vaccine (10 μg PA + CpG + chitosan) survived the spore challenge (Huang et al. 2007). If the survival results from both studies are combined and compared, nasal powder vaccination (with 19/19 rabbits surviving) can be concluded superior to nasal liquid vaccination (9/14 survived) using the Fisher's Exact test ($P = 0.0084$). Powder PA vaccine formulations were also shown to have superior storage stability at 25 and 40°C when compared to liquid PA formulations (Huang et al. 2007). Collectively, these studies demonstrate that nasal delivery of a dry powder anthrax vaccine provides a needle-free immunization regimen that is superior to liquid formulations in both storage stability and protective efficacy.

A dry powder anthrax vaccine formulated with MPL and chitosan has also generated protection against lethal anthrax spore challenge in rabbits (Klas et al. 2008; Wimer-Mackin et al. 2006). Rabbits immunized on days 0 and 28 with a dry powder vaccine formulation containing 90 μg PA, 25 μg MPL, 14 mg chitosan and 18 μg of a *B. anthracis* capsule peptide in mannitol were completely protected against spore challenge on day 85 (Wimer-Mackin et al. 2006). Inclusion of chitosan was required for maximal immune responses (Wimer-Mackin et al. 2006). This group later reported that a single dry powder immunization with 150 μg PA, 50 μg MPL and chitosan protected 80% of rabbits against a lethal anthrax spore challenge (Klas et al. 2008). A nasal liquid vaccine formulation was not tested to determine if the dry vaccine had superior protective efficacy. In addition, the ability of these powder vaccines to induce antigen-specific mucosal IgA responses was not reported (Klas et al. 2008; Wimer-Mackin et al. 2006).

6.2 Influenza Virus Vaccines

Studies with influenza antigens have also demonstrated the feasibility and potential efficacy of mucosally delivered dry powder influenza vaccines (Amorij et al. 2008; 2007a, b; Coucke et al. 2009; Garmise et al. 2006, 2007; Huang et al. 2004; Maa et al. 2004). Multiple groups have clearly demonstrated that preparation of inactivated influenza as a dry powder provides a formulation that maintains stability and potency after storage at room temperature or 40°C (Amorij et al. 2007; Garmise et al. 2007; Huang et al. 2004; Maa et al. 2004). For example, after 4–8 weeks of storage at 25°C and 25–50% relative humidity, liquid influenza formulations lost >60% of their original HA titer while powder formulations maintained HA titers at 100% up to 12 weeks (Garmise et al. 2007; Huang et al. 2004). Others have reported that a dry powder influenza vaccine formulated with trehalose maintained nearly 80% of its original HA titer when stored for 26 weeks at 45°C (Amorij et al. 2007). Such vaccine formulations would be highly beneficial in developing countries.

Dry influenza vaccines have effectively induced antigen-specific immune responses after mucosal delivery in mice (Amorij et al. 2007), rats (Garmise et al. 2007; Huang et al. 2004) and rabbits (Coucke et al. 2009). Pulmonary immunization of mice via insufflation of powder containing 5 μg HA on days 0, 14 and 28 induced HAI activity and HA-specific IgG and IgA titers in serum that were significantly greater than those in mice given IM or nasal immunizations with liquid containing the same HA dose (Amorij et al. 2007). Maximal influenza-specific nasal and lung IgG and IgA responses as well as cell-mediated IFN-γ responses in spleen were detected in mice nasally immunized with the dry powder vaccine (Amorij et al. 2007). The observation that pulmonary HA delivery as a powder induced responses superior to those induced by pulmonary liquid vaccine suggests that the immunogenic properties of a vaccine may be influenced by the powder formulation. Mucosal vaccination with a powder may target antigen to immune inductive tissues or APC that are not as effectively contacted by liquid vaccine formulations. In addition, the use of powder formulations may alter the mucosal residence time of antigen when compared to a liquid vaccine, and this may influence the immunogenicity of the vaccine. Additional studies are needed to determine the mechanisms responsible for the enhanced immunogenicity of powder vaccines in the respiratory tract.

Nasal immunization studies in rats using powder influenza vaccine formulations have evaluated the ability of mucoadhesives to increase the immunogenicity of powder vaccines (Garmise et al. 2007; Huang et al. 2004). The inclusion of chitosan in a powder influenza vaccine was a crucial component of the vaccine formulation since a powder formulation lacking chitosan exhibited much lower immunogenicity based on serum IgG titers, serum HAI titers and nasal IgA titers (Huang et al. 2004). The powder vaccine formulation containing chitosan induced immune responses similar to those induced by nasal or IM immunization with the exception that IM immunization did not induce nasal IgA responses (Huang et al. 2004). It is important to note that the serum HAI and nasal IgA titers were highly variable in rats immunized with the chitosan powder formulations. The immune responses induced by IM or nasal immunization with liquid vaccine were more consistent (Huang et al. 2004). In a separate study, the use of mucoadhesives, including chitosan, did not significantly influence the serum IgG or nasal IgA responses induced in rats after nasal powder immunization (Garmise et al. 2007). These studies suggest that work is needed to optimize powder vaccine delivery methods so that more consistent immune responses are induced. It is also important to mention that the organization of the nasal cavity in mice and rats is very different from that of the nasal cavity of larger species, such as rabbits, non-human primates and humans (Brandtzaeg 2003; Harkema et al. 2006; Yeh et al. 1997). Therefore, delivery methods in rodents may not be optimal for delivery in other laboratory animals or humans.

Powder influenza vaccine formulations have also been tested in rabbits (Coucke et al. 2009). In contrast to the rodent studies above, nasal immunization of rabbits with influenza powder vaccines was not as effective as IM immunization with liquid vaccine (Coucke et al. 2009). Influenza powder vaccines induced serum anti-HA titers that were roughly 100-fold lower than those induced by IM immunization (Coucke et al. 2009). Serum HAI titers were also lower in nasal powder-vaccinated rabbits than IM immunized rabbits (Coucke et al. 2009). However, nasal immunization with dry influenza vaccine did induce serum anti-HA IgG titers that were significantly greater than those generated by nasal immunization with a liquid influenza vaccine (Coucke et al. 2009). Interestingly, like rabbits nasally immunized with anthrax powder vaccines (Huang et al. 2007), nasal immunization of rabbits with dry influenza vaccines did not generate vaccine-specific IgA in nasal secretions (Coucke et al. 2009). The lack of mucosal IgA responses in nasally immunized rabbits is in stark contrast with the potent induction of mucosal IgA antibodies in nasally immunized mice. We have also found it difficult to induce antigen-specific mucosal IgA in nasally immunized macaques, despite induction of systemic IgG responses (Egan et al. 2004). Collectively, these studies demonstrate that dry powder nasal influenza vaccines can provide increased vaccine stability in the absence of a cold chain and they are able to induce influenza-specific systemic antibody responses. However, additional studies are needed to optimize dry vaccine formulations, adjuvants and delivery methods to maximize the induction of antigen-specific serum IgG and mucosal IgA.

6.3 Measles Vaccines

Multiple studies with over 2,800 humans total (Low et al. 2008) have demonstrated that pulmonary immunization with aerosolized measles virus vaccine produces only mild side effects and is more effective than SC immunization. Thus, a logical progression for improved measles vaccination is the development of dry powder pulmonary vaccines. Indeed, recent studies suggest that formulation of live-attenuated measles into powders for pulmonary delivery is possible (Burger et al. 2008; LiCalsi et al. 2001). In fact, a powder formulation of measles vaccine with characteristics suitable for lung delivery (Burger et al. 2008) recently passed the WHO stability test (at least one log reduction in virus titer after 7 days of storage at 37°C). However, pulmonary immunization of macaques with dry measles vaccine did not induce neutralizing antibody responses comparable to those induced by injection (de Swart et al. 2007). All six macaques immunized by injection developed serum neutralizing antibodies to measles virus within 24 days, and these persisted up to 396 days. In contrast, only two of six macaques immunized with the dry powder measles vaccine had neutralizing antibodies at 24 or 93 days after vaccination, and only one of these had detectable neutralizing antibody after 396 days (de Swart et al. 2007). In this study, the dry vaccine was delivered to ketamine-anesthetized macaques intratracheally, and powder was observed in the exhaled breath of these animals after dosing (de Swart et al. 2007). Thus, the delivery method was both suboptimal and impractical for human application. Optimization of vaccine formulations and delivery methods in clinical studies (see below) may identify a dry powder immunization method that is safe and effective in humans.

6.4 Diphtheria Vaccines

Immunization of the guinea pig lung (Amidi et al. 2007) or human nasal cavity (Huo et al. 2005) with dry powder diphtheria vaccines has provided further support for the efficacy of dry vaccines. Pulmonary (intratracheal) immunization of guinea pigs with a diphtheria toxoid (DT) powder formulation containing chitosan produced significantly greater systemic neutralizing antibody responses when compared to SC injection of an alum-adjuvanted DT vaccine (Amidi et al. 2007). The inclusion of chitosan in the powder formulation was critical as pulmonary immunization with a DT powder lacking chitosan failed to induce neutralizing antibodies (Amidi et al. 2007). In addition, only guinea pigs immunized by the pulmonary route with DT powders containing chitosan developed anti-DT IgA in bronchoalveolar fluids (Amidi et al. 2007).

Nasal immunization of humans with a dry powder meningococcal polysaccharide-DT_{CRM197} conjugate vaccine has proved effective for the induction of serum meningococcal bactericidal and DT neutralizing antibodies (Huo et al. 2005). Chitosan was included in the nasal powder vaccine formulation. Nasal IgA specific for meningococcal polysaccharide and DT_{CRM197} was significantly increased in subjects nasally immunized with dry vaccine on days 0 and 28, but not in those given a single IM immunization (Huo et al. 2005). This clinical study demonstrated that a practical needle-free method of immunization using dry powders was effective in humans. The nasal delivery method involved insertion of the tip of a powder delivery syringe into a nostril as far as it would go without causing discomfort while the subjects sat in a semi-reclined position. After quickly depressing the syringe plunger to deliver powder, the syringe was removed and the subjects pressed the nostril shut for a few minutes (Huo et al. 2005). Pressing the nostril shut ensured that vaccine was not be exhaled. It also maximized contact of powder with nasal surface secretions, which reconstitute the vaccine.

7 Mucosal Delivery of Dry Powder Vaccines

While identification of effective antigen/adjuvant/mucoadhesive formulations will be a critical step in the development of dry powder vaccines for humans, the development of reliable, reproducible and practical delivery methods are equally important steps in this pathway. Optimization of delivery methods will be critical for development of cost-effective, mucosal dry powder vaccines. Several questions must be addressed for nasal or pulmonary dry powder vaccination in humans. For example, what is the ideal particle size, the optimal body position or the optimal vaccine dose for consistent induction of immune responses? Numerous nasal immunization studies with liquid vaccines in mice have also demonstrated that variables such as volume and anesthesia significantly influence the outcome of immunization. Nasal immunization of mice with large vaccine volumes (Eyles et al. 2001, 1999; Pickett et al. 2000; Southam et al. 2002; Thompson et al. 1999) and/or administration of anesthetics before nasal immunization (Janakova et al. 2002; Sloat and Cui 2006; Southam et al. 2002) has been associated with induction of greater immune responses due to vaccine introduction in the lungs. But this can literally drown the mouse, and hence should be avoided.

Comprehensive studies to define the parameters of effective dry vaccination in non-human primates or humans have not yet been performed. Pulmonary delivery

of insulin powder has been used in non-human primates as a surrogate for vaccine delivery (Grainger et al. 2004). Absorption of insulin was compared after delivery as a powder in the lung (using a Penn Century insufflator), as a liquid in the trachea, and as a liquid injected SC (Grainger et al. 2004). Insulin bioavailability from the inhaled powder was similar to that observed after SC injection, but greater than that after tracheal liquid delivery (Grainger et al. 2004). However, there were too few animals for a thorough dose-response comparison of dry powder delivery versus instilled or injected liquids. There was also significant animal-to-animal variation after powder insufflation to the lung (Grainger et al. 2004).

The use of preclinical animal models to optimize dry powder vaccine delivery for humans is problematic. The insulin powder insufflation study was performed in sedated cynomolgus macaques that were maintained in supine position with a Penn Century insufflator inserted into the trachea via an oropharyngeal tube (Grainger et al. 2004). Analogous anesthesia and delivery methods were used in non-human primates to evaluate a dry powder measles vaccine (de Swart et al. 2007). Similar to the insulin study, all six macaques immunized by injection developed neutralizing antibodies in serum, while powder vaccination induced these antibodies in only two of six macaques (de Swart et al. 2007). In both studies, powder was observed in the exhaled breath after completion of the delivery procedure (de Swart et al. 2007; Grainger et al. 2004), suggesting that additional studies are needed to optimize methods of dry powder vaccination. However, this may be difficult in macaques because dry powder vaccination in these animals requires both anesthesia and tracheal tubes for vaccine delivery. In addition, powder dosing in macaques may not be comparable to powder dosing in humans due to differences in size, physiology and the inability to communicate instructions to the monkeys (de Swart et al. 2007). In contrast to powder drug delivery where the goal may simply be absorption, powder vaccination may require delivery to a particular region of the nasal cavity or lung for maximal induction of antigen-specific immune responses. Clinical studies to optimize mucosal delivery of dry powder vaccines in humans are needed.

8 Evaluating Safety of Respiratory Tract Vaccines

Dry powder delivery to the nasal cavity raises more safety concerns than simple liquid formulations, which may explain the small number of studies performed and the limited success of some nasal dry powder products. Mucosal irritation or damage can be influenced by the stabilizer/sugar, mucoadhesive compound and excipients used in the formulation, or the application dose, frequency and individual tolerance. Local irritation, burning and stinging have been reported with nasal application of surfactants such as Laureth-9, bile salts and sodium taurodihydrofusidate (Illum and Davis 1992). A slight nasal itch occurred when β-cyclodextrin was used (Merkus et al. 1999; Merkus et al. 1996). Others reported nasal burning and sinusitis when glycocholate and methylcellulose were used to enhance nasal absorption of insulin (Lalej-Bennis et al. 2001). Discomfort can readily be communicated by humans, but the signs are more difficult to discern in animals unless there is obvious struggling, sneezing, salivating, head shaking and nose rubbing (Hsieh 1994). However, there are other methods available that can provide more definitive measures of local mucosal toxicity.

The standard method to assess local side effects is histological evaluation of mucosal membranes and submucosa immediately after exposure to formulations. Metaplasia and infiltration of inflammatory cells are indicative of mucosal toxicity (Callens et al. 2001; Harkema et al. 2006; Ugwoke et al. 2000). Several in vitro cell studies have been described for toxicological investigation of nasal absorption enhancers and surfactants (Chandler et al. 1995). Classical mucoadhesives, such as chitosan and carboxymethylcellulose (CMC), have been examined using Caco-2 epithelial cells or a human nasal cell culture system to monitor cytotoxicity and ciliotoxicity indicated by ciliary beat frequency (CBF) (Thanou et al. 1999; Ugwoke et al. 2000). Results showed that chitosan had marginal effects on CBF of Caco-2 cells, whereas CMC had mild-to-moderate cilio-inhibition in human nasal epithelial cell suspensions. However, the aforementioned methods can be invasive and time consuming. Thus, instead of measuring protein markers by conventional nasal perfusion methods (Hirai et al. 1981; Marttin et al. 1995), Callens et al. (2001) developed a non-invasive method using nasal lavage. The amount of total protein, cytosolic lactate dehydrogenase (LDH) and membrane-bound alkaline phosphatase (ALP) was monitored in rabbit nasal lavage as an indication of mucosal toxicity by DDWM/Carbopol® 974 P (Callens et al. 2001). The mucosal toxicity of the formulation was also evaluated with an alternative animal model (Adriaens and Remon 1999), which utilizes the slug *Arion lusitanicus*. The results showed a significant release of LDH after administration of positive control DDWM/Benzalkonium chloride or DDWM/Carbopol® 974 P (90:10). However, the latter remained constant after repeated treatment. The LDH released from the slug body wall was not significant for the DDWM/Carbopol® 974 P group, though this treatment induced more mucus secretions. These findings were supported by a histological study, which led to the conclusion that the 90:10 formulation of DDWM/Carbopol® 974 P had negligible toxicity on the nasal mucosa. In another study, a slug mucosal irritation test was used to evaluate the toxicity of a dry powder influenza vaccine that contained a spray-dried mixture of Amioca®/Carbopol® 974P (Coucke et al. 2009). The results indicated that a mixture containing 50–100% of Carbopol® 974P with influenza virus can be classified as mildly damaging (Coucke et al. 2009).

Enterotoxin-based immunogens or adjuvants that can bind nerves in the human nasal cavity have also been confirmed unsafe due to the risk of inflammatory reactions that may be Bell's Palsy (Couch 2004; Lewis et al. 2009; Mutsch et al. 2004; van Ginkel et al. 2005). However, immunization in the human respiratory tract can clearly be done safely and effectively with other products. For example, the live-attenuated, nasally administered influenza vaccine FluMist is FDA approved and safe (Ambrose et al. 2011). Aerosol delivery of measles vaccine

(Arora et al. 2002) produced only mild side effects and was more effective than SC immunization. Nonetheless, as with any new vaccine, careful studies will be required to demonstrate that nasal or pulmonary vaccines are safe in humans.

9 Conclusion

The storage, stability and immunogenicity of mucosally administered dry powder vaccines in preclinical and clinical studies provide encouraging support that dry vaccines may soon be able to provide a needle-free method of immunization for humans. While dry powder immunization studies in animals are important, the development of safe and effective dry vaccines for humans will depend on their performance in clinical studies designed to optimize formulations and delivery methods while evaluating safety. Developments in the toxicological assessment of nasally applied products have been promising. However, no standardized method has been proposed by regulatory agencies. Nevertheless, mucosal and mucociliary toxicity studies will be necessary to ensure successful development of dry vaccines for delivery in the respiratory tract. As with all medications and vaccines used in humans, we must keep a keen eye on the safety of these products during their development.

References

Adriaens E, Remon JP (1999) Gastropods as an evaluation tool for screening the irritating potency of absorption enhancers and drugs. Pharm Res 16:1240–1244

Alpar HO, Eyles JE, Williamson ED et al (2001) Intranasal vaccination against plague, tetanus and diphtheria. Adv Drug Deliv Rev 51:173–201

Ambrose CS, Levin MJ, Belshe RB (2011) The relative efficacy of trivalent live attenuated and inactivated influenza vaccines in children and adults. Influenza Other Respi Viruses 5:62–75

Amidi M, Romeijn SG, Borchard G et al (2006) Preparation and characterization of protein-loaded N-trimethyl chitosan nanoparticles as nasal delivery system. J Control Release 111:107–116

Amidi M, Pellikaan HC, Hirschberg H et al (2007) Diphtheria toxoid-containing microparticulate powder formulations for pulmonary vaccination: preparation, characterization and evaluation in guinea pigs. Vaccine 25:6818–6829

Amorij JP, Meulenaar J, Hinrichs WL et al (2007a) Rational design of an influenza subunit vaccine powder with sugar glass technology: preventing conformational changes of haemagglutinin during freezing and freeze-drying. Vaccine 25:6447–6457

Amorij JP, Saluja V, Petersen AH et al (2007b) Pulmonary delivery of an inulin-stabilized influenza subunit vaccine prepared by spray-freeze drying induces systemic, mucosal humoral as well as cell-mediated immune responses in BALB/c mice. Vaccine 25:8707–8717

Amorij JP, Huckriede A, Wilschut J et al (2008) Development of stable influenza vaccine powder formulations: challenges and possibilities. Pharm Res 25:1256–1273

Arora P, Sharma S, Garg S (2002) Permeability issues in nasal drug delivery. Drug Discov Today 7:967–975

Baker DJ, Jeram J, Reid LA (2002) Failure of the vaccine cold chain following modification of a domestic refrigerator. N Z Med J 115:U251

Barton GM, Medzhitov R (2002) Control of adaptive immune responses by toll-like receptors. Curr Opin Immunol 14:380–383
Bateman ND, Whymark AD, Clifton NJ et al (2002) A study of intranasal distribution of azelastine hydrochloride aqueous nasal spray with different spray techniques. Clin Otolaryngol Allied Sci 27:327–330
Bates DV, Fish BR, Hatch TF et al (1966) Deposition and retention models for internal dosimetry of the human respiratory tract. Task group on lung dynamics. Health Phys 12:173–207
Baumann U (2008) Mucosal vaccination against bacterial respiratory infections. Expert Rev Vaccines 7:1257–1276
Bhuyan AL (2000) Immunisation and the cold chain. J Indian Med Assoc 98:26–27, 29
Boyaka PN, Tafaro A, Fischer R et al (2003) Effective mucosal immunity to anthrax: neutralizing antibodies and Th cell responses following nasal immunization with protective antigen. J Immunol 170:5636–5643
Bradney CP, Sempowski GD, Liao HX et al (2002) Cytokines as adjuvants for the induction of anti-human immunodeficiency virus peptide immunoglobulin G (IgG) and IgA antibodies in serum and mucosal secretions after nasal immunization. J Virol 76:517–524
Brandtzaeg P (2003) Immunology of tonsils and adenoids: everything the ENT surgeon needs to know. Int J Pediatr Otorhinolaryngol 67:S69–S76
Brankston G, Gitterman L, Hirji Z et al (2007) Transmission of influenza A in human beings. Lancet Infect Dis 7:257–265
Burger JL, Cape SP, Braun CS et al (2008) Stabilizing formulations for inhalable powders of live-attenuated measles virus vaccine. J Aerosol Med Pulm Drug Deliv 21:25–34
Callens C, Remon JP (2000) Evaluation of starch-maltodextrin-carbopol 974 P mixtures for the nasal delivery of insulin in rabbits. J Control Release 66:215–220
Callens C, Adriaens E, Dierckens K et al (2001) Toxicological evaluation of a bioadhesive nasal powder containing a starch and carbopol 974 P on rabbit nasal mucosa and slug mucosa. J Control Release 76:81–91
Callens C, Pringels E, Remon JP (2003) Influence of multiple nasal administrations of bioadhesive powders on the insulin bioavailability. Int J Pharm 250:415–422
Cameron P (1997) Good pharmaceutical freeze-drying practice. Interpharm Press, Buffalo Grove
Carpenter JF, Crowe JH (1989) An infrared spectroscopic study of the interactions of carbohydrates with dried proteins. Biochemistry 28:3916–3922
Casella CR, Mitchell TC (2008) Putting endotoxin to work for us: monophosphoryl lipid A as a safe and effective vaccine adjuvant. Cell Mol Life Sci 65:3231–3240
Chandler SG, Thomas NW, Illum L (1995) Nasal absorption in the rat. IV. Membrane activity of absorption enhancers. Int J Pharm 117:139–146
Chang BS, Kendrick BS, Carpenter JF (1996a) Surface-induced denaturation of proteins during freezing and its inhibition by surfactants. J Pharm Sci 85:1325–1330
Chang BS, Reeder G, Carpenter JF (1996b) Development of a stable freeze-dried formulation of recombinant human interleukin-1 receptor antagonist. Pharm Res 13:243–249
Chen D, Endres RL, Erickson CA et al (2002) Epidermal powder immunization using non-toxic bacterial enterotoxin adjuvants with influenza vaccine augments protective immunity. Vaccine 20:2671–2679
Cheng YS, Holmes TD, Gao J et al (2001) Characterization of nasal spray pumps and deposition pattern in a replica of the human nasal airway. J Aerosol Med 14:267–280
Clements CJ, Larsen G, Jodar L (2004) Technologies that make administration of vaccines safer. Vaccine 22:2054–2058
Cooper CL, Davis HL, Morris ML et al (2004a) CPG 7909, an immunostimulatory TLR9 agonist oligodeoxynucleotide, as adjuvant to Engerix-B HBV vaccine in healthy adults: a double-blind phase I/II study. J Clin Immunol 24:693–701
Cooper CL, Davis HL, Morris ML et al (2004b) Safety and immunogenicity of CPG 7909 injection as an adjuvant to fluarix influenza vaccine. Vaccine 22:3136–3143
Cooper CL, Davis HL, Angel JB et al (2005) CPG 7909 adjuvant improves hepatitis B virus vaccine seroprotection in antiretroviral-treated HIV-infected adults. AIDS 19:1473–1479

Costantino HR, Langer R, Klibanov AM (1994) Moisture-induced aggregation of lyophilized insulin. Pharm Res 11:21–29

Costantino HR, Langer R, Klibanov AM (1995) Aggregation of a lyophilized pharmaceutical protein, recombinant human albumin: effect of moisture and stabilization by excipients. Biotechnology (NY) 13:493–496

Costantino HR, Andya JD, Nguyen PA et al (1998) Effect of mannitol crystallization on the stability and aerosol performance of a spray-dried pharmaceutical protein, recombinant humanized anti-IgE monoclonal antibody. J Pharm Sci 87:1406–1411

Couch RB (2004) Nasal vaccination, *Escherichia coli* enterotoxin, and Bell's palsy. N Engl J Med 350:860–861

Coucke D, Schotsaert M, Libert C et al (2009) Spray-dried powders of starch and crosslinked poly(acrylic acid) as carriers for nasal delivery of inactivated influenza vaccine. Vaccine 27:1279–1286

Croyle MA, Roessler BJ, Davidson BL et al (1998) Factors that influence stability of recombinant adenoviral preparations for human gene therapy. Pharm Dev Technol 3:373–383

Cui Z, Sloat BR (2006) Topical immunization onto mouse skin using a microemulsion incorporated with an anthrax protective antigen protein-encoding plasmid. Int J Pharm 317:187–191

Czerkinsky C, Anjuere F, McGhee JR et al (1999) Mucosal immunity and tolerance: relevance to vaccine development. Immunol Rev 170:197–222

Daubenberger CA (2007) TLR9 agonists as adjuvants for prophylactic and therapeutic vaccines. Curr Opin Mol Ther 9:45–52

Davis SS (2001) Nasal vaccines. Adv Drug Deliv Rev 51:21–42

de Swart RL, LiCalsi C, Quirk AV et al (2007) Measles vaccination of macaques by dry powder inhalation. Vaccine 25:1183–1190

Dean HJ, Chen D (2004) Epidermal powder immunization against influenza. Vaccine 23:681–686

Duddu SP, Zhang G, Dal Monte PR (1997) The relationship between protein aggregation and molecular mobility below the glass transition temperature of lyophilized formulations containing a monoclonal antibody. Pharm Res 14:596–600

Egan MA, Chong SY, Hagen M et al (2004) A comparative evaluation of nasal and parenteral vaccine adjuvants to elicit systemic and mucosal HIV-1 peptide-specific humoral immune responses in cynomolgus macaques. Vaccine 22:3774–3788

Elson CO (1996) Cholera toxin as a mucosal adjuvant. In: Kiyono H, Ogra PL, McGhee JR (eds) Mucosal vaccines. Academic, New York, pp 59–72

Eriksson JH, Hinrichs WL, de Jong GJ et al (2003) Investigations into the stabilization of drugs by sugar glasses: III. The influence of various high-pH buffers. Pharm Res 20:1437–1443

Eyles JE, Williamson ED, Alpar HO (1999) Immunological responses to nasal delivery of free and encapsulated tetanus toxoid: studies on the effect of vehicle volume. Int J Pharm 189:75–79

Eyles JE, Bramwell VW, Williamson ED et al (2001) Microsphere translocation and immunopotentiation in systemic tissues following intranasal administration. Vaccine 19: 4732–4742

Fink AL (1995) Molten globules. Methods Mol Biol 40:343–360

Fox KC (1995) Biopreservation. Putting proteins under glass. Science 267:1922–1923

Franks F (1994) Long-term stabilization of biologicals. Biotechnology (NY) 12:253–256

Freytag LC, Clements JD (2005) Mucosal adjuvants. Vaccine 23:1804–1813

Garmise RJ, Hickey AJ (2008) Calibration of the andersen cascade impactor for the characterization of nasal products. J Pharm Sci 97:3462–3466

Garmise RJ, Mar K, Crowder TM et al (2006) Formulation of a dry powder influenza vaccine for nasal delivery. AAPS Pharm Sci Tech 7:E19

Garmise RJ, Staats HF, Hickey AJ (2007) Novel dry powder preparations of whole inactivated influenza virus for nasal vaccination. AAPS Pharm Sci Tech 8:E81

Giudice EL, Campbell JD (2006) Needle-free vaccine delivery. Adv Drug Deliv Rev 58:68–89

Gold MS, Kemp AE, Osbourne M (1998) Counting the cost of disrupting the vaccine cold chain. Med J Aust 168:471–472

Gomez G, Pikal MJ, Rodriguez-Hornedo N (2001) Effect of initial buffer composition on pH changes during far-from-equilibrium freezing of sodium phosphate buffer solutions. Pharm Res 18:90–97

Grainger CI, Alcock R, Gard TG et al (2004) Administration of an insulin powder to the lungs of cynomolgus monkeys using a Penn century insufflator. Int J Pharm 269:523–527

Hageman MJ (1988) The role of moisture in protein stability. Drug Dev Ind Pharm 14:2047–2070

Hagen SJ, Hofrichter J, Eaton WA (1995) Protein reaction kinetics in a room-temperature glass. Science 269:959–962

Halperin SA, Van Nest G, Smith B et al (2003) A phase I study of the safety and immunogenicity of recombinant hepatitis B surface antigen co-administered with an immunostimulatory phosphorothioate oligonucleotide adjuvant. Vaccine 21:2461–2467

Hamajima K, Sasaki S, Fukushima J et al (1998) Intranasal administration of HIV-DNA vaccine formulated with a polymer, carboxymethylcellulose, augments mucosal antibody production and cell-mediated immune response. Clin Immunol Immunopathol 88:205–210

Hancock BC, Zografi G (1994) The relationship between the glass transition temperature and the water content of amorphous pharmaceutical solids. Pharm Res 11:471–477

Harkema JR, Carey SA, Wagner JG (2006) The nose revisited: a brief review of the comparative structure, function, and toxicologic pathology of the nasal epithelium. Toxicol Pathol 34:252–269

Hawe A, Kasper JC, Friess W et al (2009) Structural properties of monoclonal antibody aggregates induced by freeze-thawing and thermal stress. Eur J Pharm Sci 38:79–87

Hirai S, Yashiki T, Matsuzawa T et al (1981) Absorption of drugs from the nasal mucosa of rat. Int J Pharm 7:317–325

Hornick RB, Eigelsbach HT (1966) Aerogenic immunization of man with live tularemia vaccine. Bacteriol Rev 30:532–538

Hsieh DS (1994) Drug permeation enhancement: theory and applications. Marcel Dekker, New York

Huang J, Garmise RJ, Crowder TM et al (2004) A novel dry powder influenza vaccine and intranasal delivery technology: induction of systemic and mucosal immune responses in rats. Vaccine 23:794–801

Huang J, Mikszta JA, Ferriter MS et al (2007) Intranasal administration of dry powder anthrax vaccine provides protection against lethal aerosol spore challenge. Hum Vaccines 3:90–93

Huo Z, Sinha R, McNeela EA et al (2005) Induction of protective serum meningococcal bactericidal and diphtheria-neutralizing antibodies and mucosal immunoglobulin A in volunteers by nasal insufflations of the Neisseria meningitidis serogroup C polysaccharide-CRM197 conjugate vaccine mixed with chitosan. Infect Immun 73:8256–8265

Hutin YJ, Chen RT (1999) Injection safety: a global challenge. Bull World Health Organ 77:787–788

Illum L, Davis SS (1992) Intranasal insulin. Clinical pharmacokinetics. Clin Pharmacokinet 23:30–41

Illum L, Jabbal-Gill I, Hinchcliffe M et al (2001) Chitosan as a novel nasal delivery system for vaccines. Adv Drug Deliv Rev 51:81–96

Janakova L, Bakke H, Haugen IL et al (2002) Influence of intravenous anesthesia on mucosal and systemic antibody responses to nasal vaccines. Infect Immun 70:5479–5484

Jenkins MK, Khoruts A, Ingulli E et al (2001) In vivo activation of antigen-specific CD4 T cells. Ann Rev Immunol 19:23–45

Jiang ZH, Koganty RR (2003) Synthetic vaccines: the role of adjuvants in immune targeting. Curr Med Chem 10:1423–1439

Jiang G, Joshi SB, Peek LJ et al (2006) Anthrax vaccine powder formulations for nasal mucosal delivery. J Pharm Sci 95:80–96

Jordan GM, Yoshioka S, Terao T (1994) The aggregation of bovine serum albumin in solution and in the solid state. J Pharm Pharmacol 46:182–185

Jovanovic N, Bouchard A, Hofland GW et al (2004) Stabilization of proteins in dry powder formulations using supercritical fluid technology. Pharm Res 21:1955–1969

Kasel JA, Fulk RV, Togo Y et al (1968) Influenza antibody in human respiratory secretions after subcutaneous or respiratory immunization with inactivated virus. Nature 218:594–595

Kendal AP, Snyder R, Garrison PJ (1997) Validation of cold chain procedures suitable for distribution of vaccines by public health programs in the USA. Vaccine 15:1459–1465

Kimbell JS, Segal RA, Asgharian B et al (2007) Characterization of deposition from nasal spray devices using a computational fluid dynamics model of the human nasal passages. J Aerosol Med 20:59–74

Klas SD, Petrie CR, Warwood SJ et al (2008) A single immunization with a dry powder anthrax vaccine protects rabbits against lethal aerosol challenge. Vaccine 26:5494–5502

Klinman DM, Xie H, Little SF et al (2004) CpG oligonucleotides improve the protective immune response induced by the anthrax vaccination of rhesus macaques. Vaccine 22:2881

Kompella UB, Koushik K (2001) Preparation of drug delivery systems using supercritical fluid technology. Crit Rev Ther Drug Carrier Syst 18:173–199

Kueltzo LA, Wang W, Randolph TW et al (2008) Effects of solution conditions, processing parameters, and container materials on aggregation of a monoclonal antibody during freeze-thawing. J Pharm Sci 97:1801–1812

Kurita K (2006) Chitin and chitosan: functional biopolymers from marine crustaceans. Mar Biotechnol (NY) 8:203–226

Lalej-Bennis D, Boillot J, Bardin C et al (2001) Six month administration of gelified intranasal insulin in 16 type 1 diabetic patients under multiple injections: efficacy vs subcutaneous injections and local tolerance. Diabetes Metab 27:372–377

Lazzell V, Waldman RH, Rose C et al (1984) Immunization against influenza in humans using an oral enteric-coated killed virus vaccine. J Biol Standard 12:315–321

Levine MM (2003) Can needle-free administration of vaccines become the norm in global immunization? Nat Med 9:99

Lewis DJM, Huo Z, Barnett S et al (2009) Transient facial nerve paralysis (bell's palsy) following intranasal delivery of a genetically detoxified mutant of *Escherichia coli* heat labile toxin. PLoS One 4:e6999

Li S, Patapoff TW, Overcashier D et al (1996) Effects of reducing sugars on the chemical stability of human relaxin in the lyophilized state. J Pharm Sci 85:873–877

LiCalsi C, Maniaci MJ, Christensen T et al (2001) A powder formulation of measles vaccine for aerosol delivery. Vaccine 19:2629–2636

Lien E, Ingalls RR (2002) Toll-like receptors. Crit Care Med 30:S1–S11

Logullo P, de Carvalho HB, Saconi R et al (2008) Fear of injections is a reason for not to vaccinate their children, say caretakers. Vaccine 26:141

Low N, Kraemer S, Schneider M et al (2008) Immunogenicity and safety of aerosolized measles vaccine: systematic review and meta-analysis. Vaccine 26:383–398

Lu D, Hickey AJ (2007) Pulmonary vaccine delivery. Expert Rev Vaccines 6:213–226

Luykx DM, Casteleijn MG, Jiskoot W et al (2004) Physicochemical studies on the stability of influenza haemagglutinin in vaccine bulk material. Eur J Pharm Sci 23:65–75

Maa YF, Nguyen PA, Sweeney T et al (1999) Protein inhalation powders: spray drying vs spray freeze drying. Pharm Res 16:249–254

Maa YF, Ameri M, Shu C et al (2004) Influenza vaccine powder formulation development: spray-freeze-drying and stability evaluation. J Pharm Sci 93:1912–1923

Mahler HC, Muller R, Friess W et al (2005) Induction and analysis of aggregates in a liquid IgG1-antibody formulation. Eur J Pharm Biopharm 59:407–417

Mahler HC, Friess W, Grauschopf U et al (2009) Protein aggregation: pathways, induction factors and analysis. J Pharm Sci 98:3043–3057

Mann JF, Acevedo R, Campo JD et al (2009) Delivery systems: a vaccine strategy for overcoming mucosal tolerance? Expert Rev Vaccines 8:103–112

Marttin E, Verhoef JC, Romeijn SG et al (1995) Effects of absorption enhancers on rat nasal epithelium in vivo: release of marker compounds in the nasal cavity. Pharm Res 12:1151–1157

McAllister C, Karymov MA, Kawano Y et al (2005) Protein interactions and misfolding analyzed by AFM force spectroscopy. J Mol Biol 354:1028–1042
McCluskie MJ, Davis HL (1999) CpG DNA as mucosal adjuvant. Vaccine 18:231–237
McGowen AL, Hale LP, Shelburne CP et al (2009) The mast cell activator compound 48/80 is safe and effective when used as an adjuvant for intradermal immunization with Bacillus anthracis protective antigen. Vaccine 27:3544–3552
McLachlan JB, Shelburne CP, Hart JP et al (2008) Mast cell activators: a new class of highly effective vaccine adjuvants. Nat Med 14:536–541
McNeela EA, Jabbal-Gill I, Illum L et al (2004) Intranasal immunization with genetically detoxified diphtheria toxin induces T cell responses in humans: enhancement of Th2 responses and toxin-neutralizing antibodies by formulation with chitosan. Vaccine 22:909–914
Merkus FWHM, Schipper NGM, Verhoef JC (1996) The influence of absorption enhancers on intranasal insulin absorption in normal and diabetic subjects. J Control Release 41:69–75
Merkus FW, Verhoef JC, Marttin E et al (1999) Cyclodextrins in nasal drug delivery. Adv Drug Deliv Rev 36:41–57
Mikszta JA, Sullivan VJ, Dean C et al (2005) Protective immunization against inhalational anthrax: a comparison of minimally invasive delivery platforms. J Infect Dis 191:278–288
Mills KH, Cosgrove C, McNeela EA et al (2003) Protective levels of diphtheria-neutralizing antibody induced in healthy volunteers by unilateral priming-boosting intranasal immunization associated with restricted ipsilateral mucosal secretory immunoglobulin A. Infect Immun 71:726–732
Mitchell JP, Nagel MW, Nichols S et al (2006) Laser diffractometry as a technique for the rapid assessment of aerosol particle size from inhalers. J Aerosol Med 19:409–433
Modlin RL (2002) Mammalian toll-like receptors. Ann Allergy Asthma Immunol 88:543–548
Molina MC, Armstrong TK, Zhang Y et al (2004) The stability of lyophilized lipid/DNA complexes during prolonged storage. J Pharm Sci 93:2259–2273
Mutsch M, Zhou W, Rhodes P et al (2004) Use of the inactivated intranasal influenza vaccine and the risk of Bell's palsy in Switzerland. New Engl J Med 350:896–903
Naini V, Byron PR, Phillips EM (1998) Physicochemical stability of crystalline sugars and their spray-dried forms: dependence upon relative humidity and suitability for use in powder inhalers. Drug Dev Ind Pharm 24:895–909
Nally JE, Artiushin S, Sheoran AS et al (2000) Induction of mucosal and systemic antibody specific for SeMF3 of streptococcus equi by intranasal vaccination using a sucrose acetate isobutyrate based delivery system. Vaccine 19:492–497
Newman SP, Moren F, Clarke SW (1987a) Deposition pattern from a nasal pump spray. Rhinology 25:77–82
Newman SP, Moren PF, Clarke SW (1987b) The nasal distribution of metered dose inhalers. J Laryngol Otol 101:127–132
Newman SP, Steed KP, Hardy JG et al (1994) The distribution of an intranasal insulin formulation in healthy volunteers: effect of different administration techniques. J Pharm Pharmacol 46:657–660
Nordone SK, Peacock JW, Kirwan SM et al (2006) Capric acid and hydroxypropylmethylcellulose increase the immunogenicity of nasally administered peptide vaccines. AIDS Res Hum Retroviruses 22:558–568
Oh YK, Park JS, Yoon H et al (2003) Enhanced mucosal and systemic immune responses to a vaginal vaccine coadministered with RANTES-expressing plasmid DNA using in situ-gelling mucoadhesive delivery system. Vaccine 21:1980–1988
Oksanen CA, Zografi G (1990) The relationship between the glass transition temperature and water vapor absorption by poly(vinylpyrrolidone). Pharm Res 7:654–657
Oliveira ML, Areas AP, Ho PL (2007) Intranasal vaccines for protection against respiratory and systemic bacterial infections. Expert Rev Vaccines 6:419–429
Orii Y, Morita M (1977) Measurement of the pH of frozen buffer solutions by using pH indicators. J Biochem 81:163–168

Park JS, Oh YK, Kang MJ et al (2003) Enhanced mucosal and systemic immune responses following intravaginal immunization with human papillomavirus 16 L1 virus-like particle vaccine in thermosensitive mucoadhesive delivery systems. J Med Virol 70:633–641

Peng Z, Wang H, Mao X et al (2001) CpG oligodeoxynucleotide vaccination suppresses IgE induction but may fail to down-regulate ongoing IgE responses in mice. Int Immunol 13:3–11

Persing DH, Coler RN, Lacy MJ et al (2002) Taking toll: lipid A mimetics as adjuvants and immunomodulators. Trends Microbiol 10:S32–S37

Pickett TE, Pasetti MF, Galen JE et al (2000) In vivo characterization of the murine intranasal model for assessing the immunogenicity of attenuated salmonella enterica serovar typhi strains as live mucosal vaccines and as live vectors. Infect Immun 68:205–213

Pikal MJ (1999) Mechanisms of protein stabilization during freeze-drying and storage: the relative importance of thermodynamic stabilization and glassy state relaxation dynamics. In: Rey Louis, May JC (eds) Freeze-drying/lyophilization of pharmaceutical and biological products Vol 96. Marcel Dekker, New York, pp 161–198

Pikal MJ, Dellerman KM, Roy ML et al (1991) The effects of formulation variables on the stability of freeze-dried human growth hormone. Pharm Res 8:427–436

Porgador A, Staats HF, Faiola B et al (1997) Intranasal immunization with CTL epitope peptides from HIV-1 or ovalbumin and the mucosal adjuvant cholera toxin induces peptide-specific CTLs and protection against tumor development in vivo. J Immunol 158:834–841

Prestrelski SJ, Tedeschi N, Arakawa T et al (1993) Dehydration-induced conformational transitions in proteins and their inhibition by stabilizers. Biophys J 65:661–671

Prestrelski SJ, Pikal KA, Arakawa T (1995) Optimization of lyophilization conditions for recombinant human interleukin-2 by dried-state conformational analysis using Fourier-transform infrared spectroscopy. Pharm Res 12:1250–1259

Pringels E, Callens C, Vervaet C et al (2006) Influence of deposition and spray pattern of nasal powders on insulin bioavailability. Int J Pharm 310:1–7

Reid SD, Penna G, Adorini L (2000) The control of T cell responses by dendritic cell subsets. Curr Opin Immunol 12:114–121

Schagger H, von Jagow G (1991) Blue native electrophoresis for isolation of membrane protein complexes in enzymatically active form. Anal Biochem 199:223–231

Schild GC, Wood JM, Newman RW (1975) A single-radial-immunodiffusion technique for the assay of influenza haemagglutinin antigen. Proposals for an assay method for the haemagglutinin content of influenza vaccines. Bull World Health Organ 52:223–231

Schule S, Friess W, Bechtold-Peters K et al (2007) Conformational analysis of protein secondary structure during spray-drying of antibody/mannitol formulations. Eur J Pharm Biopharm 65:1–9

Schule S, Schulz-Fademrecht T, Garidel P et al (2008) Stabilization of IgG1 in spray-dried powders for inhalation. Eur J Pharm Biopharm 69:793–807

Sesardic D, Dobbelaer R (2004) European union regulatory developments for new vaccine adjuvants and delivery systems. Vaccine 22:2452

Setia S, Mainzer H, Washington ML et al (2002) Frequency and causes of vaccine wastage. Vaccine 20:1148–1156

Seto WH, Tsang D, Yung R et al (2003) Effectiveness of precautions against droplets and contact in prevention of nosocomial transmission of severe acute respiratory syndrome (SARS). Lancet 361:1519–1520

Sewall H (1925) The role of epithelium in experimental immunization. Science 62:293–299

Seya T, Akazawa T, Tsujita T et al (2006) Role of toll-like receptors in adjuvant-augmented immune therapies. Evid Based Complement Alternat Med 3:31–38

Shalaev EY, Zografi G (1996) How does residual water affect the solid-state degradation of drugs in the amorphous state? J Pharm Sci 85:1137–1141

Shoyele SA, Cawthorne S (2006) Particle engineering techniques for inhaled biopharmaceuticals. Adv Drug Deliv Rev 58:1009–1029

Shriver JW (2009) Protein-structure, stability and interactions. Humana Press, New York

Singh M, Briones M, O'Hagan DT (2001) A novel bioadhesive intranasal delivery system for inactivated influenza vaccines. J Control Release 70:267–276

Sloat BR, Cui Z (2006) Evaluation of the immune response induced by a nasal anthrax vaccine based on the protective antigen protein in anaesthetized and non-anaesthetized mice. J Pharm Pharmacol 58:439–447

Smart JD (2005) The basics and underlying mechanisms of mucoadhesion. Adv Drug Deliv Rev 57:1556–1568

Soane RJ, Frier M, Perkins AC et al (1999) Evaluation of the clearance characteristics of bioadhesive systems in humans. Int J Pharm 178:55–65

Southam DS, Dolovich M, O'Byrne PM et al (2002) Distribution of intranasal instillations in mice: effects of volume, time, body position, and anesthesia. Am J Physiol Lung Cell Mol Physiol 282:L833–L839

Spiers ID, Eyles JE, Baillie LW et al (2000) Biodegradable microparticles with different release profiles: effect on the immune response after a single administration via intranasal and intramuscular routes. J Pharm Pharmacol 52:1195–1201

Sreerama N, Woody RW (2000) Estimation of protein secondary structure from circular dichroism spectra: comparison of CONTIN, SELCON, and CDSSTR methods with an expanded reference set. Anal Biochem 287:252–260

Sreerama N, Woody RW (2004a) Computation and analysis of protein circular dichroism spectra. Methods Enzymol 383:318–351

Sreerama N, Woody RW (2004b) On the analysis of membrane protein circular dichroism spectra. Protein Sci 13:100–112

Staats HF, Ennis FA Jr (1999) IL-1 is an effective adjuvant for mucosal and systemic immune responses when coadministered with protein immunogens. J Immunol 162:6141–6147

Staats HF, McGhee JR (1996) Application of basic principles of mucosal immunity to vaccine development. In: Kiyono H, Ogra PL, McGhee JR (eds) Mucosal vaccines. Academic, New York, pp 17–39

Staats HF, Jackson RJ, Marinaro M et al (1994) Mucosal immunity to infection with implications for vaccine development. Curr Opin Immunol 6:572–583

Staats HF, Nichols WG, Palker TJ (1996) Mucosal immunity to HIV-1: systemic and vaginal antibody responses after intranasal immunization with the HIV-1 C4/V3 peptide T1SP10 MN(A). J Immunol 157:462–472

Staats HF, Montgomery SP, Palker TJ (1997) Intranasal immunization is superior to vaginal, gastric, or rectal immunization for the induction of systemic and mucosal anti-HIV antibody responses. AIDS Res Hum Retroviruses 13:945–952

Staats HF, Bradney CP, Gwinn WM et al (2001) Cytokine requirements for induction of systemic and mucosal CTL after nasal immunization. J Immunol 167:5386–5394

Staats HF, Alam SM, Scearce RM et al (2007) In vitro and in vivo characterization of anthrax anti-protective antigen and anti-lethal factor monoclonal antibodies after passive transfer in a mouse lethal toxin challenge model to define correlates of immunity. Infect Immun 75:5443–5452

Strickley RG, Anderson BD (1997) Solid-state stability of human insulin. II. Effect of water on reactive intermediate partitioning in lyophiles from pH 2–5 solutions: stabilization against covalent dimer formation. J Pharm Sci 86:645–653

Sullivan VJ, Mikszta JA, Laurent P et al (2006) Noninvasive delivery technologies: respiratory delivery of vaccines. Exp Opin Drug Deliv 3:87–95

Telko MJ, Hickey AJ (2005) Dry powder inhaler formulation. Respir Care 50:1209–1227

Tellier R (2006) Review of aerosol transmission of influenza A virus. Emerg Infect Dis 12:1657–1662

Teloni R, von Hunolstein C, Mariotti S et al (1994) Antibody classes & subclasses induced by mucosal immunization of mice with *Streptococcus pyogenes* M6 protein & oligodeoxynucleotides containing CpG motifs. Indian J Med Res 119:126–130

Tengvall S, Josefsson A, Holmgren J et al (2005) CpG oligodeoxynucleotide augments HSV-2 glycoprotein D DNA vaccine efficacy to generate T helper 1 response and subsequent protection against primary genital herpes infection in mice. J Rep Immunol 68:53

Thanou MM, Verhoef JC, Romeijn SG et al (1999) Effects of N-trimethyl chitosan chloride, a novel absorption enhancer, on caco-2 intestinal epithelia and the ciliary beat frequency of chicken embryo trachea. Int J Pharm 185:73–82

Thomas TC, McNamee MG (1990) Purification of membrane proteins. Methods Enzymol 182:499–520

Thompson AH, McRoberts JG, Crowe SR et al (1999) Optimal induction of upper respiratory tract immunity to reovirus 1/L by combined upper and lower respiratory tract inoculation. Vaccine 17:1404–1415

Uddowla S, Freytag LC, Clements JD (2007) Effect of adjuvants and route of immunizations on the immune response to recombinant plague antigens. Vaccine 25:7984–7993

Ugwoke MI, Agu RU, Jorissen M et al (2000) Toxicological investigations of the effects carboxymethylcellulose on ciliary beat frequency of human nasal epithelial cells in primary suspension culture and in vivo on rabbit nasal mucosa. Int J Pharm 205:43–51

Ugwoke MI, Verbeke N, Kinget R (2001) The biopharmaceutical aspects of nasal mucoadhesive drug delivery. J Pharm Pharmacol 53:3–21

US Department of Health and Human Services, Food and Drug Administration, and Center for Drug Evaluation and Research (2002) Guidance for industry: nasal spray and inhalation solution, suspension, and spray drug products—chemistry, manufacturing, and controls documentation www.fda.gov/downloads/Drugs/GuidanceComplianceRegulatoryInformation/Guidances/ucm070575

Uversky VN, Permyakov EA (2007) Methods in protein structure and stability analysis. Part B, vibrational spectroscopy. Nova Biomedical Books, New York

Van Den Berg L, Rose D (1959) Effect of freezing on the pH and composition of sodium and potassium phosphate solutions; the reciprocal system KH2PO4-Na2-HPO4–H2O. Arch Biochem Biophys 81:319–329

van der Lubben IM, Verhoef JC, Borchard G et al (2001) Chitosan for mucosal vaccination. Adv Drug Deliv Rev 52:139–144

van Ginkel FW, Jackson RJ, Yoshino N et al (2005) Enterotoxin-based mucosal adjuvants alter antigen trafficking and induce inflammatory responses in the nasal tract. Infect Immun 73:6892–6902

Van Hoeven N, Pappas C, Belser JA et al (2009) Human HA and polymerase subunit PB2 proteins confer transmission of an avian influenza virus through the air. Proc Natl Acad Sci USA 106:3366–3371

Waldman RH, Mann JJ, Small PA Jr (1969) Immunization against influenza. Prevention of illness in man by aerosolized inactivated vaccine. JAMA 207:520–524

Wang W (1999) Instability, stabilization, and formulation of liquid protein pharmaceuticals. Int J Pharm 185:129–188

Wang W (2000) Lyophilization and development of solid protein pharmaceuticals. Int J Pharm 203:1–60

Weeratna RD, Brazolot Millan CL, McCluskie MJ et al (2001) CpG ODN can re-direct the Th bias of established Th2 immune responses in adult and young mice. FEMS Immunol Med Microbiol 32:65

Weers JG, Tarara TE, Clark AR (2007) Design of fine particles for pulmonary drug delivery. Expert Opin Drug Deliv 4:297–313

Wigley FM, Wood SH, Waldman RH (1969) Aerosol immunization of humans with tetanus toxoid. J Immunol 103:1096–1098

Wimer-Mackin S, Hinchcliffe M, Petrie CR et al (2006) An intranasal vaccine targeting both the bacillus anthracis toxin and bacterium provides protection against aerosol spore challenge in rabbits. Vaccine 24:3953–3963

Wood JM, Schild GC, Newman RW et al (1977) An improved single radial-immunodiffusion technique for the assay of influenza haemagglutinin antigen: application for potency determinations of inactivated whole virus and subunit vaccines. J Biol Stand 5:237–247

Xiao BG, Link H (1997) Mucosal tolerance: a two-edged sword to prevent and treat autoimmune diseases. Clin Immunol Immunopathol 85:119–128

Xu W, Tamura T, Takatsu K (2008) CpG ODN mediated prevention from ovalbumin-induced anaphylaxis in mouse through B cell pathway. Int Immunopharmacol 8:351–361

Yeh HC, Brinker RM, Harkema JR et al (1997) A comparative analysis of primate nasal airways using magnetic resonance imaging and nasal casts. J Aerosol Med 10:319–329

Yoshioka S, Stella VJ (2002) Stability of drugs and dosage forms. Kluwer Academic Publisher, Boston, MA

Yoshioka S, Aso Y, Izutsu K et al (1993) Aggregates formed during storage of beta-galactosidase in solution and in the freeze-dried state. Pharm Res 10:687–691

Zohrabian A, Hayes EB, Petersen LR (2006) Cost-effectiveness of West Nile virus vaccination. Emerg Infect Dis 12:375–380

Mucosal Immunity and HIV-1 Infection: Applications for Mucosal AIDS Vaccine Development

Igor M. Belyakov and Jeffrey D. Ahlers

Abstract Natural transmission of human immunodeficiency virus type 1 (HIV-1) occurs through gastrointestinal and vaginal mucosa. These mucosal tissues are major reservoirs for initial HIV replication and amplification, and the sites of rapid $CD4^+$ T cell depletion. In both HIV-infected humans and SIV-infected macaques, massive loss of $CD4^+$ $CCR5^+$ memory T cells occurs in the gut and vaginal mucosa within the first 10–14 days of infection. Induction of local HIV-specific immune responses by vaccines may facilitate effective control of HIV or SIV replication at these sites. Vaccines that induce mucosal responses, in particular $CD8^+$ cytotoxic T lymphocytes (CTL), have controlled viral replication at mucosal sites and curtailed systemic dissemination. Thus, there is strong justification for development of next generation vaccines that induce mucosal immune effectors against HIV-1 including $CD8^+$ CTL, $CD4^+$ T helper cells and secretory IgA. In addition, further understanding of local innate mechanisms that impact early viral replication will greatly inform future vaccine development. In this review, we examine the current knowledge concerning mucosal AIDS vaccine development. Moreover, we propose immunization strategies that may be able to elicit an effective immune response that can protect against AIDS as well as other mucosal infections.

I. M. Belyakov (✉)
Midwest Research Institute, 110 Thomas Johnson Drive, Suite 170, Frederick, MD 21702, USA
e-mail: igorbelyakov@yahoo.com

J. D. Ahlers
National Institute of Allergy and Infectious Diseases, National Institutes of Health, 6700 Rockledge Drive, Bethesda, MD 20817, USA

Current Topics in Microbiology and Immunology (2012) 354: 157–179
DOI: 10.1007/82_2010_119

Published Online: 4 January 2011

Contents

1 Introduction

Gastrointestinal (GI) and vaginal mucosal tissues are major sites of HIV entry and initial infection (Veazey et al. 1998; Berzofsky et al. 2001; Belyakov and Berzofsky 2004; Neutra and Kozlowski 2006; Wilkinson and Cunningham 2006; Morrow et al. 2007; Belyakov and Ahlers 2008; Ahlers and Belyakov 2009a; Belyakov and Ahlers 2009b). An early sign of immunodeficiency virus infection is depletion of $CD4^+$ $CCR5^+$ memory T-cells in the mucosa (Brenchley et al. 2004; Li et al. 2005; Mehandru et al. 2004; Veazey et al. 1998, 2003). Dysfunction of the mucosal immune system during the early stages of AIDS leads to major structural abnormalities in the gut of infected individuals and to the development of opportunistic infections (Clayton et al. 2001; Heise et al. 1994; Kotler et al. 1984; Sharpstone et al. 1999). Subsequent systemic immune activation is considered a hallmark of the disease. Thus, AIDS can be considered primarily as a disease of the mucosal immune system (Belyakov and Berzofsky 2004). There is substantial evidence indicating that virus replication is rapid in the mucosa, eliminating $CD4^+$ target cells before dissemination into blood 2–7 days later (Spira et al. 1996; Zhang et al. 1999). Thus, the induction of $CD8^+$ CTL and $CD4^+$ T helper cells in concert with protective antibodies will be important criteria for an effective HIV vaccine (Kozlowski et al. 1997; Murphey-Corb et al. 1999; Baba et al. 2000; Barouch et al. 2000; Amara et al. 2001; Shiver et al. 2002; Kozlowski and Neutra 2003; McMichael 2006; Manrique et al. 2009; Sui et al. 2010).

2 Role of Mucosal $CD8^+$ CTL in Protection Against Local Viral Infection

Initially, studies pertaining to the mucosal immunology of HIV infection focused on induction of envelope specific antibody responses and the role of secretory IgA (S-IgA) and IgG in viral control (Funkhouser et al. 1993; Mazzoli et al. 1997). Failure to detect an early neutralizing antibody response in infected individuals, and the possibility that infection was primarily amplified by cell-to-cell spread, suggested that an effective antibody response was subverted by HIV infection. Furthermore, S-IgA antibodies were infrequently detected in mucosal secretions of HIV-infected individuals (Mestecky and Jackson 1994). In contrast, a major role for $CD8^+$ CTL in initial virus control was suggested in seminal studies showing that the depletion of peripheral $CD8^+$ cells in SIV-infected macaques significantly increased virus loads (Castro et al. 1992; Jin et al. 1999; Schmitz et al. 1999). However, evidence of a role for mucosal $CD8^+$ CTL in control of immunodeficiency virus infection was limited (Gallichan and Rosenthal 1996; Porgador et al. 1997; Belyakov et al. 1998a, b; Berzofsky et al. 1999; Berzofsky et al. 2004; Belyakov and Ahlers 2008; Ahlers and Belyakov 2009a).

Early studies in our laboratory attempted to understand the role of mucosal $CD8^+$ T cells in reducing mucosal viral loads and delaying the appearance of virus in the blood. We asked whether immunization with CD4Th-CD8 epitope peptide constructs through different mucosal routes (e.g., intrarectal, intragastric, intranasal) could elicit HIV-specific $CD8^+$ CTL in small intestinal Peyer's patches (PP) or lamina propria (Belyakov et al. 1998b). Mice were immunized with 4 doses of the synthetic HIV-1 Th-CTL envelope peptide construct, PCLUS3-18IIIB, on day 0, 7, 14 and 21 in combination with cholera toxin (CT) mucosal adjuvant. In a comparison of the three mucosal routes of immunization, only intrarectal (I.R.) immunization induced long-lasting, antigen-specific $CD8^+$ CTL memory in both the inductive PP and lamina propria effector sites as well as in the spleen. The CTL responses in spleen after I.R. immunization were similar to those induced by subcutaneous (S.C.) immunization (Belyakov et al. 1998b). In contrast, S.C. immunization with PCLUS3-18IIIB induced systemic $CD8^+$ CTL responses with little evidence of mucosal $CD8^+$ T cell responses (Belyakov et al. 1998b).

Strong long-lasting mucosal $CD8^+$ CTL responses can also be generated by mucosal immunization with recombinant vaccinia virus vectors (Belyakov et al. 1998d, 1999; Wyatt et al. 2008). In a follow up study, we demonstrated the mucosal immunogenicity of replication-defective modified vaccinia Ankara (MVA) virus expressing the HIV89.6 gp160 envelope protein in mice (Belyakov et al. 1998d). A single I.R. immunization with MVA89.6 generated antigen-specific $CD8^+$ CTL in both PP and intestinal lamina propria, at least as efficiently as a replication-competent recombinant vaccinia virus expressing 89.6 gp160 (Belyakov et al. 1998d). Furthermore, $CD8^+$ CTL responses were detected in PP up to 6 months after I.R. immunization with MVA89.6 and were slightly higher than those after immunization with WR89.6 virus (Belyakov et al. 1998d). In contrast, intraperitoneal (I.P.) immunization with MVA89.6 induced CTL in the PP but not in the intestinal lamina propria. The magnitude of the response in PP of I.P. immunized animals was modest compared to the spleen, and this result was reproducible in three independent experiments (Belyakov et al. 1998d).

Transcutaneous immunization has also been shown to induce immune responses in the GI tract (Glenn et al. 1998; Scharton-Kersten et al. 2000). The application of antigen and adjuvant directly onto the skin has induced robust IgG and S-IgA responses, as well as $CD8^+$ CTL in PP and lamina propria (Glenn et al.

2000; Gockel et al. 2000; Belyakov et al. 2004b). In addition, studies have demonstrated protection against mucosal challenge with toxin or live virus following transcutaneous immunization (Glenn et al. 1998; Gockel et al. 2000; Scharton-Kersten et al. 2000; Belyakov et al. 2004b). Transcutaneous vaccination targets antigen to bone marrow-derived Langerhan's dendritic cells (DC) resident in the outer epidermal layers of skin. In a recent study, we demonstrated that activated DC carrying skin-derived antigen migrate from the skin to PP and present antigen directly to resident lymphocytes (Belyakov et al. 2004). By using an in vivo pulsed antigen-presenting cell (APC)/T cell co-culture model for tracking migrating APC by flow cytometry, we demonstrated that $CD11c^+$ DC carrying skin-derived antigens can be isolated from PP inductive sites in intestinal mucosa within 24 h following transcutaneous immunization with HIV peptide vaccine and CT mucosal adjuvant (Belyakov et al. 2004). The ex vivo treatment of bone marrow-derived $CD11c^+$ DC with vitamin D3, CT, or forskolin has been shown to increase the ability of DC to migrate to inductive mucosal sites and to induce mucosal immune responses (Enioutina et al. 2000).

Direct evidence supporting the ability of local $CD8^+$ CTL to mediate protection against mucosal viral transmission has been difficult to obtain (Belyakov et al. 1998a). Furthermore, previous studies demonstrating protection against mucosal viral challenge had not elucidated immune mechanisms involved in protection (Marx et al. 1993). A number of studies have shown a role for $CD8^+$ CTL in protection against mucosal infections, such as influenza (Gao et al. 1991; Ulmer et al. 1993). However, understanding the role of $CD8^+$ CTL at mucosal sites of infection in control and resolution of infection where antibody plays a prominent role in protection is complex (Eichelberger et al. 1991; Lukacher et al. 1984; Taylor and Askonas 1986). In an early study, we were able to demonstrate CTL-mediated protection against mucosal viral challenge and showed that $CD8^+$ CTLs present at the mucosal site of challenge were required for protection (Belyakov et al. 1998a). Using a novel model mucosal viral challenge system with recombinant vaccinia virus that expresses HIV-1 gp160 in infected cells but not in the virus particle (in order to eliminate the contribution of antibody-mediated responses), we found that I.R. immunization with the synthetic HIV envelope peptide vaccine, PCLUS3-18IIIB, induced a mucosal $CD8^+$ CTL response that protected mice against vaccinia-gp160 challenge up to 6 months after mucosal immunization (Belyakov et al. 1998a). Protection was attributed to a specific T cell response against gp160 since mice were not protected against challenge with vaccinia virus expressing an unrelated protein (Belyakov et al. 1998a). Importantly, protection against I.R. challenge with vaccinia-gp160 was dependent on $CD8^+$ CTL as it was abrogated by treatment of I.R. immunized mice with anti-CD8 antibody (Belyakov et al. 1998a). Because S.C. HIV peptide immunization, which elicited a similar level of $CD8^+$ CTL in the spleen but not in the mucosa, did not protect, we concluded that protection against mucosal challenge requires local $CD8^+$ CTL. Local mucosal (but not systemic) delivery of IL-12 with CT in the vaccine formulation significantly increased mucosal and systemic HIV-specific CTL activity as well as the level of protection (Belyakov et al. 1998a).

Furthermore, we showed that the effect of IL-12 was dependent on induction of IFN-γ, as no effect of IL-12 in enhanced protection was seen in IFN-γ knock-out mice. This was the first study to demonstrate that mucosal $CD8^+$ CTL can mediate protection following local virus challenge in the mucosa (Belyakov et al. 1998a).

It is important to note that mucosal T cell responses and partial protection can be achieved with systemic immunization routes (Kaufman et al. 2008; Lin et al. 2007; Pal et al. 2006; Tatsis et al. 2007). However, it is the authors' opinion that optimal mucosal immune responses and protective immunity are achieved through oral, nasal, rectal, or vaginal mucosal immunization routes (Ahlers and Belyakov 2009a; Belyakov and Ahlers 2008, 2009). Also, it is important to state that mucosal DC are the main target for mucosal vaccination and systemic immunization may have a limited effect on these DC. DC precursors that are recruited to mesenteric lymph nodes (MLN) during inflammation are fully capable of secreting IL-12 and are potent inducers of Th1 IFN-γ responses. A recent study identified a population of $CD11c^{hi}$ $CD11b^{hi}$ lamina propria DC that express toll-like receptor (TLR)-5 and produce proinflammatory cytokines such as IL-6 and IL-12, but not IL-23 or IL-10, in response to flagellin (Uematsu et al. 2008). Understanding the unique properties of mucosal DC and the mucosal milieu in regulating local T and B cell responses and "mucosal memory" will be important for the delivery of vaccines that can provide protection against mucosal infections. Although the magnitude, quality of response, and tissue residency of cells that migrate to mucosal sites following systemic immunization needs further investigation, the targeting of mucosal DC for induction of local immune responses by mucosal vaccination has proven more effective for containing mucosal infections. Thus, next generation HIV-1 vaccines and vaccines against other mucosal pathogens will require formulations and delivery strategies which can effectively induce frontline mucosal immune responses and memory (Belyakov and Ahlers 2009a).

3 Cytokine and Adjuvants for Enhancing Mucosal CTL Responses

Cytokines and mucosal adjuvants are two major factors that can significantly augment mucosal $CD8^+$ CTL responses and protective efficacy of mucosal vaccines (Table 1) (Beagley and Elson 1992; Belyakov et al. 1999a; Belyakov et al. 2000; Staats et al. 2001; O'Neill et al. 2002; Ahlers et al. 2003; Belyakov et al. 2004a; Zhu et al. 2008; Ahlers and Belyakov 2009b; Zhu et al. 2010). Identification of cytokines, chemokines, and immunomodulatory molecules that augment mucosal CTL responses and resistance to mucosal viral challenge has largely been empirical (Belyakov et al. 1998c; Belyakov et al. 2004c; Belyakov et al. 2006a, b). We asked whether the combination of GM-CSF, which recruits DC to inductive sites, and IL-12, which drives $CD4^+$ Th1 function and $CD8^+$ CTL responses, could enhance mucosal immunogenicity and protective efficacy of an HIV-1 peptide vaccine given with mucosal adjuvants CT or LT(R192G). CT, one of the most

Table 1 Strategies for optimizing HIV vaccines

Strategy	Mechanism of activity	References
Mucosal route of immunization for induction of CTL in the mucosa	Protection against mucosal viral transmission was accomplished by establishing $CD8^+$ CTL in the mucosal tissue prior to exposure. Generation of functional $CD8^+$ CTL and compartmentalized immunity by mucosal vaccination was associated with the preservation of $CD4^+$ T cells in the colonic lamina propria after mucosal challenge with pathogenic virus	Barnett et al. (2008), Belyakov et al. (1998a, b, d, 1999, 2000, 2001a, 2006b, 2007a), Bruhl et al. (1998), Caputo et al. (2008), Egan et al. (2004), Kaneko et al. (2000), Li et al. (2008), Manrique et al. (2009), Mercier et al. (2007), Pinczewski et al. (2005), Ranasinghe et al. (2006), Sharpe et al. (2003), Shata et al. (2001), Vajdy et al. (2001)
Heterologous mucosal prime/boost	High quality $CD8^+$ CTL responses were generated in the intestinal mucosa after mucosal priming with HIV gp160 envelope DNA vaccine and mucosal boosting with recombinant viral vector expressing the same envelope gene. A single systemic immunization with rMVA was sufficient for induction of high-avidity $CD8^+$ CTL in systemic lymphoid organs, whereas a single mucosal immunization with rMVA was not able to elicit high-avidity $CD8^+$ CTL in the mucosa. A heterologous mucosal DNA prime-viral vector mucosal boost strategy was needed to induce functional HIV-1-specific $CD8^+$ CTL in intestinal mucosa	Allen et al. (2000), Amara et al. (2001), Belyakov et al. (2008), Eo et al. (2001), Evans et al. (2003), Gherardi et al. (2003), Gherardi et al. (2004), Hanke et al. (1998), Masopust et al. (2006), Neeson et al. (2006), Peacock et al. (2004), Ranasinghe et al. (2006), Ranasinghe et al. (2007), Sharpe et al. (2003), Zhou et al. (2007), Huang et al. (2007)

(continued)

Table 1 (continued)

Strategy	Mechanism of activity	References
Generation of high avidity CTL	High-avidity CTL are readily activated by low concentrations of peptide/MHC presented on target cells, while low avidity CTL require higher concentrations of peptide to become fully activated and exert effector function. Strong costimulation skew CTL toward higher avidity cells. High-avidity CTL exert selective pressure on HIV during the acute phase of infection, resulting in the emergence of escape variants. Vaccines that induce high-avidity mucosal CTL reduce dissemination of virus from the mucosa to the blood	Alexander-Miller et al. (1996), Belyakov et al. (2006b, 2007a, b, 2008), Bennett et al. (2007), Dzutsev et al. (2007), Estcourt et al. (2002), O'Connor et al. (2002), Oh et al. (2003), Ranasinghe et al. (2007), Sedlik et al. (2000), Snyder et al. (2003), Yoshizawa et al. (2003)
Inclusion of cytokines, chemokines, costimulatory molecules, and TLR ligands that enhance vaccine efficacy	Cytokine and chemokine combinations and TLR-triggering can help recruit monocytes, macrophages and neutrophils to local lymph nodes. TLR fusion proteins may help target antigen to the appropriate APC, stimulate maturation of DC, steer cellular immune responses toward Th1-type, and enhance mucosal S-IgA and IgG antibodies and isotype balance. Synergistic combinations of cytokines and immunomodulating molecules may be required for protection against mucosal challenge with virus. Mucosal adjuvant LT(R192G) alone was as effective as CT plus IL-12. GM-CSF synergized with LT(R192G). A triple cytokine combination of GM-CSF, IL-12, and TNF-α was synergistic for induction of $CD8^+$ CTL and for antiviral protection. Choice of adjuvants affects the interplay of cytokines and chemokines in regulation of mucosal CTL	Ahlers et al. (2001a, b, 2003), Belyakov et al. (1998c, 2000), Biragyn et al. (2002), Lena et al. (2002), O'Neill et al. (2002), Staats et al. (2001), Staats and Ennis 1999), Trumpfheller et al. (2008)

(continued)

Table 1 (continued)

Strategy	Mechanism of activity	References
Counteracting Treg mechanisms that dampen immune responses	Depletion of Treg with anti-CD25 antibody significantly enhanced $CD8^+$ T cell immunodominant responses in both the acute and memory phases of the immune response. The depletion of $CD4^+$ T cells enhanced long-lasting CD8-mediated protective immunity upon protein vaccination. In vivo inactivation experiments attributed enhancement primarily to MHC class II-restricted $CD4^+$ Treg cells which suppress the differentiation process towards effector memory $CD8^+$ T cells. Controlling suppressor effects at the time of vaccination may produce more effective long-term immunity	Denning et al. (2007), Heit et al. (2008), Shevach 2002), and Suvas et al. (2003)
Push–pull approach to maximize vaccine efficacy	A synergistic enhancement of vaccine mediated $CD8^+$ CTL generation and antiviral protection by GM-CSF and the costimulatory molecule CD40L, combined with the relief of suppression mediated by $CD4^+$ Treg cells, including $CD4^+$ NKT cells may provide optimum induction of $CD8^+$ CTL. Cytokines, costimulatory molecule agonists, and TLR synergies in combination with antibodies that block IL-10 or IL-13 produced by Type II NKT cells may provide optimum long term memory and protection	Ahlers et al. (2002) and Sutmuller et al. (2001)

commonly used mucosal adjuvants in experimental animals, is unsuitable for humans because of potent toxicity associated with a massive luminal secretory response (Xu-Amano et al. 1993; Marinaro et al. 1995; Elson 1996; Braun et al. 1999). A number of studies have introduced mutations into CT in an attempt to eliminate the toxicity associated with the ADP-ribosyltransferase activity of the A subunit and induction of cAMP in cells. These efforts have only been partially successful since induction of cAMP has been shown to be necessary for adjuvant activity. Dickinson and Clements constructed the LT(R192G) attenuated derivative of *Escherichia coli* heat-labile enterotoxin (LT) using site-directed mutagenesis (Dickinson and Clements 1995). They found that a single amino acid substitution of Glycine for Arginine at position 192 within the disulfide-subtended region of the LT A subunit separating A1 from A2 was effective for reducing toxicity while retaining significant adjuvant properties (Dickinson and Clements 1995; Dickinson and Clements 1996; Morris et al. 2000).

Using either CT or LT(R192G) and the HIV PCLUS3-18IIIB envelope peptide construct, we were able to demonstrate a synergistic effect between these mucosal adjuvants and the combination of GM-CSF and IL-12 for generating mucosal $CD8^+$ CTL in I.R. immunized mice (Belyakov et al. 2000). Furthermore, I.R. immunization with the HIV peptide plus LT(R192G) proved to be as effective for induction of HIV-specific $CD8^+$ CTL in PP and intestinal lamina propria as native LT or CT (Belyakov et al. 2000). After just two mucosal immunizations, the combination of the two cytokines synergistically enhanced the $CD8^+$ CTL response to the HIV-1 peptide vaccine (Belyakov et al. 2000). Co-administration of GM-CSF and IL-12 with peptide also markedly enhanced protection against mucosal challenge with vaccinia-gp160 when compared to animals immunized with each cytokine alone (Belyakov et al. 2000). However, supplementation of peptide vaccine with LT(R192G) and both cytokines afforded the greatest protection. The LT(R192G) adjuvant may produce a more favorable cytokine profile since, in contrast to CT, it did not inhibit IL-12 production (Belyakov et al. 2000). Also, much less IL-4 was induced by LT(R192G) than CT. Thus, the selection of mucosal adjuvant may be critical for influencing the cytokine environment and the induction of mucosal T cell responses that prevent viral transmission. It is important to note that different strategies from those used to elicit optimal cellular responses may be required for induction of humoral responses at mucosal sites. New HIV vaccine design incorporating $CD4^+$ and $CD8^+$ T cell epitopes with appropriate envelope immunogen structures and TLR agonists and the utilization of mucosal delivery strategies that target mucosal DC may induce both high-avidity $CD8^+$ CTL and local IgA and IgG neutralizing antibodies.

In a subsequent study, we demonstrated that GM-CSF, IL-12 and TNF-α also act synergistically in the induction of CD8+ CTL following systemic immunization (Ahlers et al. 2001a). The combination of IL-12 and TNF-α was essential for the optimal development of Th1 responses to provide help for $CD8^+$ CTL induction in vivo, while GM-CSF increased the number and activity of antigen-presenting DC in draining lymph nodes where the immune response was initiated (Ahlers et al. 2001a). Most importantly, significant improvement in protection against viral challenge was achieved when the triple combination of cytokines (GM-CSF, IL-12 and TNF-α) was co-administered with peptide vaccine (Ahlers et al. 2001a).

The increased magnitude in CTL responses and protection against viral infection afforded by synergistic combinations of cytokines could be further improved using a "push–pull" approach to counteract natural negative regulatory mechanisms which dampen Th1-type immune responses (Table 1) (Sutmuller et al. 2001; Ahlers et al. 2002). In a recent study, we showed that both T regulatory (Treg) and Natural Killer-T (NKT) cells suppress vaccine-induced immune responses (Ahlers et al. 2002). We found that relief of suppression through in vivo depletion of regulatory $CD4^+$ cells, including $CD4^+$ NKT cells, or blockade of IL-13 with an IL-13 receptor competitive inhibitor significantly improved vaccine-mediated $CD8^+$ T cell responses and protection against surrogate viral challenge. These results were confirmed in CD1-deficient animals that lack NKT cells (Ahlers et al. 2002). We reasoned that in mice in which $CD4^+$ T cells were depleted by antibody, the combination of GM-CSF and CD40L might substitute for $CD4^+$ T cell help. We deduced that GM-CSF would recruit more professional APC to the draining lymph nodes where soluble CD40L would provide maturation and activation signals (Ahlers et al. 2002). Indeed, GM-CSF and CD40L given with HIV peptide vaccine did act synergistically to enhance CTL responses in CD4-depleted mice. The improved CTL responses achieved by this push–pull strategy translated to significant protection against vaccinia-gp160 challenge (Ahlers et al. 2002). Thus, mucosal vaccination strategies that utilize both synergistic combinations of Th1-promoting cytokines and approaches that inhibit negative regulatory mechanisms could significantly enhance protective immunity against mucosal HIV transmission.

4 Mucosal Vaccination for Induction of Protective CTL in the Mucosa

Immune correlates of protection against HIV-1 are still not very well understood (Acierno et al. 2006; Ahlers, 2009 #8052; McMichael 2006; Neutra and Kozlowski 2006; Belyakov et al. 2008). However, accumulating experimental evidence suggests that mucosal immune responses (including S-IgA, IgG and $CD8^+$ CTL) in combination with circulating HIV neutralizing antibodies, $CD8^+$ CTL and $CD4^+$ T helper cells, and innate immune responses can exert varying degrees of control of HIV or SIV replication (Baba et al. 2000; Mascola et al. 2000; Bafica et al. 2004; Acierno et al. 2006; McMichael 2006). Disappointing results of the Merck vaccine trial underscore the importance of eliciting frontline mucosal immune responses that can significantly reduce virus load in the intestinal mucosa and subsequent viral dissemination to blood and peripheral lymphoid tissues.

We next asked whether mucosal $CD8^+$ CTL induced by mucosal immunization of rhesus macaques could impact the course of mucosal pathogenic retroviral infection similar to our studies in the surrogate viral challenge model in mice (Belyakov et al. 2001a). We found that SIV-specific CTL could be induced in the colon and mesenteric lymph nodes by I.R. immunization of monkeys with a synthetic HIV envelope/SIV gag, pol peptide vaccine and LT(R192G) adjuvant (Belyakov et al. 2001a). The SIV-specific intestinal CD8$^+$ CTL were able to traffic to systemic lymphoid tissues. Interestingly, S.C. immunized monkeys also developed significant CD8$^+$ CTL in the mesenteric lymph nodes. However, after rectal infection with chimeric simian–human immunodeficiency virus (SHIV)-ku2, the monkeys immunized by the I.R. route demonstrated a more rapid decline in blood and intestinal virus loads and a significantly lower viral load set point in blood when compared to S.C. immunized animals or adjuvant only controls. We speculated that more CD8$^+$ CTL induced by I.R. immunization were in the right place at the time of I.R. challenge with SHIVku2 (Belyakov et al. 2001a). The numbers of CD4$^+$ and CD8$^+$ T cells in I.R. immunized animals were also better preserved after SHIV challenge when compared to S.C. immunized animals. Thus, CD8$^+$ CTL induced at sites of mucosal challenge can significantly reduce immunodeficiency virus infection in primates, and mucosal immunization may be optimal to parenteral immunization for generating these cells. Rhesus macaques immunized by the intranasal route with a T cell-inducing SIV DNA/MVA vaccine have similarly demonstrated better control of rectal SIVmac251 infection when compared to macaques given the same vaccine by the I.M. route (Manrique et al. 2009). These studies provide strong rationale for the development of mucosal vaccines that generate HIV-specific CTL and T helper cells at sites of HIV exposure in humans.

5 Functional CD8$^+$ CTL for Preventing Immunodeficiency Virus Infection

5.1 Prime-Boost Strategies for Generating High-Avidity CTL

CD8$^+$ T cells that can be activated after recognition of peptide/MHC class I at low peptide concentration are defined as high-avidity CD8$^+$ CTL, whereas those that require high peptide concentrations are termed low-avidity CD8$^+$ CTL (Alexander-Miller et al. 1996; Snyder et al. 2003; Belyakov et al. 2006b; Belyakov et al. 2007b; Ahlers and Belyakov 2010c). It is well known today that high-avidity CD8$^+$ CTL are more effective for preventing viral infections (Alexander-Miller et al. 1996; Belyakov et al. 2006b, 2007a; Estcourt et al. 2002; Gallimore et al. 1998) and eliminating tumors (Yee et al. 1999; Zeh et al. 1999). Also, a functional impairment of HIV-specific CD8$^+$ CTL has been associated with clinical AIDS progression (Acierno et al. 2006; Ahlers and Belyakov 2010a; Appay et al. 2000; Hel et al. 2001; McKay et al. 2002). Thus, immunization strategies that generate high-avidity CD8$^+$ T cells in mucosal and systemic lymphoid tissues could significantly impact initial virus infection and progression of disease. Different combinations of heterologous prime-boost immunization protocols are currently being investigated in multiple experimental and clinical trials for HIV-1, other infectious diseases and cancer (Belshe et al. 1998; Allen et al. 2000; Barouch et al. 2000; Amara et al. 2000; Shiver et al. 2002; Gherardi et al. 2003; Dale et al. 2006) (Table 1).

In our studies, we employed a prime-boost immunization strategy consisting of a DNA prime and a rMVA or recombinant adenovirus (rAd) virus boost, all encoding an HIV-1 envelope protein, to evaluate immunization routes for ability to induce mucosal as well as systemic HIV-specific $CD8^+$ CTL in mice (Belyakov et al. 2008). A systemic I.M. prime-boost approach induced a strong CTL response in the spleen specific for the immunodominant CTL envelope epitope P18-I10 (measured by ^{51}Cr-release assay, 7 days after in vitro stimulation with P18-I10-peptide) and high-avidity CTL (determined by IFN-γ ELISPOT assay using titrated concentrations of P18-I10 peptide). However, the HIV-specific CTL responses in Peyer's patches were very low after I.M. DNA-MVA prime-boost immunizations (Belyakov et al. 2008). When the prime and boost routes were distinct, the delivery site of the boost had a greater impact than the site of DNA priming. For example, I.M. DNA prime and I.R. MVA boost was more effective than I.R. DNA prime and I.M. MVA boost for eliciting high-avidity $CD8^+$ CTL in the intestine. The optimal CTL response in the gut was observed after I.R. priming with HIV DNA vaccine and I.R. boosting with MVA (Belyakov et al. 2008). The I.R. prime-boost strategy also induced a very strong systemic P18-I10-specific CTL response. A single I.M. immunization with MVA was sufficient to elicit high-avidity $CD8^+$ CTL in systemic lymphoid organs (Belyakov et al. 2008). However, a single I.R. immunization with MVA was not able to elicit high-avidity $CD8^+$ CTL in the mucosa. These results indicate that a mucosal prime-mucosal boost strategy might be crucial to induce optimal cellular immunity in the mucosa. The requirement of a booster vaccination for induction of functionally active CTL in mucosal tissues using mucosal immunization routes may also be more stringent than that for generating high-avidity CTL in systemic tissues using systemic immunization routes (Belyakov et al. 2008).

5.2 Vaccine-Induced Mucosal High-Avidity $CD8^+$ CTL Preventing Virus Dissemination from Mucosa

It is a strongly debated subject whether mucosal or systemic $CD8^+$ CTL are necessary to prevent or reduce virus dissemination from the initial mucosal infection site to systemic tissues (Belyakov et al. 2004a; Belyakov and Berzofsky 2004; Belyakov et al. 2006b; Neutra and Kozlowski 2006; Belyakov and Ahlers 2008; Kaufman et al. 2008; Ahlers and Belyakov 2010b; Ahlers and Belyakov 2010c). Also, the role of CTL avidity in control of mucosal AIDS virus transmission is unknown. To address these questions, we used rhesus macaques to compare a peptide-based vaccine, a viral vector-based vaccine, and a combination peptide-prime/viral vector boost regimen (Belyakov et al. 2006b). We chose a prime-boost strategy with replication-incompetent recombinant NYVAC poxvirus expressing HIV envelope and SIV gag, pol proteins because similar systemic prime-viral vector boost strategies have been shown to elicit strong systemic CD8$^+$ CTL responses (Amara et al. 2001; Hanke et al. 1998; Hel et al. 2002; Shiver et al. 2002). The peptide vaccine contained a mixture of HIV and SIV CTL epitopes presented by Mamu-A*01, the class I antigen expressed by the macaques selected for this study (Belyakov et al. 2006b). All vaccines were delivered I.R. with a combination of GM-CSF, IL-12 and CpG oligodeoxynucleotides (ODN) as adjuvants. Four weeks after the last immunization, all macaques were challenged I.R. with SHIVku2 and monitored for plasma viral loads and CD8$^+$ CTL responses. Two weeks after the last immunization, we analyzed avidity of mucosal CD8$^+$ CTL in the MLN. To examine avidity, the T cell responses were evaluated by plotting specific lysis versus epitope concentration on peptide-coated target cells (Belyakov et al. 2001b; Belyakov et al. 2006b). We found that both vaccination regimens which included the peptide vaccine, GM-CSF, IL-12, and CpG ODN led to similar avidity, whereas I.R. NYVAC immunization alone produced CTL responses of lower magnitude and avidity. Thus, the peptide immunization and a combination of cytokines and CpG ODN improved CTL avidity and functionality, whereas boosting with NYVAC improved the magnitude of the CD8$^+$ CTL responses but not the quality. The prime-boost regimen was necessary to obtain responses with both the highest magnitude and avidity.

Next, we performed I.R. challenge and measured acute-phase peak viremia in blood as an indicator of systemic dissemination (Belyakov and Ahlers 2008; Belyakov et al. 2006b). We found that macaques given the peptide prime-poxvirus boost exhibited a significant (2.5 week) delay in peak viremia compared to macaques immunized with peptide or poxvirus alone. We interpreted this delay in the peak viremia to most likely reflect a temporary local mucosal control of initial virus replication by high-avidity CD8$^+$ CTL preventing rapid dissemination of virus from the intestinal mucosa into the bloodstream. At day 17 after challenge, when viral loads were near their peak, we found a strong inverse correlation between viremia and the numbers of antigen-specific CD8$^+$ T cells in the colon but not those in the blood. In addition, the animals that had CD8$^+$ CTL with the highest avidity in MLN were those that demonstrated the best viral control (Belyakov et al. 2006b). Thus, we demonstrated for the first time that a peptide-prime and poxvirus-boost vaccine that induced high levels of high-avidity mucosal CD8$^+$ CTL can delay dissemination of I.R. administered pathogenic SHIVku2 in macaques, and that such protection correlates better with mucosal rather than systemic CD8$^+$ CTL (Belyakov et al. 2006b).

5.3 *Localization of High Quality CD8$^+$ CTL at Sites of Vaccine Delivery*

A number of recent studies have demonstrated that antigen-specific CD8$^+$ CTL and partial protection against mucosal challenge with pathogenic SHIV can be achieved after systemic vaccination (Horner et al. 2001; Pal et al. 2006; Stevceva et al. 2002;

Vogel et al. 2003). However, as we and others have shown, mucosal vaccination can be even more effective for the clearance of virus from the major site of replication in the mucosa (Belyakov et al. 2006b, 2007a). The mechanism of protection generated by mucosal vaccination is not well understood. For example, the localization of $CD8^+$ effector and memory T cells after mucosal vaccination has not been well characterized. However, for many mucosal intracellular pathogens (including HIV and Herpes), an effective vaccine strategy will require induction and long-term maintenance of antigen-specific B cells, $CD4^+$ Th cells and CTL at the site of viral transmission. In one study, we performed mucosal versus systemic immunization and compared $CD8^+$ CTL avidity in lymphoid tissues proximal and distal to the site of immunization (Belyakov et al. 2007a). We observed a novel compartmentalization of functional HIV-specific $CD8^+$ CTL in tissue most proximal to the site of immunization (Belyakov et al. 2007a). In this study, mice were immunized with MVA by the S.C. or I.R. immunization routes. To determine the extent of compartmentalization, we measured vaccinia B8R peptide-specific $CD8^+$ T cells by tetramer staining (Tscharke et al. 2005) and by IFN-γ production using ELISPOT with cells from the spleen, small intestinal epithelium, and lamina propria (Belyakov et al. 2007a). We found that both systemic and mucosal routes of immunization generated vaccinia-specific $CD8^+$ T cells in both systemic and mucosal compartments, when measured as total numbers of B8R tetramer-positive $CD8^+$ T cells. However, when we characterized the functional activity of the cells by IFN-γ production, the cell distribution was asymmetric (Belyakov et al. 2007a). The S.C. vaccination with MVA induced a significant number of IFN-γ-producing cells in the spleen, but not in the gut, while I.R. immunization generated greater numbers of IFN-γ secreting $CD8^+$ T cells in the intestinal epithelium and lamina propria. Thus, mucosal immunization produced a much higher ratio of IFN-γ-secreting cells to the total B8R-tetramer positive cells in the gut when compared to systemic immunization (Belyakov et al. 2007a). We also found that I.R. immunization induced more IL-12-producing DC in the colon, while S.C. vaccination induced more IL-12-producing DC in axillary lymph nodes (ALN). Thus, differences in local DC activation could account for the differences in functional T cells in proximal versus distal tissues (Belyakov et al. 2007a) (Fig. 1).

We also characterized the function and avidity of CTL in mucosal MLN and systemic ALN of Mamu-A*01+ rhesus macaques after I.R. and S.C. vaccination with an HIV–SIV Th-CTL peptide vaccine by using a functional ^{51}Cr release assay with different concentrations of peptide (Kuroda et al. 1998)-coated target cells and ELISPOT assay for IFN-γ secretion (Belyakov et al. 2007a). We observed that after I.R. immunization, specific lysis by MLN cells was very high against both low and high concentrations of CTL peptide on target cells, indicating a large proportion of high-avidity $CD8^+$ CTL. In contrast, S.C. vaccination induced greater levels of high-avidity $CD8^+$ CTL in ALN and was less effective for induction of functional $CD8^+$ CTL in MLN. Moreover, we found a strong inverse correlation between the number of high-avidity $CD8^+$ CTL in the mucosal compartment and viral load in the colon 200 days after I.R. challenge with SHIVku-2 (Belyakov et al. 2007a). There was also a strong positive correlation between the percentage of $CD4^+$ T cells

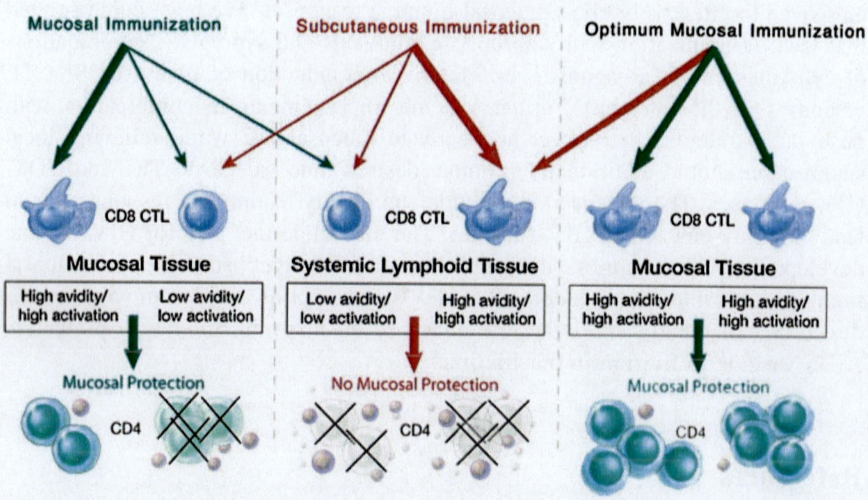

Fig. 1 Avidity of CTL in relation to vaccination route and protection. High-avidity CD8$^+$ CTL are optimal to low-avidity CTL for containing immunodeficiency virus infection. Suboptimal mucosal immunization (e.g., with vaccine lacking adjuvants) can induce high-avidity CTL at the vaccination site but it also produces low-avidity CD8$^+$ CTL or T cell anergy, which results in limited mucosal protection. Systemic immunization produces high-avidity CTL in systemic tissues but not mucosal tissues, allowing rapid CD4$^+$ T cell depletion and viral spread to the periphery. Optimal mucosal immunization establishes high-avidity CD8$^+$ CTL in both mucosal and peripheral lymphoid tissues. Multiple variables influence the quality of the CTL response achieved by mucosal vaccination including: dose, frequency, the use of synergistic combinations of mucosal adjuvants, cytokines, chemokines, and TLR ligands to enhance vaccine efficacy. Furthermore, heterologous prime-boost strategies and push–pull approaches will be needed to maximize vaccine efficacy

in colonic lamina propria and the number of high-avidity antigen-specific CD8$^+$ CTL in the same location (Belyakov et al. 2007a). Thus, a mucosal AIDS vaccine reduced viral load and the depletion of CD4$^+$ T cells in the intestinal mucosa. Control of mucosally transmitted immunodeficiency virus infection can be generated by local mucosal immunization, and the mechanism for this control can be attributed to the focusing of high quality cellular responses at sites of viral exposure (Belyakov et al. 2007a). The additional induction of mucosal and systemic antibodies should improve protection even more significantly by working in concert with CTL to prevent viral entry and replication in mucosal tissues.

6 Conclusion

Local mucosal CD8$^+$ CTL and antibody may completely prevent HIV transmission at mucosal surfaces or potentially control virus replication within mucosal tissues prior to systemic dissemination. We believe that a number of approaches can be employed to effectively elicit mucosal immune responses. We have demonstrated that local immunization with appropriate adjuvants and synergistic combinations of cytokines and TLR agonists are effective for induction of potent $CD8^+$ CTL responses in the intestine. Further vaccine improvements in combination with push–pull strategies that target and activate mucosal DC while relieving local suppression should additionally promote desired mucosal $CD4^+$ Th1 and $CD8^+$ CTL responses. The enhanced magnitude and quality of immune responses could lead to highly efficacious HIV vaccines. The next important step for HIV vaccine development will be to move these new design and delivery strategies for mucosal immunization into Phase 1 clinical trials. We are optimistic that moving in this direction will greatly accelerate the efforts of so many in bringing a protective AIDS vaccine to fruition in our lifetime.

References

Acierno PM, Schmitz JE, Gorgone DA et al (2006) Preservation of functional virus-specific memory CD8+ T lymphocytes in vaccinated, simian human immunodeficiency virus-infected rhesus monkeys. J Immunol 176:5338–5345

Ahlers JD, Belyakov IM (2009a) Strategies for optimizing targeting and delivery of mucosal HIV vaccines. Eur J Immunol 39:2657–2669

Ahlers JD, Belyakov IM (2009b) Strategies for recruiting and targeting dendritic cells for optimizing HIV vaccines. Trends Mol Med 15:263–274

Ahlers JD, Belyakov IM (2010a) Lessons learned from natural infection: focusing on the design of protective T cell vaccines for HIV/AIDS. Trends Immunol 31:120–130

Ahlers JD, Belyakov IM (2010b) Memories that last forever: strategies for optimizing vaccine T-cell memory. Blood 115:1678–1689

Ahlers JD, Belyakov IM (2010c) New paradigms for generating effective CD8+ T cell responses against HIV-1/AIDS. Discov Med 9:528–537

Ahlers JD, Belyakov IM, Matsui S et al (2001a) Mechanisms of cytokine synergy essential for vaccine protection against viral challenge. Int Immunol 13:897–908

Ahlers JD, Belyakov IM, Matsui S et al (2001b) Signals delivered through TCR instruct IL-12R expression: IL-12 and TNFα synergize for IL-12R expression at low antigen dose. Int Immunol 13:1433–1442

Ahlers JD, Belyakov IM, Terabe M et al (2002) A push-pull approach to maximize vaccine efficacy: abrogating suppression with an IL-13 inhibitor while augmenting help with GM-CSF and CD40L. Proc Natl Acad Sci USA 99:13020–13025

Ahlers JD, Belyakov IM, Berzofsky JA (2003) Cytokine, chemokine and costimulatory molecule modulation to enhance efficacy of HIV vaccines. Curr Mol Med 3:285–301

Alexander-Miller MA, Leggatt GR, Berzofsky JA (1996) Selective expansion of high or low avidity cytotoxic T lymphocytes and efficacy for adoptive immunotherapy. Proc Natl Acad Sci USA 93:4102–4107

Allen TM, Vogel TU, Fuller DH et al (2000) Induction of AIDS virus-specific CTL activity in fresh, unstimulated peripheral blood lymphocytes from rhesus macaques vaccinated with a DNA prime/modified vaccinia virus Ankara boost regimen. J Immunol 164:4968–4978

Amara RR, Villinger F, Altman JD et al (2001) Control of a mucosal challenge and prevention of AIDS by a multiprotein DNA/MVA vaccine. Science 292:69–74

Appay V, Nixon DF, Donahoe SM et al (2000) HIV-specific CD8(+) T cells produce antiviral cytokines but are impaired in cytolytic function. J Exp Med 192:63–75

Baba TW, Liska V, Hofmann-Lehmann R et al (2000) Human neutralizing monoclonal antibodies of the IgG1 subtype protect against mucosal simian-human immunodeficiency virus infection. Nat Med 6:200–206

Bafica A, Scanga CA, Schito M et al (2004) Influence of coinfecting pathogens on HIV expression: evidence for a role of Toll-like receptors. J Immunol 172:7229–7234

Barnett SW, Srivastava IK, Kan E et al (2008) Protection of macaques against vaginal SHIV challenge by systemic or mucosal and systemic vaccinations with HIV-envelope. AIDS 22:339–348

Barouch DH, Santra S, Schmitz JE et al (2000) Control of viremia and prevention of clinical AIDS in rhesus monkeys by cytokine-augmented DNA vaccination. Science 290:486–492

Beagley KW, Elson CO (1992) Cells and cytokines in mucosal immunity and inflammation. Gastroenterol Clin North Am 21:347–366

Belshe RB, Gorse GJ, Mulligan MJ, Evans TG, Keefer MC, Excler JL, Duliege AM, Tartaglia J, Cox WI, McNamara J, Hwang KL, Bradney A, Montefiori D, Weinhold KJ (1998) Induction of immune responses to HIV-1 by canarypox virus (ALVAC) HIV-1 and gp120 SF-2 recombinant vaccines in uninfected volunteers. NIAID AIDS Vaccine Evaluation Group. Aids 12:2407–2415

Belyakov IM, Ahlers JD (2008) Functional CD8(+) CTLs in mucosal sites and HIV infection: moving forward toward a mucosal AIDS vaccine. Trends Immunol 29:574–585

Belyakov IM, Ahlers JD (2009b) What role does the route of immunization play in the generation of protective immunity against mucosal pathogens? J Immunol 183:6883–6892

Belyakov IM, Ahlers JD (2009a) Comment on "trafficking of antigen-specific CD8+ T lymphocytes to mucosal surfaces following intramuscular vaccination". J Immunol 182: 1779–1780

Belyakov IM, Ahlers JD, Berzofsky JA (2004a) Mucosal AIDS vaccines: current status and future directions. Expert Rev Vaccines 3: Suppl 65–73

Belyakov IM, Berzofsky JA (2004b) Immunobiology of mucosal HIV infection and the basis for development of a new generation of mucosal AIDS vaccines. Immunity 20:247–253

Belyakov IM, Clements JD, Ahlers JD, Strober W, Berzofsky JA (1999a) Approaches to improve engineered HIV vaccine which induce mucosal immunity. J Human Virol 2:217–210

Belyakov IM, Ahlers JD, Brandwein BY et al (1998a) The importance of local mucosal HIV-specific CD8+ cytotoxic T lymphocytes for resistance to mucosal-viral transmission in mice and enhancement of resistance by local administration of IL-12. J Clin Invest 102:2072–2081

Belyakov IM, Derby MA, Ahlers JD et al (1998b) Mucosal immunization with HIV-1 peptide vaccine induces mucosal and systemic cytotoxic T lymphocytes and protective immunity in mice against intrarectal recombinant HIV-vaccinia challenge. Proc Natl Acad Sci USA 95:1709–1714

Belyakov IM, Kelsall B, Strober W et al (1998c) Use of rIL-12 for enhancing the mucosal cytotoxic T lymphocyte response to a peptide HIV vaccine. J Invest Med 46:216A

Belyakov IM, Klinman D, Kuznetsov VA, Moniuszko M, Ahlers JD, Kelsall B, Strober W, Franchini G, Berzofsky JA (2004c) Progress on new mucosalvaccine stategies for HIV. FASEB Journal 18:A821–A821

Belyakov IM, Wyatt LS, Ahlers JD et al (1998d) Induction of mucosal CTL response by intrarectal immunization with a replication-deficient recombinant vaccinia virus expressing HIV 89.6 envelope protein. J Virol 72:8264–8272

Belyakov IM, Moss B, Strober W et al (1999) Mucosal vaccination overcomes the barrier to recombinant vaccinia immunization caused by preexisting poxvirus immunity. Proc Natl Acad Sci USA 96:4512–4517

Belyakov IM, Ahlers JD, Clements JD et al (2000) Interplay of cytokines and adjuvants in the regulation of mucosal and systemic HIV-specific cytotoxic T lymphocytes. J Immunol 165:6454–6462

Belyakov IM, Hel Z, Kelsall B et al (2001a) Mucosal AIDS vaccine reduces disease and viral load in gut reservoir and blood after mucosal infection of macaques. Nat Med 7:1320–1326

Belyakov IM, Wang J, Koka R et al (2001b) Activating CTL precursors to reveal CTL function without skewing the repertoire by in vitro expansion. Eur J Immunol 31:3557–3566

Belyakov IM, Hammond SA, Ahlers JD et al (2004) Transcutaneous immunization induces mucosal CTL and protective immunity by migration of primed skin dendritic cells. J Clin Invest 113:998–1007

Belyakov IM, Isakov D, Zhu Q et al (2006a) Enhancement of CD8+ T cell immunity in the lung by CpG ODN increases protective efficacy of a Modified Vaccinia Ankara vaccine against lethal poxvirus infection even in CD4-deficient host. J Immunol 177:6336–6343

Belyakov IM, Kuznetsov VA, Kelsall B et al (2006b) Impact of vaccine-induced mucosal high avidity CD8+ CTLs in delay of AIDS-viral dissemination from mucosa. Blood 107:3258–3264

Belyakov IM, Isakov D, Zhu Q et al (2007a) A novel functional CTL avidity/activity compartmentalization to the site of mucosal immunization contributes to protection of macaques against simian/human immunodeficiency viral depletion of mucosal CD4+ T cells. J Immunol 178:7211–7221

Belyakov IM, Kozlowski S, Mage M et al (2007b) Role of {alpha}3 domain of class I MHC molecules in the activation of high- and low-avidity CD8+ CTLs. Int Immunol 19:1413–1420

Belyakov IM, Ahlers JD, Nabel GJ et al (2008) Generation of functionally active HIV-1 specific CD8(+) CTL in intestinal mucosa following mucosal, systemic or mixed prime-boost immunization. Virology 381:106–115

Bennett MS, Ng HL, Dagarag M et al (2007) Epitope-dependent avidity thresholds for cytotoxic T-lymphocyte clearance of virus-infected cells. J Virol 81:4973–4980

Berzofsky JA, Ahlers JD, Belyakov IM (2001) Strategies for designing and optimizing new generation vaccines. Nature Reviews Immunology 1:209–219

Berzofsky JA, Ahlers JD, Derby MA, Pendleton CD, Arichi T, Belyakov IM (1999) Approaches to improve engineered vaccines for human immunodeficiency virus (HIV) and other viruses that cause chronic infections. Immunol Rev 170:151–172

Berzofsky JA, Ahlers J, Janik J et al (2004) Progress on new vaccine strategies against chronic viral infections. J Clin Invest 114:450–462

Biragyn A, Belyakov IM, Chow YH et al (2002) DNA vaccines encoding human immunodeficiency virus-1 glycoprotein 120 fusions with proinflammatory chemoattractants induce systemic and mucosal immune responses. Blood 100:1153–1159

Braun MC, He J, Wu C-Y, Kelsall BL (1999) Cholera toxin suppresses interleukin (IL)-12 production and IL-12 receptor B1 and B2 chain expression. J Exp Med 189:541–552

Brenchley JM, Schacker TW, Ruff LE et al (2004) CD4+ T cell depletion during all stages of HIV disease occurs predominantly in the gastrointestinal tract. J Exp Med 200:749–759

Bruhl P, Kerschbaum A, Eibl MM et al (1998) An experimental prime-boost regimen leading to HIV type 1-specific mucosal and systemic immunity in BALB/c mice. AIDS Res Hum Retroviruses 14:401–407

Caputo A, Brocca-Cofano E, Castaldello A et al (2008) Characterization of immune responses elicited in mice by intranasal co-immunization with HIV-1 Tat, gp140 DeltaV2Env and/or SIV Gag proteins and the nontoxicogenic heat-labile Escherichia coli enterotoxin. Vaccine 26:1214–1227

Castro BA, Homsy J, Lennette E et al (1992) HIV-1 expression in chimpanzees can be activated by CD8+ cell depletion or CMV infection. Clin Immunol Immunopathol 65:227–233

Clayton F, Kapetanovic S, Kotler DP (2001) Enteric microtubule depolymerization in HIV infection: a possible cause of HIV-associated enteropathy. AIDS 15:123–124

Dale CJ, Thomson S, De Rose R et al (2006) Prime-boost strategies in DNA vaccines. Methods Mol Med 127:171–197

Denning TL, Wang YC, Patel SR et al (2007) Lamina propria macrophages and dendritic cells differentially induce regulatory and interleukin 17-producing T cell responses. Nat Immunol 8:1086–1094

Dickinson BL, Clements JD (1995) Dissociation of *Escherichia coli* heat-labile enterotoxin adjuvanticity from ADP-ribosyltransferase activity. Infect Immun 63:1617–1623

Dickinson BL, Clements JD (1996) Use of Escherichia coli heat-liable enterotoxin asan oral adjuvant. In: Mucosal Vaccines. Academic Press, New York, pp 73–87

Dzutsev AH, Belyakov IM, Isakov DV et al (2007) Avidity of CD8 T cells sharpens immunodominance. Int Immunol 19:497–507

Egan MA, Chong SY, Rose NF et al (2004) Immunogenicity of attenuated vesicular stomatitis virus vectors expressing HIV type 1 Env and SIV Gag proteins: comparison of intranasal and intramuscular vaccination routes. AIDS Res Hum Retroviruses 20:989–1004

Eichelberger M, Allan W, Zijlstra M et al (1991) Clearance of influenza virus respiratory infection in mice lacking class I major histocompatibility complex-restricted CD8+ T cells. J Exp Med 174:875–880

Elson CO (1996) Cholera toxin as a mucosal adjuvant. In: Kiyono H, McGhee JR, Ogra PL (eds) Mucosal Vaccines. Academic Press, San Diego, pp 59–72

Enioutina EY, Visic D, Daynes RA (2000) The induction of systemic and mucosal immune responses to antigen-adjuvant compositions administered into the skin: alterations in the migratory properties of dendritic cells appears to be important for stimulating mucosal immunity. Vaccine 18:2753–2767

Eo SK, Gierynska M, Kamar AA et al (2001) Prime-boost immunization with DNA vaccine: mucosal route of administration changes the rules. J Immunol 166:5473–5479

Estcourt MJ, Ramsay AJ, Brooks A et al (2002) Prime-boost immunization generates a high frequency, high-avidity CD8(+) cytotoxic T lymphocyte population. Int Immunol 14:31–37

Evans DT, Chen LM, Gillis J et al (2003) Mucosal priming of simian immunodeficiency virus-specific cytotoxic T-lymphocyte responses in rhesus macaques by the Salmonella type III secretion antigen delivery system. J Virol 77:2400–2409

Funkhouser A, Clements ML, Slome S et al (1993) Antibodies to recombinant gp160 in mucosal secretions and sera of persons infected with HIV-1 and seronegative vaccine recipients. AIDS Res Hum Retroviruses 9:627–632

Gallichan WS, Rosenthal KL (1996) Long-lived cytotoxic T lymphocyte memory in mucosal tissues after mucosal but not systemic immunization. J Exp Med 184:1879–1890

Gallimore A, Dumrese T, Hengartner H et al (1998) Protective immunity does not correlate with the hierarchy of virus-specific cytotoxic T cell responses to naturally processed peptides. J Exp Med 187:1647–1657

Gao X-M, Zheng B, Liew FY et al (1991) Priming of influenza virus-specific cytotoxic T lymphocytes vivo by short synthetic peptides. J Immunol 147:3268–3273

Gherardi MM, Najera JL, Perez-Jimenez E et al (2003) Prime-boost immunization schedules based on influenza virus and vaccinia virus vectors potentiate cellular immune responses against human immunodeficiency virus Env protein systemically and in the genitorectal draining lymph nodes. J Virol 77:7048–7057

Gherardi MM, Perez-Jimenez E, Najera JL et al (2004) Induction of HIV immunity in the genital tract after intranasal delivery of a MVA vector: enhanced immunogenicity after DNA prime-modified vaccinia virus Ankara boost immunization schedule. J Immunol 172:6209–6220

Glenn GM, Scharton-Kersten T, Vassell R et al (1998) Transcutaneous immunization with cholera toxin protects mice against lethal mucosal toxin challenge. J Immunol 161:3211–3214

Glenn GM, Taylor DN, Li X et al (2000) Transcutaneous immunization: a human vaccine delivery strategy using a patch. Nat Med 6:1403–1406

Gockel CM, Bao S, Beagley KW (2000) Transcutaneous immunization induces mucosal and systemic immunity: a potent method for targeting immunity to the female reproductive tract. Mol Immunol 37:537–544

Hanke T, Blanchard TJ, Schneider J et al (1998) Enhancement of MHC class I-restricted peptide-specific T cell induction by a DNA prime/MVA boost vaccination regime. Vaccine 16:439–445

Heise C, Miller CJ, Lackner A et al (1994) Primary acute simian immunodeficiency virus infection of intestinal lymphoid tissue is associated with gastrointestinal dysfunction. J Infect Dis 169:1116–1120

Heit A, Gebhardt F, Lahl K et al (2008) Circumvention of regulatory CD4(+) T cell activity during cross-priming strongly enhances T cell-mediated immunity. Eur J Immunol 38:1585–1597

Hel Z, Nacsa J, Kelsall BL et al (2001) Impairment of Gag-specific D8^{+} T-cell function in mucosal and sytemic compartments of SIV_{mac251}- and $SHIV_{KU2}$-infected macaques. J Virol 75:11483–11495

Hel Z, Nacsa J, Tryniszewska E et al (2002) Containment of simian immunodeficiency virus infection in vaccinated macaques: correlation with the magnitude of virus-specific pre- and postchallenge CD4+ and CD8+ T cell responses. J Immunol 169:4778–4787

Horner AA, Datta SK, Takabayashi K et al (2001) Immunostimulatory DNA-based vaccines elicit multifaceted immune responses against HIV at systemic and mucosal sites. J Immunol 167:1584–1591

Huang X, Xu J, Qiu C et al (2007) Mucosal priming with PEI/DNA complex and systemic boosting with recombinant TianTan vaccinia stimulate vigorous mucosal and systemic immune responses. Vaccine 25:2620–2629

Jin X, Bauer DE, Tuttleton SE et al (1999) Dramatic rise in plasma viremia after CD8+ T cell depletion in simian immunodeficiency virus-infected macaques. J Exp Med 189:991–998

Kaneko H, Bednarek I, Wierzbicki A et al (2000) Oral DNA vaccination promotes mucosal and systemic immune responses to HIV envelope glycoprotein. Virology 267:8–16

Kaufman DR, Liu J, Carville A et al (2008) Trafficking of antigen-specific CD8+ T lymphocytes to mucosal surfaces following intramuscular vaccination. J Immunol 181:4188–4198

Kotler DP, Gaetz HP, Lange M et al (1984) Enteropathy associated with the acquired immunodeficiency syndrome. Ann Intern Med 101:421–428

Kozlowski PA, Neutra MR (2003) The role of mucosal immunity in prevention of HIV transmission. Curr Mol Med 3:217–228

Kozlowski PA, Cu-Uvin S, Neutra MR, Flanigan TP (1997) Comparison of the oral, rectal, and vaginal immunization routes for induction of antibodies in rectal and genital tract secretions of women. Infect Immun. 65:1387–1394

Kuroda MJ, Schmitz JE, Barouch DH et al (1998) Analysis of Gag-specific cytotoxic T lymphocytes in simian immunodeficiency virus-infected rhesus monkeys by cell staining with a tetrameric major histocompatibility complex class I-peptide complex. J Exp Med 187:1373–1381

Lena P, Villinger F, Giavedoni L et al (2002) Co-immunization of rhesus macaques with plasmid vectors expressing IFN-gamma, GM-CSF, and SIV antigens enhances anti-viral humoral immunity but does not affect viremia after challenge with highly pathogenic virus. Vaccine 20(Suppl 4):A69–A79

Li Q, Duan L, Estes JD et al (2005) Peak SIV replication in resting memory CD4+ T cells depletes gut lamina propria CD4+ T cells. Nature 434:1148–1152

Li Z, Zhang M, Zhou C et al (2008) Novel vaccination protocol with two live mucosal vectors elicits strong cell-mediated immunity in the vagina and protects against vaginal virus challenge. J Immunol 180:2504–2513

Lin SW, Cun AS, Harris-McCoy K et al (2007) Intramuscular rather than oral administration of replication-defective adenoviral vaccine vector induces specific CD8+ T cell responses in the gut. Vaccine 25:2187–2193

Lukacher AE, Braciale VL, Braciale TJ (1984) In vivo effector function of influenza virus-specific cytotoxic T lymphocyte clones is highly specific. J Exp Med 160:814–826

Manrique M, Kozlowski PA, Wang SW et al (2009) Nasal DNA-MVA SIV vaccination provides more significant protection from progression to AIDS than a similar intramuscular vaccination. Mucosal Immunol 2:536–550

Marinaro M, Staats HF, Hiroi T, Jackson RJ, Coste M, Boyaka PN, Okahashi N, Yamamoto M, Kiyono H, Bluethmann H, Fujihashi K, McGhee JR (1995) Mucosal adjuvant effect of cholera toxin in mice results from induction of T helper 2 (Th2) cells and IL-4. J.Immunol. 155:4621–4629

Marx PA, Compans RW, Gettie A et al (1993) Protection against vaginal SIV transmission with microencapsulated vaccine. Science 260:1323–1327

Mascola JR, Stiegler G, VanCott TC et al (2000) Protection of macaques against vaginal transmission of a pathogenic HIV-1/SIV chimeric virus by passive infusion of neutralizing antibodies. Nat Med 6:207–210

Masopust D, Ha SJ, Vezys V et al (2006) Stimulation history dictates memory CD8 T cell phenotype: implications for prime-boost vaccination. J Immunol 177:831–839

Mazzoli S, Trabattoni D, Lo Caputo S et al (1997) HIV-specific mucosal and cellular immunity in HIV-seronegative partners of HIV-seropositive individuals. Nat Med 3:1250–1257

McKay PF, Schmitz JE, Barouch DH et al (2002) Vaccine protection against functional CTL abnormalities in simian human immunodeficiency virus-infected rhesus monkeys. J Immunol 168:332–337

McMichael AJ (2006) HIV vaccines. Annu Rev Immunol 24:227–255

Mehandru S, Poles MA, Tenner-Racz K et al (2004) Primary HIV-1 infection is associated with preferential depletion of CD4+ T lymphocytes from effector sites in the gastrointestinal tract. J Exp Med 200:761–770

Mercier GT, Nehete PN, Passeri MF et al (2007) Oral immunization of rhesus macaques with adenoviral HIV vaccines using enteric-coated capsules. Vaccine 25:8687–8701

Mestecky J, Jackson S (1994) Reassessment of the impact of mucosal immunity in infection with the human immunodeficiency virus (HIV) and design of relevant vaccines. J Clin Immunol 14:259–272

Morris CB, Cheng E, Thanawastien A et al (2000) Effectiveness of intranasal immunization with HIV-gp160 Env CTL epitope peptide (E7) in combination with the mucosal adjuvant LT(R192G). Vaccine 18:1944–1951

Morrow G, Vachot L, Vagenas P et al (2007) Current concepts of HIV transmission. Curr HIV/AIDS Rep 4:29–35

Murphey-Corb M, Wilson LA, Trichel AM et al (1999) Selective induction of protective MHC class I restricted CTL in the intestinal lamina propria of rhesus monkeys by transient SIV infection of the colonic mucosa. J Immunol 162:540–549

Neeson P, Boyer J, Kumar S et al (2006) A DNA prime-oral Listeria boost vaccine in rhesus macaques induces a SIV-specific CD8 T cell mucosal response characterized by high levels of alpha4beta7 integrin and an effector memory phenotype. Virology 354:299–315

Neutra MR, Kozlowski PA (2006) Mucosal vaccines: the promise and the challenge. Nat Rev Immunol 6:148–158

O'Connor DH, Allen TM, Vogel TU et al (2002) Acute phase cytotoxic T lymphocyte escape is a hallmark of simian immunodeficiency virus infection. Nat Med 8:493–499

Oh S, Hodge JW, Ahlers JD et al (2003) Selective induction of high avidity CTL by altering the balance of signals from antigen presenting cells. J Immunol 170:2523–2530

O'Neill E, Martinez I, Villinger F et al (2002) Protection by SIV VLP DNA prime/protein boost following mucosal SIV challenge is markedly enhanced by IL-12/GM-CSF co-administration. J Med Primatol 31:217–227

Pal R, Venzon D, Santra S et al (2006) Systemic immunization with an ALVAC-HIV-1/protein boost vaccine strategy protects rhesus macaques from CD4+ T-cell loss and reduces both systemic and mucosal SHIVKU2 RNA levels. J Virol 80:3732–3742

Peacock JW, Nordone SK, Jackson SS et al (2004) Gender differences in human immunodeficiency virus type 1-specific CD8 responses in the reproductive tract and colon following nasal peptide priming and modified vaccinia virus Ankara boosting. J Virol 78:13163–13172

Pinczewski J, Zhao J, Malkevitch N et al (2005) Enhanced immunity and protective efficacy against SIVmac251 intrarectal challenge following ad-SIV priming by multiple mucosal routes and gp120 boosting in MPL-SE. Viral Immunol 18:236–243

Porgador A, Staats HF, Faiola B et al (1997) Intranasal immunization with CTL epitope peptides from HIV-1 or ovalbumin and the mucosal adjuvant cholera toxin induces peptide-specific CTLs and protection against tumor development in vivo. J Immunol 158:834–841

Ranasinghe C, Medveczky JC, Woltring D et al (2006) Evaluation of fowlpox-vaccinia virus prime-boost vaccine strategies for high-level mucosal and systemic immunity against HIV-1. Vaccine 24:5881–5895

Ranasinghe C, Turner SJ, McArthur C et al (2007) Mucosal HIV-1 pox virus prime-boost immunization induces high-avidity CD8+ T cells with regime-dependent cytokine/granzyme B profiles. J Immunol 178:2370–2379
Scharton-Kersten T, Yu J, Vassell R et al (2000) Transcutaneous immunization with bacterial ADP-ribosylating exotoxins, subunits, and unrelated adjuvants. Infect Immun 68:5306–5313
Schmitz JE, Kuroda MJ, Santra S et al (1999) Control of viremia in simian immunodeficiency virus infection by CD8+ lymphocytes. Science 283:857–860
Sedlik C, Dadaglio G, Saron MF et al (2000) In vivo induction of a high-avidity, high-frequency cytotoxic T-lymphocyte response is associated with antiviral protective immunity. J Virol 74:5769–5775
Sharpe S, Hanke T, Tinsley-Bown A et al (2003) Mucosal immunization with PLGA-microencapsulated DNA primes a SIV-specific CTL response revealed by boosting with cognate recombinant modified vaccinia virus Ankara. Virology 313:13–21
Sharpstone D, Neild P, Crane R et al (1999) Small intestinal transit, absorption, and permeability in patients with AIDS with and without diarrhoea. Gut 45:70–76
Shata MT, Reitz MS Jr, DeVico AL et al (2001) Mucosal and systemic HIV-1 Env-specific CD8(+) T-cells develop after intragastric vaccination with a Salmonella Env DNA vaccine vector. Vaccine 20:623–629
Shevach EM (2002) CD4+ CD25+ suppressor T cells: more questions than answers. Nat Rev Immunol 2:389–400
Shiver JW, Fu TM, Chen L et al (2002) Replication-incompetent adenoviral vaccine vector elicits effective anti-immunodeficiency virus immunity. Nature 415:331–335
Snyder JT, Alexander-Miller MA, Berzofsky JA et al (2003) Molecular mechanisms and biological significance of CTL avidity. Curr HIV Res 1:287–294
Spira AI, Marx PA, Patterson BK et al (1996) Cellular targets of infection and route of viral dissemination after an intravaginal inoculation of simian immunodeficiency virus into rhesus macaques. J Exp Med 183:215–225
Staats HF, Ennis FA Jr (1999) IL-1 is an effective adjuvant for mucosal and systemic immune responses when coadministered with protein immunogens. J Immunol 162:6141–6147
Staats HF, Bradney CP, Gwinn WM et al (2001) Cytokine requirements for induction of systemic and mucosal CTL after nasal immunization. J Immunol 167:5386–5394
Stevceva L, Alvarez X, Lackner AA et al (2002) Both mucosal and systemic routes of immunization with the live, attenuated NYVAC/simian immunodeficiency virus SIV(gpe) recombinant vaccine result in gag-specific CD8(+) T-cell responses in mucosal tissues of macaques. J Virol 76:11659–11676
Sui Y, Zhu Q, Gagnon S et al (2010) Innate and adaptive immune correlates of vaccine and adjuvant-induced control of mucosal transmission of SIV in macaques. Proc Natl Acad Sci USA 107:9843–9848
Sutmuller RPM, Van Duivenvoorde LM, Van Elsas A et al (2001) Synergism of cytotoxic T lymphocyte-associated antigen 4 blockade and depletion of CD25+ regulatory T cells in antitumor therapy reveals alternative cytotoxic T lymphocyte responses. J Exp Med 194:823–832
Suvas S, Kumaraguru U, Pack CD et al (2003) CD4+CD25+ T cells regulate virus-specific primary and memory CD8+ T cell responses. J Exp Med 198:889–901
Tatsis N, Lin SW, Harris-McCoy K et al (2007) Multiple immunizations with adenovirus and MVA vectors improve CD8+ T cell functionality and mucosal homing. Virology 367:156–167
Taylor PM, Askonas BA (1986) Influenza nucleoprotein-specific cytotoxic T-cell clones are protective in vivo. Immunology 58:417–420
Trumpfheller C, Caskey M, Nchinda G et al (2008) The microbial mimic poly IC induces durable and protective CD4+ T cell immunity together with a dendritic cell targeted vaccine. Proc Natl Acad Sci USA 105:2574–2579
Tscharke DC, Karupiah G, Zhou J et al (2005) Identification of poxvirus CD8+ T cell determinants to enable rational design and characterization of smallpox vaccines. J Exp Med 201:95–104

Uematsu S, Fujimoto K, Jang MH et al (2008) Regulation of humoral and cellular gut immunity by lamina propria dendritic cells expressing Toll-like receptor 5. Nat Immunol 9:769–776

Ulmer JB, Donnelly JJ, Parker SE et al (1993) Heterologous protection against influenza by injection of DNA encoding a viral protein. Science 259:1745–1749

Vajdy M, Gardner J, Neidleman J et al (2001) Human immunodeficiency virus type 1 Gag-specific vaginal immunity and protection after local immunizations with sindbis virus-based replicon particles. J Infect Dis 184:1613–1616

Veazey RS, DeMaria M, Chalifoux LV et al (1998) Gastrointestinal tract as a major site of CD4+ T cell depletion and viral replication in SIV infection. Science 280:427–431

Veazey RS, Marx PA, Lackner AA (2003) Vaginal CD4+ T cells express high levels of CCR5 and are rapidly depleted in simian immunodeficiency virus infection. J Inf Dis 187:769–776

Vogel TU, Reynolds MR, Fuller DH et al (2003) Multispecific vaccine-induced mucosal cytotoxic T lymphocytes reduce acute-phase viral replication but fail in long-term control of simian immunodeficiency virus SIVmac239. J Virol 77:13348–13360

Wilkinson J, Cunningham AL (2006) Mucosal transmission of HIV-1: first stop dendritic cells. Curr Drug Targets 7:1563–1569

Wyatt LS, Belyakov IM, Earl PL et al (2008) Enhanced cell surface expression, immunogenicity and genetic stability resulting from a spontaneous truncation of HIV Env expressed by a recombinant MVA. Virology 372:260–272

Xu-Amano J, Kiyono H, Jackson RJ, Staats HF, Fujihashi K, Burrows PD, Elson CO, Pillai S, McGhee JR (1993) Helper T cell subsets for immunoglobulin A responses: oral immunization with tetanus toxoid and cholera toxin as adjuvant selectively induces Th2 cells in mucosa associated tissues. J Exp Med 178:1309–1320

Yee C, Savage PA, Lee PP et al (1999) Isolation of high avidity melanoma-reactive CTL from heterogeneous populations using peptide-MHC tetramers. J Immunol 162:2227–2234

Yoshizawa I, Mizuochi T, Ogata A et al (2003) Studies on the generation and maintenance of mucosal cytotoxic T lymphocytes against human immunodeficiency virus type 1 Gag in mice. AIDS Res Hum Retroviruses 19:469–479

Zeh HJ 3rd, Perry-Lalley D, Dudley ME et al (1999) High avidity CTLs for two self-antigens demonstrate superior in vitro and in vivo antitumor efficacy. J Immunol 162:989–994

Zhang Z-Q, Schuler T, Zupancic M et al (1999) Sexual transmission and propagation of SIV and HIV in resting and activated CD4+ T cells. Science 286:1353–1357

Zhou Q, Hidajat R, Peng B et al (2007) Comparative evaluation of oral and intranasal priming with replication-competent adenovirus 5 host range mutant (Ad5hr)-simian immunodeficiency virus (SIV) recombinant vaccines on immunogenicity and protective efficacy against SIV(mac251). Vaccine 25:8021–8035

Zhu Q, Egelston C, Vivekanandhan A et al (2008) Toll-like receptor ligands synergize through distinct dendritic cell pathways to induce T cell responses: implications for vaccines. Proc Natl Acad Sci USA 105:16260–16265

Zhu Q, Egelston C, Gagnon S et al (2010) Using 3 TLR ligands as a combination adjuvant induces qualitative changes in T cell responses needed for antiviral protection in mice. J Clin Invest 120:607–616

Mucosal Vaccines for Biodefense

N. J. Mantis, L. A. Morici and C. J. Roy

Abstract Bioterrorism is the deliberate release of biological toxins, pathogenic viruses, bacteria, parasites, or other infectious agents into the public sphere with the objective of causing panic, illness, and/or death on a local, regional, or possibly national scale. The list of potential biological agents compiled by the Centers for Disease Control and Prevention is long and diverse. However, a trait common to virtually all the potential bioterrorism agents is the fact that they are likely to be disseminated by either aerosol or in food/water supplies with the intention of targeting the mucosal surfaces of the respiratory or gastrointestinal tracts, respectively. In some instances, inhalation or ingestion would mimic the natural route by which humans are exposed to these agents. In other instances, (*e.g.*, the inhalation of a toxin is normally associated with food borne illness), it would represent an unnatural route of exposure. For most potential bioterrorism agents, the respiratory or gastrointestinal mucosa may simply serve as a route of entry by which they gain access to the systemic compartment where intoxication/replication occurs. For others, however, the respiratory or gastrointestinal mucosa is the primary tissue associated with pathogenesis, and therefore, the tissue for which countermeasures must be developed.

N. J. Mantis (✉)
Division of Infectious Diseases, Wadsworth Center, NYDOH, 120 New Scotland Ave, Albany NY 12208, USA
e-mail: nmantis@wadsworth.org

L. A. Morici
Department of Microbiology and Immunology, Tulane University School of Medicine, 1430 Tulane Ave, New Orleans LA 70112, USA

C. J. Roy
Infectious Disease Aerobiology, Tulane National Primate Research Center, 18703 Three Rivers Rd, Covington LA 70433, USA

Current Topics in Microbiology and Immunology (2012) 354: 181–195
DOI: 10.1007/82_2011_122

Published Online: 3 April 2011

Contents

1 Introduction

"The ability of our nation to detect and counter bioterrorism depends to a large degree on the information generated by biomedical research on disease-causing microorganisms and the immune system's response to them." *Dr. Anthony Fauci, Director, National Institutes of Allergy and Infectious Disease, National Institutes of Health, USA.*

In 1999, the Centers for Disease Control (CDC) convened a special expert panel to identify known biological weapons or potential biological threat agents ("biothreats") which, if used for nefarious purposes, posed a significant threat to civilian populations (Rotz et al. 2002). The panel established a list of potential bioterrorism agents, including toxins, viruses, bacteria, and protozoa, that were classified into three categories (A, B, and C). The classification system was based on the following four criteria: (i) the potential to cause morbidity and mortality in healthy individuals; (ii) the potential to be disseminated within the public sphere; (iii) the perceived threat and potential to elicit fear or panic; (iv) the capacity of local, state, and federal public health networks to respond and control an event. In response to the Public Health Security and Bioterrorism Preparedness and Response Act of 2002, the Department of Health and Human Services (DHHS) and the United States Department of Agriculture (USDA) expanded this original list to include emerging infectious diseases, as well as threats to livestock and economically important crops. The members of this expanded list are collectively referred to as Select Agents and Toxins, the possession and use of which is now regulated by the National Select Agent Registry under the auspices of the CDC. The National Institutes of Health (NIH), specifically the National Institute of Allergy and Infectious Diseases (NIAID), considers a subset of the select agents as "Priority Pathogens" for which there is a particular need for countermeasures, including vaccines. A complete list of these agents with their respective designations (Category A–C) is presented in Table 1.

Table 1 Category A–C Biothreats

Toxins
Botulinum neurotoxins[a,A]
Shigatoxin[a]
Tetrodotoxin[a]
T-2 toxin[a]
Staphylococcal enterotoxins[a,B]
Ricin[a,A]
Diacetoxyscirpenol[a]
Conotoxins[a]
Abrin[a]
Saxitoxin[a]
Shiga-like ribosome inactivating proteins[a]
Clostridium perfringens epsilon toxin[a,B]
Viruses
Eastern equine encephalitis[a,B]
Hendra virus[b]
Variola major (smallpox)[a,A]
Variola minor (alastrim)[a,A]
Monkeypox[a,A]
Filoviruses
Ebola virus[a,A]
Marburg virus[a,A]
Arenaviruses
Junin[a,A]
Machupo[a,A]
Guanarito[a,A]
Flexal[a,A]
Sabia[a,A]
Lassa[a,A]
Japanese encephalitis virus[B]
Venezuelan equine encephalitis[b,B]
Dengue[A]
LaCrosse[B]
California encephalitis[B]
Western equine encephalitis[B]
Bunyaviruses
Hantaviruses[A]
Rift Valley Fever[b,A]
Chikungunya[C]
Hepatitis A[B]
Yellow fever[C]
Rabies[C]
Nipah virus[b]
Tick-borne encephalitis complex (flavivirus)
Central European tick-borne encephalitis[a]
Kyasanur forest disease[a,B]
Omsk hemorrhagic fever[a]
Far eastern tick-borne encephalitis[a]
Russian spring/summer encephalitis[a]
Avian influenza virus (highly pathogenic)[c]
Reconstructed 1918 influenza virus[a]
Cercopithecine herpesvirus 1 (Herpes B virus)[a]
Severe acute respiratory syndrome (SARS)[C]
Caliciviruses[B]
Influenza[C]
West nile virus[B]
Crimean-congo hemorrhagic fever[a,C]
Bacteria/Rickettsia
Bacillus anthracis[b,A]
Brucella abortus[b,B]
Brucella melitensis[b,B]
Brucella suis[b,B]
Burkholderia mallei[b,B]
Burkholderia pseudomallei[b,B]
Coxiella burnetii[a,B]
Francisella tularensis[a,A]
Yersinia pestis[a,A]
Rickettsia prowazekii[a,B]
Rickettsia rickettsii[a]
Pathogenic vibrios[B]
Shigella species[B]
Salmonella species[B]
Listeria monocytogenes[B]
Yersinia enterolitica[B]
Campylobacter jejuni[B]
Multi-drug resistant tuberculosis[C]
Other Rickettsias[C]
Chlamydia psittaci[A]
Diarrheagenic *E. coli*[B]
Botulinum toxin-producing species of *Clostridium*[a]
Protozoa
Cryptosporidium parvum[B]
Cyclospora cayatanensis[B]
Entamoeba histolytica[B]
Toxoplasma[B]
Giardia lamblia[B]

(continued)

Table 1 (continued)

Fungi
Coccidioides posadasii[a]
Coccidioides immitis[a]
Microsporidia[B]

Listing of the biological agents considered to be a threat to human health as a compilation from a number of sources including the 1) select agents and toxins provided by the U.S. Department of Health and Human Services (DHHS), Centers for Disease Control and Prevention (CDC) and the U.S. Department of Agriculture (USDA) and 2) the priority pathogens from the National Institutes of Health/National Institute of Allergy and Infectious Diseases (NIAID) (www3.niaid.nih.gov/topics/BiodefenseRelated/Biodefense/research/CatA.htm)

[a] Select Agents and Toxins designated by DHHS/CDC

[b] Overlap select agents and toxins that are designated and regulated by both DHHS/CDC and the U.S. Department of Agriculture (USDA)

[c] Select agents designated and regulated by the USDA

[A, B, C] NIH/NIAID priority pathogens group A, B or C

1.1 Category A Agents

The CDC Category A agents include four pathogens that are highly infectious as aerosols. These are *Bacillus anthracis*, *Yersinia pestis*, smallpox (variola major) and *Francisella tularensis*. Among these, smallpox poses the greatest threat to public safety due to its highly pathogenic nature, its capacity to spread person-to-person, and the fact that herd immunity to the virus has waned since routine vaccination was discontinued more than three decades ago (Artenstein 2008). Anthrax also poses a significant and real threat to public health because *B. anthracis* spores are highly infectious, though the disease itself is not communicable. Also among the list of Category A agents is botulinum neurotoxin (BoNT), one of the most lethal known biological toxins. While BoNT can be aerosolized and is highly toxic following inhalation, the CDC's primary concern is the possible use of the toxin to contaminate food/water supplies (Sobel et al. 2002). The toxin is extremely potent via the oral route (~LD_{50} of 0.001 μg/kg) and has a long history as a bioweapon. Botulinum neurotoxin has been produced in large scale quantities by numerous governments as well as terrorist organizations (Sobel et al. 2002).

1.2 Category B Agents

The Category B agents are defined as being moderately easy to disseminate, capable of inflicting moderate morbidity/low mortality and requiring specific enhancements to standard diagnostic capacity, as well as enhanced disease surveillance. Whereas, the Category A agents are primarily threats by aerosol, the majority of the Category B agents target the gastrointestinal tract. These include food and water safety threats (e.g., *Salmonella* and *Shigella* species, pathogenic vibrios, enterotoxigenic *E. coli*), as well as toxins (e.g., ricin, staphylococcal enterotoxin B). In general, the Category B agents are not communicable from person to person but tend to be relatively easy to disperse at doses sufficient to be highly debilitating, and to necessitate prolonged medical attention. Many of the food/water safety threats are endemic in developing countries and are already a focus of ongoing biomedical research.

1.3 Category C Agents

At present, the Category C agents are not considered as high risk, but rather as emerging diseases that may pose a threat to public health in the future. The CDC restricts this category to Nipah virus and hantavirus, whereas the NIAID Category C priority pathogens include yellow fever, influenza, rabies, tick-borne encephalitis viruses, severe acute respiratory syndrome associated coronavirus (SARS-CoV), as well as certain other types of drug/antibiotic-resistant pathogens, such as tuberculosis-causing mycobacteria. In addition, the NIAID Category C agents include pathogens commonly found circulating in the general population (*e.g.*, Hepatitis A), and which possess the potential to cause morbidity among the larger population.

2 Assessing the Risk Posed by Biothreat Agents

It is generally assumed that biothreat agents will be disseminated by one of the two routes: aerosol or introduction into food/water supplies. Aerosol dissemination of pathogenic organisms, from either a point source such as a contaminated letter sent through the postal service, or from a planned aerial attack remain the greatest type of biological threat to the general public. No other modality of dispersion, except perhaps the widespread contamination of drinking water, could do more harm than aerosol dissemination of an infectious or toxic agent (Henderson 1999). Indeed, when engineered with the intent of causing mass casualties, biological agents pose health risks similar in magnitude to chemical or nuclear threats. Past weapons programs in the US and in the former Union of Soviet Socialist Republics (USSR) developed industrial processes for producing biological preparations that were optimized for aerosol delivery using sophisticated drying, milling, and packaging processes (Kortepeter et al. 2001). These preparations were designed for dispersion as highly respirable particles containing extremely large concentrations of stable, viable biological agent. Although many of the known biological weapons programs have been discontinued, aerosol delivery of an infectious or highly toxic biological agent continues to be a potential threat that rivals other weapons of mass destruction in terms of potential morbidity and mortality, as well as widespread panic.

The actual efficiency of aerosol to disseminate biological agents depends on the sophistication of the sample preparation, as well as biological and physical stressors in the environment. The infectivity of many of these pathogens is highly dependent on their size, hydrophobicity, and aggregation, as well as environmental conditions such as humidity and temperature. Humidity and temperature can affect particle size, which in turn determines the degree to which particles can penetrate the lungs. Highly respirable aerosols produced with a homogenous size distribution, commonly associated with sophisticated biological weapons, target the lower airways and alveolar spaces of the lung. Naturally-produced infectious aerosols, on the other hand, tend to be heterogeneous with respect to size, and will deposit throughout the respiratory tract. These physical differences not only dictate the degree of mucosal exposure associated with an aerosol, but may also impact the nature of the ensuing disease.

The network of food production, processing, and distribution in the US is vast and potentially vulnerable to deliberate contamination with toxins or infectious agents (Sobel and Watson 2009). The vulnerability of the food supply at the national level is evidenced by the fact that food-borne outbreaks caused by a single source of *Salmonella* or shiga toxin-producing *E. coli* O157:H7 (STEC) are not uncommon. For example, just the past two years, two Salmonella outbreaks have accounted for more than 2,000 illnesses (and nine deaths) in 44 states and certain provinces in Canada (Maki 2009). The first Salmonella outbreak occurred between April and August 2008 and was linked to contaminated peppers (and possibly tomatoes) that originated in Mexico and were subsequently processed in the southwest US. The second outbreak, due to *S. typhimurium*, occurred between October 2008 and March 2009, and was traced to a single peanut processing plant in Georgia (www.cdc.gov/salmonella). The actual number of cases associated with these outbreaks is likely to be 20–30 times greater than the number of cases reported (Maki 2009). Contamination of water supplies has had a similar impact on public health. In 1993, an outbreak of waterborne cryptosporidium in Milwaukee, WI affected an estimated 403,000 people (Leclerc et al. 2002). Enteric infections also pose a significant threat at the local level, in which a food or water source directly accessible to consumers is deliberately adulterated. The best example of such an incident occurred in 1984 in The Dalles, OR, where members of a religious commune intentionally contaminated salad bars at public restaurants with *S. typhimurium* (Torok et al. 1997). That incident resulted in more than 700 individuals contracting gastroenteritis.

3 Assessing Degrees of Mucosal Involvement

From the perspective of vaccine development for biodefense, it is important to differentiate between biological agents that elicit mucosal infections and pathophysiology, and those agents that simply exploit mucosal tissues as a means to gain access to the systemic compartment. In the former case, mucosal immunity is likely to be essential in preventing and clearing infections. Therefore, vaccines against these agents must truly involve mucosa-associated lymphoid tissues. In situations where the mucosa functions solely as a port of entry, systemic immunity is likely to be sufficient to control infection. One such example is anthrax. While *B. anthracis* spores are highly infectious by aerosol, the vegetative bacteria generally do not proliferate locally. Rather, following inhalation, the bacteria disseminate systemically via the lymphatics and circulatory system. Once within the systemic compartment, *B. anthracis* germinates and produces two toxins which account for the lethality associated with infection (Leppla et al. 2002). Protective immunity to *B. anthracis* is associated primarily with anti-toxin serum IgG antibodies. Mucosal defense is of little (if any) importance in controlling anthrax. On the other hand, mucosal immunity is likely to be important in controlling infections caused by two other Category A bacterial pathogens, notably *Y. pestis* and *F. tularensis*, which cause mucosal and systemic complications following inhalation (Metzger et al. 2007).

For many of the Category A–C agents, transmission via the respiratory tract is considered an "unnatural" route of infection and the actual involvement of the mucosa in the pathogenesis of infection may not be currently known. As a consequence, initial host interaction and the subsequent pathophysiology will not necessarily coincide with established clinical outcomes associated with infection by the natural route. In addition, there may be no clinical data that adequately define aerosol-related disease or how it differs from the natural route of infection. An example of one such agent is Staphylococcal enterotoxin B (SEB). As a member of the superantigen family of toxins, SEB forms "bridges" between Major Histocompatibility Class II molecules on antigen presenting cells and T cell receptors on specific subsets of $CD4^+$ and $CD8^+$ T cells. As a consequence of SEB binding, T cells release massive amounts of proinflammatory cytokines and undergo hyper-proliferation which ultimately results in their depletion (Kappler et al. 1989; White et al. 1989). Staphylococcal enterotoxin B is clinically associated with food poisoning, as ingestion of microgram quantities of the toxin are sufficient to evoke violent vomiting, diarrhea, fever, and, in severe cases, lethal shock (Bergdoll 1983). Despite being classified as an enterotoxin, SEB is extremely pathogenic following aerosol challenge. Rhesus monkeys administered SEB as an aerosol suffered from vomiting and diarrhea within hours, and died about two days later (Tseng et al. 1993; Mattix et al. 1995). Postmortem analysis indicated that the animals likely succumbed to severe pulmonary edema triggered by SEB-mediated T cell proliferation in the respiratory mucosa (Mattix et al. 1995).

In the case of alpha viruses, the pathogenesis associated with infection is highly dependent on the route of exposure, at least in experimental animal models. It is hypothesized that exposure to aerosols induce disease directly via the olfactory bulb, whereas experimental infection via injection generally causes a disseminated viremia prior to nervous system engagement and encephalitis. These different manifestations of clinical symptoms and outcome following different routes of exposure have been demonstrated for the Venezuelan and Eastern equine encephalitis viruses (Ryzhikov et al. 1991). Correspondingly, immunity to the alpha viruses may depend on the route of exposure. While serum IgG antibodies may be effective for neutralizing virus following exposure via subcutaneous injection (similar to a natural exposure), these antibodies may not control viral spread following aerosol challenge. Cell-mediated immunity (CMI) rather than humoral immunity may be more important following aerosol challenge. Thus, induction of secretory antibodies at the respiratory mucosal barrier may not necessarily be an important aspect of rational vaccine design and development against these viruses (Pratt et al. 2003).

A final group of biothreat agents are those which are broadly toxic and potentially lethal irrespective of the route of exposure. In this case, systemic immunity may suffice to protect against lethality but may not prevent localized tissue damage in the mucosa. One such example is ricin toxin, which elicits both local and systemic inflammation and cell death following injection, inhalation or ingestion (Wilhelmsen and Pitt 1996; Mantis 2005; Yoder et al. 2007). Ricin is a bipartite toxin capable of intoxicating all known cell types. The ricin toxin B subunit (RTB) is a lectin with specificity for β-1,3 linked galactose and N-acetylgalactosamine residues. The A subunit (RTA) is an RNA *N*-glycosidase whose substrate is a conserved adenine residue within the so-called sarcin/ricin loop of eukaryotic 28S ribosomal RNA. Monkeys exposed to lethal doses of ricin by aerosol suffered peribronchovascular edema, mixed inflammatory cell infiltrates, and widespread necrosis in the airways and alveoli (Wilhelmsen and Pitt 1996). Death occurred 36–48 h post exposure. In a rodent model, serum IgG was sufficient to prevent death of animals after a lethal aerosol challenge, but not sufficient to prevent toxin-induced lung lesions (Griffiths et al. 1995). Although these studies need to be confirmed in a nonhuman primate model, the data suggest that vaccine development strategies must aim at eliciting both systemic and mucosal immunity to confer complete protection against certain selective agents such as ricin.

4 Inherent Challenges in Development of Mucosal Vaccines for Biodefense

The development of vaccines is, in general, an extremely challenging and expensive undertaking. It is estimated that a single vaccine takes 10–15 years to reach licensure and at a cost exceeding hundreds of million of dollars (Levine 2006). The development of vaccines for biodefense faces additional hurdles, including the following:

(i) The requirement for specialized containment facilities for biothreat research and animal studies, especially aerosol challenges.

BSL-3 facilities are absolutely required to perform research using fully virulent strains of the CDC Category A agents (e.g., *B. anthracis*, *Y. pestis*, and *F. tularensis*). Smallpox requires BSL-4 containment; this virus is held by only two laboratories in the world. Most Category B agents can be used safely under BSL-2 conditions, but generally not in aerosolized form. Ricin, abrin, SEB, epsilon toxin,

for example, are 10–1,000 fold more toxic via inhalation when compared to ingestion or transdermal exposure, and therefore, require BSL3 facilities for animal challenge studies (Mantis 2005).

In an effort to enable research on Category A and B priority pathogens, NIAID has established a national network of regional (RBL) and national (NBL) biodefense laboratories (Fig. 1) as part of the Regional Centers of Excellence (RCEs) for Biodefense and Emerging Infectious Diseases. These RCEs provide services and resources to the scientific community in all aspects of biodefense research, including BSL3 containment laboratory access, preclinical development activities, expertise in immunological, proteomic and genomic techniques, high throughput small molecule screening, and aerobiology facilities (Fig. 2). As of 2008, there were six RBLs scattered throughout the US, with seven more under construction. In addition, there were two NBLs nearing completion: one at the University of Texas Medical Branch at Galveston, and one at Boston University Medical Center. The RBLs and NBLs are designed to serve as regional and national centers for collaborative research on pathogenesis, therapeutics, diagnostics, and vaccines.

(ii) Lack of established animal models, especially involving mucosal challenge. While immunity to many Category A–B agents has been studied for decades, in most cases these models have involved systemic not mucosal exposure. Many of the animal models that have been developed are limited to rodents; there are very few large animal models (rabbit, nonhuman primate) available for efficacy/evaluation studies. Even fewer models exist that appropriately describe the pathophysiology in terms of cellular/molecular mechanisms of the disease process.

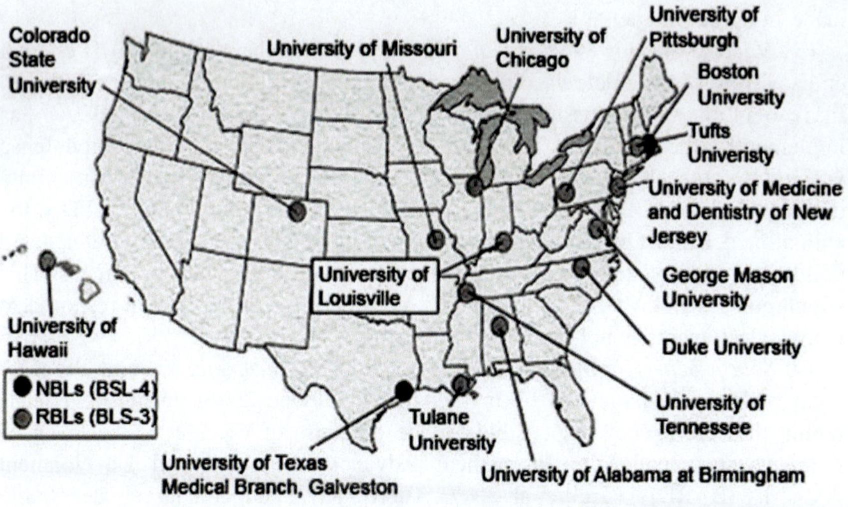

Fig. 1 Locations of NIAID-Sponsored Regional and National Biodefense Laboratories in the United States. Image from www3.niaid.nih.gov/LabsAndResources/resources/dmid/NBL_RBL/site.htm

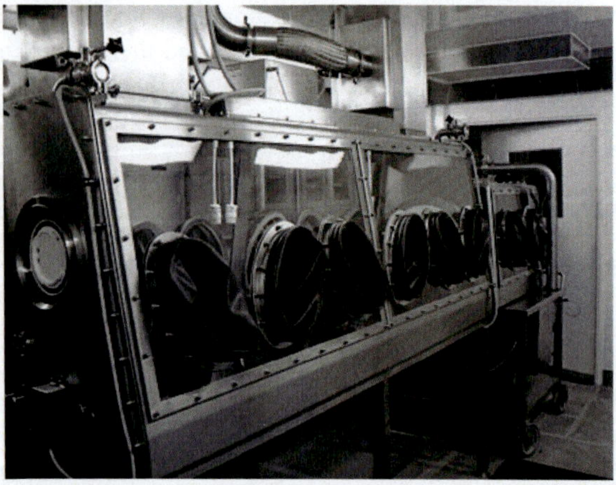

Fig. 2 Class III biological safety cabinets for biodefense research available at RBLs. The NIAID-sponsored RBLs provide full containment for infectious aerosol challenge studies with primates, as well as instrumentation for specialized bioaerosol characterization studies

The lack of relevant animal models represents a major developmental hurdle for testing and comparing biodefense vaccines, and therapeutics.

(iii) Limited (or no) access to clinical samples. The natural incidence of infection by most Category A and many Category B select agents is low or so sporadic that obtaining clinical samples for research purposes is not technically feasible. For example, in 2006 there were 20 cases of food borne botulism, 95 cases of tularemia, 17 cases of plague, and 1 incident of anthrax (www.cdc.gov/mmWR/PDF/wk/mm5553). With these infection rates, it is virtually impossible to obtain sufficient numbers of clinical samples from individuals at specific time points following infection, or to correlate clinical outcomes with observations made in animal models.

(iv) Vaccine efficacy trials may not be feasible. In general, Phase II-III clinical efficacy trials of candidate vaccines for biothreat agents are not feasible or ethical. In recognition of this issue, the Food and Drug Administration (FDA) has implemented the so-called "animal rule" which enables candidate biodefense vaccines to proceed towards licensure based on efficacy studies in relevant animal models (Crawford 2002; Sullivan et al. 2009). However, according to the FDA, the animal models must mimic the pathogenesis of human disease, and the defined end point(s) of efficacy studies must correlate with the desired effects in humans. This stipulation is somewhat of a "catch-22", considering that the human response to many select agents is not known (see above).

(v) Sole procurer of biodefense vaccines is US government. Vaccine development is driven in large part by market forces (Levine 2006). In the biodefense realm, the sole agency responsible for the purchase of vaccines is the US government, specifically the Biomedical Advanced Research and Development Authority (BARDA) (Trull et al. 2007). The BARDA budget is largely devoted to end stage acquisition, not development. Therefore, the costs of vaccine development must be covered by private investment or NIAID grants/contracts, which are highly competitive.

(vi) Vaccines must have unusually long shelf lives. It is anticipated that most biodefense vaccines will be administered to limited and specific populations of individuals (*e.g.* emergency responders, healthcare providers, politicians). The public at large will receive such vaccines only in the event of a local, regional, or national health emergency. Therefore, following acquisition by BARDA (see above), most vaccines will simply be stockpiled. From the perspective of vaccine development, this poses significant challenges, as the vaccine formulations must be impervious (possibility over periods of years) to chemical inactivation, protein unfolding, denaturation, and aggregation.

5 *Yersinia pestis* as a Case Study in Biodefense Vaccine Development

The causative agent of plague, *Yersinia pestis*, represents a hallmark pathogen for which both mucosal and systemic immunity is essential for protection. The *Y. pestis* organism is a gram-negative bacillus that can be transmitted by flea-bite or by aerosol. Depending on the mode of transmission and success of infection, three forms of the disease may manifest: bubonic, septicemic, and/or pneumonic plague. Upon flea-bite, the bacterium is introduced into the bloodstream and eventually seeds the nearest lymph nodes. The bacterium is ingested by nonactivated macrophages that are unable to control the growth of the organism. Inflammation produced in response to bacterial proliferation causes a characteristic swelling, or bubo, the classical feature of bubonic plague. Eventually, bacteria can disseminate throughout the bloodstream leading to septicemic plague and the colonization of additional sites. Pneumonic plague can result from dissemination to the lung alveoli or from the inhalation of aerosolized organisms. Pneumonic plague has a very rapid onset (1–3 days). It is highly contagious and approaches a 100% fatality rate if left untreated. Host immune responses ultimately fail to control the growth and dissemination of the organism. Without early antibiotic treatment, death can result from either pneumonia or endotoxin-induced septicemic shock (Cornelius et al. 2007). Due to the intrinsic virulence of *Y. pestis*, its ease of transmission by aerosol, and the lack of a vaccine, this bacterium poses a significant threat to biodefense and is classified as a Category A priority pathogen.

The extensive research aimed at producing an effective vaccine against plague has revealed significant contribution of mucosal immunity in protection against the respiratory form of the disease. It has long been recognized that serum antibodies generated against whole-killed *Y. pestis* can prevent bubonic and septicemic forms of the disease (Smiley 2008). However, the inability of serum antibody to prevent pneumonic plague led to the hypothesis that local mucosal immunity in the lung may be essential for protection. This has been substantiated numerous prime/boost immunization studies with recombinant capsule F1 and low calcium response (Lcr) V subunit antigens using murine models of bubonic and pneumonic plague.

Parenteral vaccination with rF1-V can protect mice against subcutaneous and aerosol challenge with *Y. pestis* (Titball and Williamson 2001). In this instance, the protection is attributed to induction of systemic F1-V specific IgG which transudate into the lungs to protect against inhaled bacteria (Williamson et al. 1997). The additional presence of antigen-specific IgA in pulmonary fluids may further contribute to protection in the respiratory tract. Survival against aerosolized *Y. pestis* was enhanced by increasing the nasal boost dosage of rF1-V, and both serum and pulmonary antibody titers to V antigen, were the best predictors of outcome (Reed and Martinez 2006). This is consistent with previous studies demonstrating that vaccination with F1 or V alone is sufficient for protection in mice against both bubonic and pneumonic plague, while vaccination with the F1-V combination provides additive protection (Titball and Williamson 2001).

In the context of a biological attack by aerosol, it is likely that systemic immunity is equally important as mucosal immunity in preventing the septicemic stage from developing after inhalation of *Y. pestis*. Mucosal immunity appears to be essential for preventing pulmonary inflammation and pneumonia, while systemic immunity is required for preventing bacterial dissemination and septicemia. This is evidenced by vaccine studies in mice that reported rapid, fulminating disease, and endotoxin-induced death in sham-vaccinated animals challenged with aerosolized *Y. pestis* (Reed and Martinez 2006). In vaccinated animals that survive the same challenge dose, both systemic and mucosal antibody titers correlate with protection. In contrast, vaccinated animals that eventually succumb to the disease display no evidence of bacterial dissemination from the lung, but develop lethal pneumonia (Reed and Martinez 2006). This could be explained by the induction of a systemic immune response in the absence of a mucosal response in these animals. The importance of systemic antibody is also exemplified by the demonstration that passive transfer of F1-V mouse antisera can protect recipient normal or SCID mice from bubonic and pneumonic challenge with *Y. pestis* (Motin et al. 1994; Anderson et al. 1996; Green et al. 1999). However, B-cell deficient mice vaccinated with live *Y. pestis* are protected against pneumonic plague unless they are additionally depleted of $CD4^+$ and $CD8^+$ T cells, IFN-γ, or TNF-α (Parent et al. 2005). Recent studies with nonhuman primates also suggest that F1-V antibodies alone may not solely correlate with protection against pneumonic plague (Smiley 2008). Thus, induction of cellular immunity may be critical to the development of an effective vaccine against plague.

Due to the likely importance of cellular immunity in preventing pneumonic plague, there is a renewed interest in the development of live-attenuated *Y. pestis* strains as vaccines (Smiley 2008). Whether such bacterial strains could be safely utilized as mucosal vaccine formulations is debatable. Future subunit vaccines for *Y. pestis* will likely utilize recombinant F1-V as the major antigenic components since no other vaccine candidates have yielded better immunogenicity and protection (Titball and Williamson 2001). However, the incorporation of additional T cell antigens may be required to achieve complete and durable immunity.

6 Conclusion

A contentious issue within the biomedical community has been the commitment of disproportionate amounts of the US NIH budget to support biodefense research (Trull et al. 2007). Opponents have argued that devotion of funds to pursue diagnostics, therapeutics, and vaccines against relatively "obscure" pathogens and toxins have been detrimental to more basic research programs aimed at preventing infectious diseases of immediate global importance. However, biodefense research should significantly impact overall worldwide health in several ways.

First, the development of vaccines, diagnostics, and therapeutics for Category A–C agents, which are generally most infectious/toxic in the respiratory and/or gastrointestinal tract, has required more basic research in mucosal innate and adaptive immunology, which will enhance our understanding of host defense against a variety of mucosal pathogens. Second, the testing of potential vaccines or therapeutics at international field sites where food- and water-borne diseases are endemic is likely to reduce deaths caused by enteric pathogens such as *S. dysenteriae* 1 and shiga toxin-producing *E. coli*. Finally, the development of vaccines for HIV, tuberculosis, and other mucosal diseases that currently cause high mortality will benefit from the identification of novel adjuvants (Guy 2007), new particle delivery platforms (Bramwell et al. 2005), and improved live-attenuated oral delivery vehicles (Galen et al. 2009).

In conclusion, the development of vaccines and other countermeasures against the diverse microbial pathogens and toxins that have been deemed potential biothreats by public health organizations, is a daunting challenge for the scientific community. Certainly, the development of vaccines against the entire list of biothreat agents is neither necessary nor realistic, but efforts towards this end should reveal new and fundamentally significant insights into innate and adaptive immunity in the mucosae, and they will undoubtedly have beneficial implications for combating infectious diseases as a whole.

Acknowledgments The authors would like to thank members of their respective laboratories for helpful discussions. NJM and CJR would like to acknowledge Dr. Robert Brey (Soligenix, Inc.) for insight into the reality of vaccine development. This work was supported by NIH grants U54AI057158, U01AI070624, U01AI075509.

References

Anderson GW Jr, Leary SE, Williamson ED et al (1996) Recombinant V antigen protects mice against pneumonic and bubonic plague caused by F1-capsule-positive and -negative strains of Yersinia pestis. Infect Immun 64:4580–4585

Artenstein AW (2008) New generation smallpox vaccines: a review of preclinical and clinical data. Rev Med Virol 18:217–231

Bergdoll MS (1983) Enterotoxins. In: Easmon CSF, Adlam C (eds) Staphylococci and staphylococcal infections, vol 2. Academic Press, New York

Bramwell VW, Eyles JE, Oya Alpar H (2005) Particulate delivery systems for biodefense subunit vaccines. Adv Drug Deliv Rev 57:1247–1265

Cornelius C, Quenee L, Anderson D et al (2007) Protective immunity against plague. Adv Exp Med Biol 603:415–424

Crawford LM (2002) New drug and biological drug. Products; evidence needed to demonstrate effectiveness of new drugs when human efficacies studies are not ethical or feasible. Federal Register 67:37988–37998

Galen JE, Pasetti MF, Tennant S et al (2009) Salmonella enterica serovar typhi live vector vaccines finally come of age. Immunol Cell Biol 87:400–412

Green M, Rogers D, Russell P et al (1999) The SCID/Beige mouse as a model to investigate protection against Yersinia pestis. FEMS Immunol Med Microbiol 23:107–113

Griffiths GD, Lindsay CD, Allenby AC et al (1995) Protection against inhalation toxicity of ricin and abrin by immunisation. Hum Exp Toxicol 14:155–164

Guy B (2007) The perfect mix: recent progress in adjuvant research. Nat Rev Microbiol 5:505–517

Henderson DA (1999) The looming threat of bioterrorism. Science 283:1279–1282

Kappler J, Kotzin B, Herron L et al (1989) V beta-specific stimulation of human T cells by staphylococcal toxins. Science 244:811–813

Kortepeter MG, Cieslak TJ, Eitzen EM (2001) Bioterrorism. J Environ Health 63:21–24

Leclerc H, Schwartzbrod L, Dei-Cas E (2002) Microbial agents associated with waterborne diseases. Crit Rev Microbiol 28:371–409

Leppla SH, Robbins JB, Schneerson R et al (2002) Development of an improved vaccine for anthrax. J Clin Invest 110:141–144

Levine MM (2006) Enteric infections and the vaccines to counter them: future directions. Vaccine 24:3865–3873

Maki DG (2009) Coming to grips with foodborne infection–peanut butter, peppers, and nationwide salmonella outbreaks. N Engl J Med 360:949–953

Mantis NJ (2005) Vaccines against the category B toxins: Staphylococcal enterotoxin B, epsilon toxin and ricin. Adv Drug Deliv Rev 57:1424–1439

Mattix ME, Hunt RE, Wilhelmsen CL et al (1995) Aerosolized staphylococcal enterotoxin B-induced pulmonary lesions in rhesus monkeys (Macaca mulatta). Toxicol Pathol 23:262–268

Metzger DW, Bakshi CS, Kirimanjeswara G (2007) Mucosal immunopathogenesis of Francisella tularensis. Ann NY Acad Sci 1105:266–283

Motin VL, Nakajima R, Smirnov GB et al (1994) Passive immunity to yersiniae mediated by anti-recombinant V antigen and protein A–V antigen fusion peptide. Infect Immun 62:4192–4201

Parent MA, Berggren KN, Kummer LW et al (2005) Cell-mediated protection against pulmonary Yersinia pestis infection. Infect Immun 73:7304–7310

Pratt WD, Davis NL, Johnston RE et al (2003) Genetically engineered, live attenuated vaccines for Venezuelan equine encephalitis: testing in animal models. Vaccine 21:3854–3862

Reed DS, Martinez MJ (2006) Respiratory immunity is an important component of protection elicited by subunit vaccination against pneumonic plague. Vaccine 24:2283–2289

Rotz LD, Khan AS, Lillibridge SR et al (2002) Public health assessment of potential biological terrorism agents. Emerg Infect Dis 8:225–230

Ryzhikov AB, Tkacheva NV, Sergeev AN et al (1991) Venezuelan equine encephalitis virus propagation in the olfactory tract of normal and immunized mice. Biomed Sci 2:607–614

Smiley ST (2008) Immune defense against pneumonic plague. Immunol Rev 225:256–271

Sobel J, Watson J (2009) Intentional terrorist contamination of food and water. In: Lutwick L, Lutwick S (eds) Beyond anthrax: the weaponization of infectious diseases. Springer, New York

Sobel J, Khan AS, Swerdlow DL (2002) Threat of a biological terrorist attack on the US food supply: the CDC perspective. Lancet 359:874–880

Sullivan NJ, Martin JE, Graham BS et al (2009) Correlates of protective immunity for Ebola vaccines: implications for regulatory approval by the animal rule. Nat Rev Microbiol 7:393–400

Titball RW, Williamson ED (2001) Vaccination against bubonic and pneumonic plague. Vaccine 19:4175–4184

Torok TJ, Tauxe RV, Wise RP et al (1997) A large community outbreak of salmonellosis caused by intentional contamination of restaurant salad bars. JAMA 278:389–395

Trull MC, du Laney TV, Dibner MD (2007) Turning biodefense dollars into products. Nat Biotechnol 25:179–184

Tseng J, Komisar JL, Chen JY et al (1993) Immunity and responses of circulating leukocytes and lymphocytes in monkeys to aerosolized staphylococcal enterotoxin B. Infect Immun 61:391–398

White J, Herman A, Pullen AM et al (1989) The V beta-specific superantigen staphylococcal enterotoxin B: stimulation of mature T cells and clonal deletion in neonatal mice. Cell 56:27–35

Wilhelmsen CL, Pitt ML (1996) Lesions of acute inhaled lethal ricin intoxication in rhesus monkeys. Vet Pathol 33:296–302

Williamson ED, Eley SM, Stagg AJ et al (1997) A sub-unit vaccine elicits IgG in serum, spleen cell cultures and bronchial washings and protects immunized animals against pneumonic plague. Vaccine 15:1079–1084

Yoder JM, Aslam RU, Mantis NJ (2007) Evidence for widespread epithelial damage and coincident production of monocyte chemotactic protein 1 in a murine model of intestinal ricin intoxication. Infect Immun 75:1745–1750

Index

Current Topics in Microbiology and Immunology (2012) 354: 197–198
DOI: 10.1007/978-3-642-23693-8